FAST FACTS

for
TRAUMA NURSING

Dawn Carpenter, DNP, ACNP-BC, CCRN, FAANP, is a practicing acute care nurse practitioner in the surgical/trauma ICU and trauma service line at Guthrie Healthcare System in Sayre, Pennsylvania, and adjunct associate clinical professor of surgery, Surgery Institute, Geisinger College of Health Professions in Danville, Pennsylvania.

Dr. Carpenter's career has spanned over 30 years as a critical care nurse, nurse practitioner, and faculty. In addition, she is also an associate professor at the University of Massachusetts Medical School, Graduate School of Nursing. She continues to mentor DNP students and is the previous coordinator of the adult gerontology acute care nurse practitioner program. She possesses a passion for educating and mentoring acute and critical care nurses and nurse practitioners as they advance their careers. Dr. Carpenter is a nationally known speaker on a variety of topics, including sepsis.

She has been actively engaged at the national level with the American Association of Critical-Care Nurses (AACN), where she routinely volunteers her time and expertise. She has been an item writer and a member of the exam development committee for the ACNPC-AG and CCRN® exams. She has been a subject matter expert for AACN for several years, advising on exam content and revising practice exam questions. Additionally, she was a member and co-chair of the Advance Practice Institute (API) planning committee and member of the nominating committee.

Alexander Menard, DNP, AGACNP-BC, is an assistant professor at the University of Massachusetts Chan Medical School, Tan Chingfen Graduate School of Nursing, where he coordinates the Adult-Gerontology Acute Care Nurse Practitioner (AG-ACNP) program. Dr. Menard has worked in critical care as a nurse and nurse practitioner for over 10 years.

He is a member of the AACN, where he volunteers his time to develop new offerings for critical care nurses and nurse practitioners, as well as a member of the National Organization of Nurse Practitioner Faculties (NONPF).

FAST FACTS
for
TRAUMA NURSING

Dawn Carpenter, DNP, ACNP-BC, CCRN, FAANP
Alexander Menard, DNP, AGACNP-BC

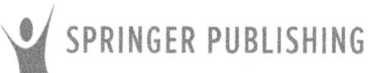

Copyright © 2025 Springer Publishing Company, LLC
All rights reserved.

No part of this publication may be reproduced, stored in a retrieval system, or transmitted in any form or by any means, electronic, mechanical, photocopying, recording, or otherwise, without the prior permission of Springer Publishing Company, LLC, or authorization through payment of the appropriate fees to the Copyright Clearance Center, Inc., 222 Rosewood Drive, Danvers, MA 01923, 978-750-8400, fax 978-646-8600, info@copyright.com or at www.copyright.com.

Springer Publishing Company, LLC
902 Carnegie Center, Princeton, NJ 08540
www.springerpub.com

Acquisitions Editor: John Zaphyr
Compositor: Transforma
Production Editor: Dennis Troutman

ISBN: 978-0-8261-6094-2
e-book ISBN: 978-0-8261-6095-9
DOI: 10.1891/9780826160959

Printed by LSI

The author and the publisher of this Work have made every effort to use sources believed to be reliable to provide information that is accurate and compatible with the standards generally accepted at the time of publication. The author and publisher shall not be liable for any special, consequential, or exemplary damages resulting, in whole or in part, from the readers' use of, or reliance on, the information contained in this book. The publisher has no responsibility for the persistence or accuracy of URLs for external or third-party Internet websites referred to in this publication and does not guarantee that any content on such websites is, or will remain, accurate or appropriate.

Library of Congress Cataloging-in-Publication Data

Names: Carpenter, Dawn, author. | Menard, Alexander, author.
Title: Fast facts for trauma nursing / Dawn Carpenter, Alexander Menard.
Other titles: Fast facts (Springer Publishing Company)
Description: Princeton, NJ : Springer Publishing Company, [2025] | Series: Fast facts | Includes bibliographical references and index. | Summary: "This book was created specifically for all levels of trauma nurses and students who care for injured patients throughout the hospital. This book presents critical information at the nurses' fingertips for quick reference in clinical settings. This book is designed to fit in the pocket for daily use by nurses in the emergency department, intensive care unit, intermediate care units, general care floors and beyond, and is based on over 30 years of experience with trauma patients and the wisdom of experienced nurse contributors. This pocket resource puts vital information at your fingertips with succinct, easy-to read bullet points, diagrams, tables, and charts, providing large amounts of data in a condensed format. Given the expansive knowledge that trauma nurses must know, it was impossible to include everything and yet be small enough for the pocket, thus selective components were chosen for inclusion"-- Provided by publisher.
Identifiers: LCCN 2024009739 | ISBN 9780826160942 (paperback) | ISBN 9780826160959 (ebook)
Subjects: MESH: Trauma Nursing--methods | Wounds and Injuries--nursing
Classification: LCC RD99.24 | NLM WY 154.2 | DDC 617/.0231--dc23/eng/20240501
LC record available at https://lccn.loc.gov/2024009739

Contact sales@springerpub.com to receive discount rates on bulk purchases.

Publisher's Note: **New and used products purchased from third-party sellers are not guaranteed for quality, authenticity, or access to any included digital components.**

Printed in the United States of America.

*This book is dedicated to all nurses who care for injured people.
I'm inspired by your commitment and dedication to the nursing profession.
You have been the nidus to publish this book.*

OTHER *FAST FACTS* BOOKS

Fast Facts on ADOLESCENT HEALTH FOR NURSING AND HEALTH PROFESSIONALS: A Care Guide (*Herrman*)

Fast Facts for the ADULT-GERONTOLOGY ACUTE CARE NURSE PRACTITIONER (*Carpenter*)

Fast Facts for the ANTEPARTUM AND POSTPARTUM NURSE: A Nursing Orientation and Care Guide (*Davidson*)

Fast Facts Workbook for CARDIAC DYSRHYTHMIAS AND 12-LEAD EKGs (*Desmarais*)

Fast Facts for the CARDIAC SURGERY NURSE: Caring for Cardiac Surgery Patients, Third Edition (*Hodge*)

Fast Facts for CAREER SUCCESS IN NURSING: Making the Most of Mentoring (*Vance*)

Fast Facts for the CATH LAB NURSE, Second Edition (*McCulloch*)

Fast Facts for the CLASSROOM NURSING INSTRUCTOR: Classroom Teaching (*Yoder-Wise, Kowalski*)

Fast Facts for the CLINICAL NURSE LEADER (*Wilcox, Deerhake*)

Fast Facts for the CLINICAL NURSE MANAGER: Managing a Changing Workplace, Second Edition (*Fry*)

Fast Facts for the CLINICAL NURSING INSTRUCTOR: Clinical Teaching, Third Edition (*Kan, Stabler-Haas*)

Fast Facts on COMBATING NURSE BULLYING, INCIVILITY, AND WORKPLACE VIOLENCE: What Nurses Need to Know (*Ciocco*)

Fast Facts About COMPETENCY-BASED EDUCATION IN NURSING: How to Teach Competency Mastery (*Wittmann-Price, Gittings*)

Fast Facts for the CRITICAL CARE NURSE, Second Edition (*Hewett*)

Fast Facts About CURRICULUM DEVELOPMENT IN NURSING: How to Develop and Evaluate Educational Programs, Second Edition (*McCoy, Anema*)

Fast Facts for DEMENTIA CARE: What Nurses Need to Know, Second Edition (*Miller*)

Fast Facts for DEVELOPING A NURSING ACADEMIC PORTFOLIO: What You Really Need to Know (*Wittmann-Price*)

Fast Facts About DIVERSITY, EQUITY, AND INCLUSION IN NURSING: Building Competencies for an Antiracism Practice (*Davis*)

Fast Facts for DNP ROLE DEVELOPMENT: A Career Navigation Guide (*Menonna-Quinn, Tortorella Genova*)

Fast Facts About EKGs FOR NURSES: The Rules of Identifying EKGs (*Landrum*)

Fast Facts for the ER NURSE: Guide to a Successful Emergency Department Orientation, Fourth Edition (*Buettner*)

Fast Facts for EVIDENCE-BASED PRACTICE IN NURSING, Third Edition (*Godshall*)

Fast Facts for the FAITH COMMUNITY NURSE: Implementing FCN/Parish Nursing (*Hickman*)

Fast Facts About FORENSIC NURSING: What You Need to Know (*Scannell*)

Fast Facts on GENETICS AND GENOMICS FOR NURSES: Practical Applications (*Subasic*)

Fast Facts for the GERONTOLOGY NURSE: A Nursing Care Guide (*Eliopoulos*)

Fast Facts About GI AND LIVER DISEASES FOR NURSES: What APRNs Need to Know (*Chaney*)

Fast Facts About the GYNECOLOGICAL EXAM: A Professional Guide for NPs, PAs, and Midwives, Second Edition (*Secor, Fantasia*)

Fast Facts in HEALTH INFORMATICS FOR NURSES (*Hardy*)

Fast Facts for HEALTH PROMOTION IN NURSING: Promoting Wellness (*Miller*)

Fast Facts for Nurses About HOME INFUSION THERAPY: The Expert's Best Practice Guide (*Gorski*)

Fast Facts for the HOSPICE NURSE: A Concise Guide to End-of-Life Care, Second Edition (*Wright*)

Fast Facts for the L&D NURSE: Labor and Delivery Orientation, Third Edition (*Groll*)

Fast Facts About LGBTQ+ CARE FOR NURSES (*Traister*)

Fast Facts for the LONG-TERM CARE NURSE: What Nursing Home and Assisted Living Nurses Need to Know (*Eliopoulos*)

Fast Facts to LOVING YOUR RESEARCH PROJECT: A Stress-Free Guide for Novice Researchers in Nursing and Healthcare (*Marshall*)

Fast Facts for MAKING THE MOST OF YOUR CAREER IN NURSING (*Redulla*)

Fast Facts for MANAGING PATIENTS WITH A PSYCHIATRIC DISORDER: What RNs, NPs, and New Psych Nurses Need to Know (*Marshall*)

Fast Facts About MEDICAL CANNABIS AND OPIOIDS: Minimizing Opioid Use Through Cannabis (*Smith, Smith*)

Fast Facts for the MEDICAL OFFICE NURSE: What You Really Need to Know (*Richmeier*)

Fast Facts for the MEDICAL–SURGICAL NURSE: Clinical Orientation (*Ciocco*)

Fast Facts for the OPERATING ROOM NURSE, Third Edition (*Criscitelli*)

Fast Facts for PATIENT SAFETY IN NURSING: How to Decrease Medical Errors and Improve Patient Outcomes (*Hunt*)

Fast Facts for PSYCHOPHARMACOLOGY FOR NURSE PRACTITIONERS (*Goldin*)

Fast Facts for the SCHOOL NURSE, Fourth Edition (*Loschiavo*)

Fast Facts About STROKE CARE FOR THE ADVANCED PRACTICE NURSE (*Morrison*)

Fast Facts for EVIDENCE-BASED PRACTICE IN NURSING, Fourth Edition (*Godshall*)

Fast Facts for the CLINICAL NURSING INSTRUCTOR, Fourth Edition (*Kan, Stabler-Haas*)

Fast Facts for TRAUMA NURSING (*Carpenter, Menard*)

CONTENTS

Reviewers	ix
Foreword	xiii
Preface	xv
Acknowledgments	xvii

SECTION I GENERAL TRAUMA PRINCIPLES

1. Trauma Systems and Trauma Center Preparedness — 3
2. Risk Factors for Trauma — 15
3. Mechanism of Injury — 23

SECTION II RESUSCITATIVE PHASE OF CARE

4. Primary Survey — 33
5. Secondary Survey — 43
6. Tertiary Survey — 57

SECTION III NURSING CARE BY SYSTEM/INJURIES

7. Neurologic Injuries and Care — 63
8. Head, Eyes, Ears, Nose, and Throat Injuries and Care — 85
9. Cardiovascular Injuries and Care — 97
10. Pulmonary Injuries and Care — 123
11. Gastrointestinal Injuries and Care — 149
12. Genitourinary and Gynecologic Injuries and Care — 165
13. Musculoskeletal Injuries and Care — 175
14. Integumentary Injuries and Care — 193

SECTION IV POSTRESUSCITATIVE PHASE OF CARE

15. Triage, Admission, and Transfer Criteria — 211
16. Best Practices in the Care of Trauma Patients — 217

SECTION V SPECIAL POPULATIONS AND CIRCUMSTANCES

17. Older Adult Trauma Patients — 235
18. Pregnant Trauma Patients — 243
19. Pediatrics — 253
20. Veterans — 259
21. Substance Use and Toxicology — 265
22. Disaster Readiness and Response — 277

SECTION VI POSTHOSPITALIZATION

23. Discharge and Follow-Up — 289
24. Injury Prevention — 297

SECTION VII ANSWER KEY

25. Study Question Answers and Rationales — 305

Index — *315*

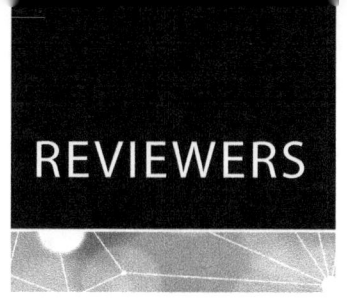

REVIEWERS

Jazzlynn Bennett, MSN, ACNPC-AG, CCRN DNP Candidate, Tan Chingfen Graduate School of Nursing, UMass Chan Medical School, Worcester, Massachusetts; Neurosurgery ICU Nurse Practitioner, Yale New Haven Hospital, Yale Bridgeport, Bridgeport, Connecticut

Dawn Carpenter, DNP, ACNP-BC, CCRN, FAANP Trauma and Surgical ICU Nurse Practitioner, Guthrie Healthcare System, Robert Packer Hospital, Sayre, Pennsylvania; Associate Professor, Faculty Doctor of Nursing Practice Program, Tan Chingfen Graduate School of Nursing, UMass Chan Medical School, Worcester, Massachusetts; Adjunct Associate Clinical Professor of Surgery, Surgery Institute, Geisinger College of Health Professions, Danville, Pennsylvania

Monee' Carter-Griffin, DNP, MAOL, APRN, ACNP-BC Director of Education and Professional Development, Critical Care Nurse Practitioner, Exceed Healthcare/Dallas Pulmonary and Critical Care, Dallas, Texas; Clinical Assistant Professor, Faculty, Adult Gerontology Acute Care Nurse Practitioner Program, College of Nursing and Health Innovation, University of Texas at Arlington, Arlington, Texas

Dianna Chamberlain, MSN, ACNPC-AG, CEN, CCRN DNP Candidate, Tan Chingfen Graduate School of Nursing, UMass Chan Medical School, Worcester, Massachusetts; Nurse Practitioner, Neuro Sciences ICU, Cedars-Sinai, Los Angeles, California

Henry Ellis, DNP, AGACNP-BC Trauma and Surgical ICU Nurse Practitioner, Surgical ICU Group, UMass Memorial Medical Center, Worcester, Massachusetts; Assistant Professor, Tan Chingfen Graduate School of Nursing, UMass Chan Medical School, Worcester, Massachusetts

Mary Fischer, PhD, MSN, WHNP-BC Assistant Professor, Tan Chingfen Graduate School of Nursing, UMass Chan Medical School, Worcester, Massachusetts; Women's Health Nurse Practitioner, Atrius Health, Newton, Massachusetts

Danielle Hebert, DNP, MBA, ANP-BC Primary Care Nurse Practitioner, UMass Community Medical Group, UMass Memorial Health, Worcester,

Massachusetts; Assistant Professor, Coordinator Adult-Gerontology Primary Care Nurse Practitioner Program, Tan Chingfen Graduate School of Nursing, UMass Chan Medical School, Worcester, Massachusetts

Johnny Isenberger, MS, ACNP-BC, CCRN Clinical Instructor, Tan Chingfen Graduate School of Nursing, UMass Chan Medical School, Worcester, Massachusetts; Surgical Critical Care Nurse Practitioner, UMass Memorial Medical Center, Worcester, Massachusetts

Vanessa Jewett, RN, EMT, TCRN Trauma Resource Nurse, Injury Prevention Coordinator, Robert Packer Hospital, Sayre, Pennsylvania

Melanie Jung, MSN, FNP-BC, CPNP-AC Pediatric Trauma Program Manager, Pediatric Surgery Nurse Practitioner, UMass Memorial Medical Center, Worcester, Massachusetts

Elizabeth A. Keller, DNP, AG-ACNP Trauma Nurse Practitioner, UMass Memorial Health System, University Campus, Worcester, Massachusetts

Jennifer Kipp, MSW, MBA Manager, Case Management and Social Work Department, Robert Packer Hospital, Sayre, Pennsylvania

Lisa LaRock, MSL, BSN, RN, PHRN, CCRN-K Senior Director, System Trauma Services, The Guthrie Clinic, Pennsylvania/New York, Trauma Program Manager, Robert Packer Hospital, Sayre, Pennsylvania

Jessica Lewis, RN, BSN Emergency Department, Professional, Nurse, Expert Level, UPMC, Muncy Hospital, Muncy, Pennsylvania

Teresa Mahan, RN, BSN, CCRN Staff Nurse, Pediatric ICU, UMass Memorial Medical Center, Worcester, Massachusetts

Lisa McNamara, MS, RN, ACNP Adult Trauma Program Director, Director of Injury Prevention, UMass Memorial Medical Center, Worcester, Massachusetts

Alexander Menard, DNP, AGACNP-BC Assistant Professor, Tan Chingfen Graduate School of Nursing, UMass Chan Medical School, Worcester, Massachusetts; Surgical Critical Care Nurse Practitioner, UMass Memorial Medical Center, Worcester, Massachusetts

Nicholas Merry, MS, AG-ACNP-BC, CCRN Staff Nurse, Massachusetts General Hospital, Boston, Massachusetts

Nichole Miller, DNP, AGACNP-BC, CCRN Assistant Professor, MSN Online-Adult Gerontology Acute Care (AGACNP) Track, Chamberlain University, Addison, Illinois

Amelia Murray, PA-C Otorhinolaryngology Physician Associate, Guthrie Healthcare System, Robert Packer Hospital, Sayre, Pennsylvania

Cindybeth S. Palmgren, MS, ANP-BC, NP-C UMass Memorial Medical Center, Lead Trauma Nurse Practitioner, Worcester, Massachusetts

Anne G. Rizzo, MD, FACS, DABS System Surgical Chair, The Guthrie Clinic; President, Surgical Services, Professor of Surgery, USUHS, VCU, GCSOM; 2nd Vice President, American College of Surgeons; Past-Chair, American Board of Surgery, Critical Care, Trauma, Burns; Special Medical Advisor to the NORTHCOM Commander, Sayre, Pennsylvania

Michael Spiros, MALD, MS, APRN, AGACNP-BC, NE-BC Department of Medicine, Nurse Manager, Oregon Health and Science University Hospital, Portland, Oregon; Adjunct Associate Professor of Nursing, School of Nursing, Oregon Health and Science University, Portland, Oregon

Raymond St. Peter, MSN, RN, CCRN NeuroTrauma Critical Care Registered Nurse, UMass Memorial Medical Center, Worcester, Massachusetts; Clinical Instructor, Graduate Entry Pathway, Tan Chingfen Graduate School of Nursing, UMass Chan Medical School, Worcester, Massachusetts; Adjunct Professor, Department of Nursing Education, Quinsigamond Community College, Worcester, Massachusetts

Jill M. Terrien, PhD, ANP-BC Associate Professor of Nursing and Medicine, Associate Dean Interprofessional and Community Partnerships, UMass Chan Medical School, Tan Chingfen Graduate School of Nursing, Worcester, Massachusetts

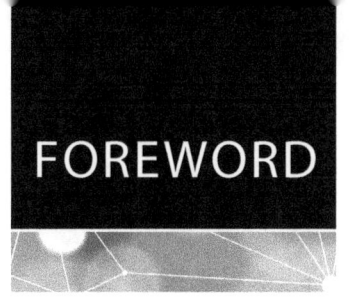

FOREWORD

Those of us who work in trauma centers on a daily basis understand that good things happen slowly, and bad things happen very quickly. A concise guide of many of these topics and situations is found in this publication, which can be accessed expediently with just-in-time information needed to optimize patient care. Our team has compiled a comprehensive review of all major topics that confront trauma caregivers. We have also included some specialty chapters that I have not seen included in such compilations before. Our chapter on veteran care is definitely unique and gives insight into the care this special population may need. This collection also includes aftercare and trauma prevention topics. Both of these are a must for trauma centers that are verified at a state or national level.

Trauma is definitely a team sport, and all members of the team are expected to participate and contribute. This compilation helps foster the team dynamics and educates to each member of the team and their roles. This will be an ongoing resource for trauma teams now and in the future.

Anne G. Rizzo, MD, FACS, DABS
System Surgical Chair, The Guthrie Clinic; President, Surgical Services, Professor of Surgery, USUHS, VCU, GCSOM; 2nd Vice President, American College of Surgeons; Past-Chair, American Board of Surgery, Critical Care, Trauma, Burns; Special Medical Advisor to the NORTHCOM Commander, Sayre, Pennsylvania

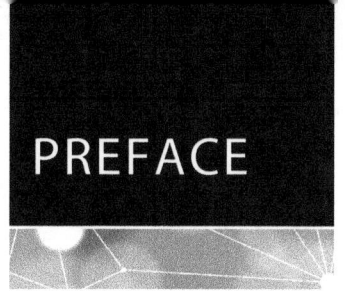

PREFACE

Welcome to the first edition of *Fast Facts for Trauma Nursing*. This book was created specifically for all levels of trauma nurses and students who care for injured patients throughout the hospital. This book presents critical information at the nurse's fingertips for quick reference in clinical settings.

This book is designed to fit in the pocket for daily use by nurses in the ED, ICU, intermediate care unit, general care floor, and beyond, and is based on over 30 years of experience with trauma patients and the wisdom of experienced nurse contributors. This pocket resource puts vital information at your fingertips with succinct, easy-to-read bullet points, diagrams, tables, and charts, providing large amounts of data in a condensed format. Given the expansive knowledge that trauma nurses must have, it was impossible to include everything and yet be small enough for the pocket; thus, selective components were chosen for inclusion.

The book is a quick access guide written by experienced trauma and critical care nurse practitioners. It is organized in a clinical system-based approach. The book provides quick-access tables, diagrams, and bullet points. It streamlines the complex information into easily understandable language. The book includes evidence-based treatments and nursing interventions for best practice and patient care.

Dawn Carpenter
Alexander Menard

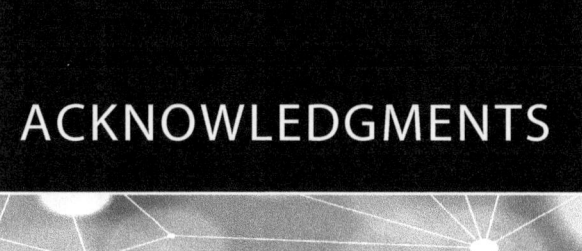

ACKNOWLEDGMENTS

We want to extend sincerest gratitude to all our colleagues at Guthrie Healthcare System, Robert Packer Hospital Level I Trauma Center, the University of Massachusetts Chan Medical School, Tan Chingfen Graduate School of Nursing, and UMass Memorial Medical Center for providing encouragement through this process.

Thank you to Springer Publishing Company for providing the opportunity to publish this book. Thank you to John Zaphyr and Brenna Croker, who have been amazingly supportive and responsive partners. We appreciate the faith you've had in us and appreciate your guidance and unwavering support. You have been essential to making this project come to fruition. It's been an absolute pleasure to work with you both!

Most importantly, I am eternally grateful to my loving husband, Andy, who has unwaveringly and selflessly supported my career. You have provided infinite love, patience, and support to help make this book a reality—I love you!!!

Dawn

I am thankful for my wife, Heather, and two children, Madelynn and Isabelle, who have continued to inspire and support.

Alex

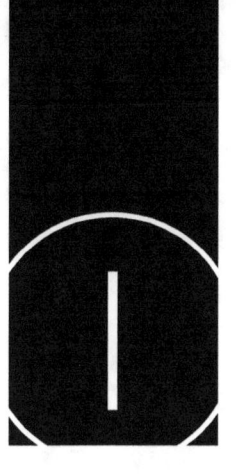

GENERAL TRAUMA PRINCIPLES

Trauma Systems and Trauma Center Preparedness
Dawn Carpenter

> Trauma is defined as an injury caused by a sudden external force to bodily tissue. A trauma system is an organized approach to care for acutely and critically injured trauma patients. Trauma systems are guided by robust trauma center standards and are accredited, designated, and verified by a state or national organization, such as the American College of Surgeons (ACS). Trauma systems require administrative and institutional commitment and support to survive and thrive. Significant resources, including people, departments, equipment, and processes, along with interagency and interfacility cooperation are essential to a trauma system. Specific criteria to stratify patients and resources are needed to allow organizations to flex to meet patient needs. Trauma systems need to constantly be in a state of team readiness to care for traumatically injured patients, including multiple patients at once. Having a standard approach to assessing and caring for trauma patients, such as Advanced Trauma Life Support (ATLS), improves survival.

In this chapter, you will learn to:
1. Differentiate among services available at each level of a trauma center.
2. Identify the different roles and responsibilities in the trauma bay.
3. Articulate the benefit of nursing certification on patient outcomes.
4. Articulate how ATLS and trauma systems came into existence.
5. Verbalize the elements of a D-MIST report.

INTRODUCTION

A trauma system is an organized approach to care for traumatically injured patients with a wide range of injuries. A trauma system coordinates specific clinical resources (facilities, personnel, and equipment) to produce optimal patient outcomes for injured patients. Trauma care involves the entire healthcare continuum, including prehospital, emergency department (ED), operative services, intensive care, acute care through discharge, and rehabilitation.

TRAUMA CENTERS

Not all hospitals meet the high standards of a trauma center. To be considered a trauma center, hospitals must be designated by either a state agency or the ACS. Either the state or the ACS verifies adherence to rigorous standards, including maintenance of a trauma registry and a structured quality improvement process. Table 1.1 details the services available at each level of trauma center. Each level plays a vital role in patient survival and enhanced outcomes. Level I and II trauma centers are expected to offer the same level of initial trauma resuscitation. A level II trauma center may transfer a patient to a level I trauma center for specific specialty care after the initial resuscitation. Many larger healthcare systems have multiple trauma centers with varying levels of care provided to geographic locations or regions.

TABLE 1.1

Trauma Center Levels

Level	Description
Level I (Academic medical center)	■ Admits ≥1,200 trauma patients per year ■ Board-certified attending trauma surgeon engages in all resuscitations and operations, and actively manages critically injured patients ■ Full range of specialists and equipment available 24/7 ■ Conducts trauma research ■ Educates general surgery residents ■ Leader in trauma education and prevention ■ Regional resource
Level II (Regional hospital)	■ Availability of all essential personnel and equipment, including neurosurgeon, 24/7 ■ Provides comprehensive trauma care ■ Provides trauma education and prevention ■ May transfer patients to level I for specific specialty care
Level III (Community hospital)	■ Has emergency resuscitation, surgery, and ICU available ■ General surgeon must be promptly available ■ Neurosurgeon not required ■ Has written transfer agreement to level I or II center
Level IV (Rural hospital)	■ Trauma-trained RN immediately available 24/7 ■ MD on-call ■ Initial evaluation/stabilization ■ Has written transfer agreement to level I or II center ■ Specializes in stabilization and rapid transfer to higher level of care
Level V (Rural clinic)	■ May not be open 24/7 ■ Trauma RN immediately available ■ MD on-call ■ Initial evaluation/stabilization, limited diagnostics ■ Has written transfer agreement to level I or II center

TRAUMA CENTER CARE TEAMS

Care of trauma patients, regardless of the facility, requires a team approach. Physicians, including trauma surgeons, emergency medicine physicians, and their senior residents, are most commonly the team leaders during trauma resuscitations, although nurse practitioners and physician assistants can also lead the resuscitation, diagnose injuries, and guide interventions. Nurses are critical to the success of trauma teams, including nurses in the ED, ICU, operating room (OR), postanesthesia care unit, and intermediate care and general care floors. Rehabilitation nurses also need to have specific knowledge to care for trauma patients, to recognize and prevent complications. Other key team members are identified in Table 1.2.

Triage of traumatically injured patients is performed by emergency medical services (EMS) teams in the field. Hospital notifications occur and triage the level of acuity to determine who requires care at a trauma center. See Table 1.3 for an example. Triage criteria can vary by hospital criteria and nomenclature. Table 1.3 lists high and moderate risk triage criteria; other institutions may refer to trauma activations on a numerical scale or other terminology.

PREPARATION

Hospitals need to be in a constant state of readiness to receive anywhere from one patient to a mass casualty situation. EDs can already be at or over capacity and still need to accommodate acutely and critically ill trauma patients. Staff knowledge, skill, and experience can affect patient outcomes. Every individual on the team needs to understand the sequence of ATLS so that the process is organized and coordinated.

TABLE 1.2

Additional Essential Trauma Center Services

Departments	Personnel	Processes

■ ORs
■ Blood bank
■ Laboratory
■ Pharmacy
■ Radiology
■ Rehabilitation
   ■ Inpatient or outpatient
■ On- or off-site
	■ Therapists
	   ■ Respiratory
	   ■ Physical
	   ■ Occupational
	   ■ Speech
	■ Dietitians
	■ Clergy/spiritual leader
	■ Psychiatrists
	■ Case manager
	■ Palliative care
	■ Social workers
	■ Substance use coaches
		■ Performance improvement
		■ Trauma prevention
		■ Follow-up and referrals

ORs, operating rooms.

TABLE 1.3

Criteria for Trauma Activation by Injury and Patient Status

Risk for Serious Injury	Injury Pattern	Patient Characteristics
High risk High risk patients should be transported to the highest level trauma center available.	<ul><li>Penetrating injury to head, neck, torso, or proximal extremities</li><li>Deformity of skull, suspected skull fracture</li><li>Suspected SCI with CSM deficits</li><li>Chest wall instability or deformity, or flail chest</li><li>Pelvis instability, suspected pelvic fracture</li><li>≥2 proximal long bone fractures</li><li>Crushed, degloved, mangled, or pulseless extremity</li><li>Amputation proximal to wrist or ankle</li><li>Active bleeding requiring a tourniquet, wound packing, or continuous pressure</li></ul>	All patients <ul><li>Respiratory distress</li><li>RR <10 or >29 BPM</li><li>Room air pulse ox <90%</li><li>Unable to follow commands</li><li>Age 0 to 9 years</li><li>SBP <70 mmHg + (2 × age in years)</li><li>Age 10 to 65 years</li><li>SBP <90 mmHg or HR > SBP</li><li>Age ≤65 years</li><li>SBP <110 mmHg or HR > SBP</li></ul>
Moderate risk Patients who meet any of these criteria (and who do not meet high risk criteria) should be transported to a trauma center; however, it does not need to be the highest level trauma center.	<ul><li>High-risk motor vehicle crash<ul><li>Partial or complete ejection</li><li>Significant intrusion</li><li>>12 inches occupant site or:</li><li>>18 inches any site</li><li>Entrapment needing extrication</li><li>Death in vehicle</li><li>Unrestrained child (age 0–9 years) with/without car seat</li><li>Vehicle telemetry data consistent with severe injury</li></ul></li><li>Rider separated from mode of transport with significant impact (motorcycle, ATV, horse, etc.)<ul><li>Pedestrian or bicycle rider thrown, run over, or significant impact</li><li>Fall from height >10 feet</li></ul></li></ul>	<ul><li>Low-level fall age <5 years or adults >65 years with significant head impact</li><li>Anticoagulant use</li><li>Suspected child abuse</li><li>Special or high-resource healthcare needs</li><li>Pregnancy >20 weeks</li><li>Burns in conjunction with trauma</li><li>Children should be triaged to pediatric-capable centers preferentially</li></ul>

BPM, breaths per minute; SCI, spinal cord injury; CSM, circulatory, sensory, motor; SBP, systolic blood pressure; HR, heart rate; RR, respiratory rate.

Source: Table modified from www.facs.org/for-medical-professionals/news-publications/news-and-articles/acs-brief/may-10-2022-issue/cot-releases-updated-national-guideline-for-field-triage-of-injured-patients/

Prehospital
EMS typically communicates with the receiving hospital to notify them of anticipated arrival to their facility so the hospital can mobilize their team and all providers can be present in the ED when the patient arrives. EMS focuses on stabilization of the cervical spine with a cervical collar and restriction of spinal motion while en route. The priority intervention is to secure the airway, control breathing, and maintain circulation. Pressure dressings, tourniquets, or pelvic binders may be applied in an attempt to prevent hemorrhage and shock. Obvious fractures or extremity deformities may be splinted as time allows. Prehospital personnel focuses on minimizing on-scene time to get the patient to definitive care rapidly.

Hospital Preparation
An ED provider who received the communication from EMS (referred to as medical command) triggers the facilities trauma activation system according to defined triage criteria set by the trauma center. The hospital trauma team responds to the ED and prepares the trauma bay for the patient's arrival. All personnel at the patient's direct bedside should wear full personal protective equipment.

The Trauma Bay
The trauma bay is a critical resource that needs to be in a continual state of readiness, as not all trauma activations afford the opportunity for advanced notice or have received prehospital care. Commonly, friends or family members bring injured patients directly to the ED. Thus, the staff and equipment must always be ready for the unexpected. The trauma bay is commonly stocked by ED support staff. The ED nurses are then responsible for double checking equipment and ensuring that disposable items are ready.

Vital equipment for trauma patients includes blood warmer and tubing, blood products in a blood refrigerator or a process to readily get blood products to the trauma bay, chest tubes with insertion equipment and suction canisters, a sterile tray with equipment to open the chest cavity, suture trays, and tracheostomy and cricothyroidotomy trays. An ultrasound machine should be kept charged and ready for use at the bedside. Warm blankets should be available, and the room temperature should be kept warm, especially in colder climates and seasons to treat/prevent hypothermia.

The availability of airway equipment including Ambu bag, oral airways, intubation equipment, GlideScope, ventilator, and difficult airway equipment is essential. Checking that all necessary equipment is readily available in the trauma bay is also extremely valuable and can be assigned to one person, considering the resources at your facility. Pharmacy ensures the medication dispensing system is stocked. A variety of analgesics, sedatives, anticoagulation reversal agents, antibiotics, and tetanus vaccines are routinely administered.

Prearrival Huddle

A prearrival huddle is commonly led by the team leader, although anyone can initiate the huddle. The purpose of the huddle is to introduce each team member and clarify their roles during the resuscitation. Information that is known about the patient is shared with the team, and instructions for anticipated patient needs are discussed. Once the patient arrives, the room should be silent so everyone can hear the EMS report and assessment findings. One person speaking at a time is critical, so everyone hears the same information. When interventions are completed, closed-loop communication is essential to ensure proper patient care and documentation.

The prearrival huddle at community hospitals (levels III and IV) is especially critical, as many patients require emergent interventions to stabilize them and plan for transfer to a higher level of care. Decision to transfer can be made based on information provided by EMS prior to patient arrival. Communications to the higher level of care can be initiated prior to patient arrival to mobilize helicopter transport and allow the receiving team to prepare.

FAST FACTS

Once the patient arrives to the trauma bay and throughout the resuscitation, the room should be silent, with only one person speaking at a time. This allows the recorder and team to adequately hear the team leader provide directions for interventions and feedback from the team when interventions are completed.

Roles

Each member in the room has an assigned role and responsibilities. Individual roles and qualifications for each role vary by hospital. See Figure 1.1 for an example of defined roles in the trauma bay. Experienced trauma nurse practitioners or physician assistants can fill any of these roles as needed or document the history and physical in the electronic health record. Not mentioned in Figure 1.1 is that an additional person is needed to contact family and be a liaison with family once they arrive. This role can be filled by a social worker, nursing supervisor, clergy, or other nurse. Other individuals that may be in the room are students (medical, nursing, respiratory, paramedic, etc.).

Team Leader

The team leader is the person directing the care. At community hospitals, the team leader will most likely be an emergency medicine physician, who may also be required to intubate or perform other procedures. The team leader will decide upon initiation of procedures or if operative intervention is required. They will also decide whether transfer to another facility is warranted.

Chapter 1 Trauma Systems and Trauma Center Preparedness 9

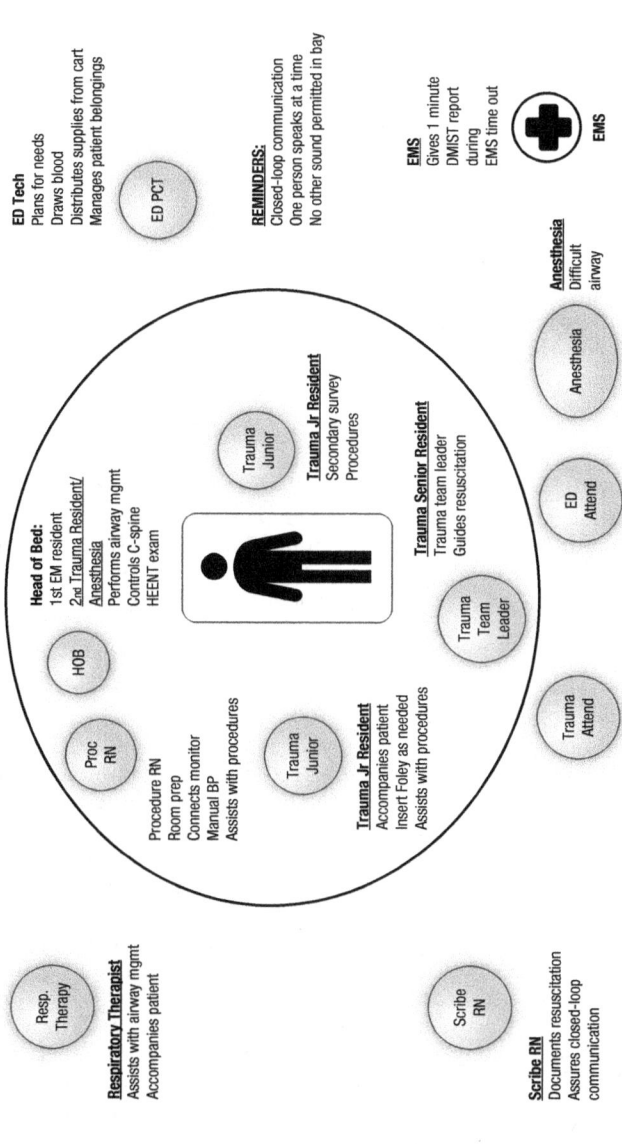

Figure 1.1 Suggested roles and responsibilities in the trauma bay.

Source: Used with permission from The Guthrie Clinic Trauma Centers, Sayre, Pennsylvania.

Nursing
Nurses are critical to the resuscitation efforts to save critically injured trauma patients. Nurses are responsible for continuous assessment and evaluation of interventions performed. Closed-loop communication is standard practice to report findings to the team leader and recorder. Common tasks completed by nurses in the trauma bay include documentation, obtaining intravenous access, monitoring, administration of medications, transfusion of blood, equipment setup, assistance with procedures, and so forth. For critically ill patients, the nurse stays with the patient at all times, including transport to the CT scanner, procedural area, the ICU, or OR.

Education
All RNs who work with trauma patients in the ED or throughout the hospital stay should receive education specific to care of trauma patients. Additional courses resulting in a certificate of completion, such as ATLS, are specific for nurses who care for trauma patients. Courses such as Advanced Trauma Care for Nurses, offered through the Society of Trauma Nurses, is an advanced course designed to increase RNs' knowledge in management of severely injured trauma patients. The ATCN course is taught in conjunction with ATLS, which team leaders are required to take. Alternatively, the Trauma Nursing Core Course is another continuing education class intended to disseminate a standardized body of trauma nursing knowledge. The Trauma Care After Resuscitation course is specifically designed for acute care, critical care, perioperative, and rehab nurses who care for patients who are admitted after they are through the ED or OR.

Certification
A national certification, the Trauma Certified Registered Nurse (TCRN) designation is an earned credential demonstrating nurses' specialized knowledge. These certifications are developed and awarded by a third-party organization that has expertise in creating and psychometrically testing the exams. Ideally, nurses who work with critically ill, complex trauma patients should hold a national certification. Certifications validate nurses' advanced knowledge and competence. These national certifications drive patients' health and enhance safety with a comprehensive credentialing process that ensures their practice is consistent with standards of excellence. National certification has been shown to reduce hospital errors, mortality rates, patient falls, and healthcare infections.

For ED nurses, the Certified Emergency Nurse (CEN) specialization equips ED nurses to treat any patient, at any time, with the latest specialty knowledge and best practices. The TCRN is for nurses who practice across the spectrum of trauma care and want to demonstrate their expertise and knowledge in trauma nursing. The certified acute or critical care RN specialization is for nurses who work in critical care, some of whom may be trauma patients.

FAST FACTS

Nurses who are nationally certified have an impact on patient health and safety. National certification has been shown to reduce hospital errors, mortality rates, patient falls, and healthcare infections.

ADVANCED TRAUMA LIFE SUPPORT

The concept of ATLS was developed in the 1970s. An orthopedic surgeon and his family were injured when a plane he was piloting in rural Nebraska crashed. His wife was killed on impact and three of his children were critically injured, whereas the surgeon sustained serious injuries. The care he and his family received at the local hospital was inadequate, and he embarked upon a journey to improve trauma care. Together with multiple healthcare and educational organizations in Nebraska, the concept of the ATLS course was born. The first ATLS course was run in 1978 and since then has expanded nationally and internationally, setting the standard for all trauma-related care.

FAST FACTS

The *golden hour* refers to the first 60 minutes after injury, when stabilizing the ABCDEs and transport to a trauma center that can provide definitive surgical intervention can prevent death.

Trauma care is guided by two primary ATLS concepts: First, treat life-threatening conditions first. Second, absence of a definitive diagnosis should not prevent initiation of required treatment. These principles guide the concepts behind the primary survey, which focuses on assessment and intervention to stabilize the ABCDEs. Primary survey includes:

A = Airway and cervical spine immobilization
B = Breathing
C = Circulation/control of bleeding/hemorrhage control
D = Disability/neurologic examination
E = Exposure (remove clothing) and environment (control body temperature)

Life-threatening injuries and conditions require immediate intervention. At any point, the decision to transfer a patient to a higher level of care can be made and the process started. The patient must be stabilized and appropriate lifesaving interventions initiated before transfer.

PATIENT ARRIVAL

Immediately upon patient arrival into the trauma bay, the team leader should ensure the primary survey is performed and intact (see Chapter 4). EMS will provide a brief report, around 1 to 2 minutes long. The report will follow the D-MIST approach (see Table 1.4).

Upon completion of the D-MIST report, the trauma team will complete the secondary survey (see Chapter 5). Chest and pelvis x-rays are required for all unstable or unresponsive patients and all patients at a level III or IV trauma center. After ensuring the patient is stable or has been stabilized since arrival, the team leader will decide upon additional testing, such as CT scans and/or additional x-rays. If the patient remains hemodynamically unstable, all sources of bleeding must be ruled out before the patient is transported to the radiology department or definitive care area. If the team identifies a source of bleeding and/or they are uncertain whether the patient has an ongoing bleeding source, they will take the patient to the operating suite or interventional radiology to manage this before completing any

TABLE 1.4

Mnemonic for EMS Report

Mnemonic: D-MIST	Information	Additional Details
D = **D**emographics	Age & gender	
M = **M**echanism of injury	What happened?	▪ Any entrapment, prolonged extrication time, intrusion into vehicle? ▪ Seatbelt use? Airbag deployment? Helmet? Other protective gear? ▪ Any LOC?
I = **I**nspection/ Injury/Illness	EMS findings	▪ Visible deformities ▪ Active bleeding ▪ Medical problems, anticoagulants
S = **S**igns & **S**ymptoms	VS, GCS, symptoms	▪ Patient complaints of pain ▪ Any symptoms prior to crash ▪ Glucose level
T = **T**reatments	What has been done PTA?	▪ Amount of IVF ▪ Any pain medications ▪ Any sedation/paralytics for intubation ▪ Antibiotics for open fractures ▪ Any transfusions ▪ Treatments from OSH, such as CT scans, blood, anticoagulation reversal

EMS, emergency medical services; GCS, Glasgow Coma Scale; IVF, intravenous fluid; LOC, loss of consciousness; OSH, outside hospital; PTA, prior to arrival; VS, vital signs.

other CT scans or movement to the patient care unit. A general rule of thumb is to have three systolic blood pressures greater than 100 mmHg before transporting a patient to radiology or a patient care unit such as the ICU. This ensures assessment and mitigation of ongoing hemorrhage.

SUMMARY

Trauma systems need to be in a constant state of readiness. Well-organized trauma teams with clearly defined roles and responsibilities expedite patient care. A quiet trauma bay enhances closed-loop communication. Having well-educated and certified nurses throughout the hospital improves patient outcomes.

REVIEW QUESTIONS

1. Nurses with national certification have been shown to:
   a. Improve errors
   b. Increase patient falls
   c. Reduce mortality rates
   d. Reduce community-acquired infections.
2. The *M* in *D-MIST report* stands for:
   a. Medical history
   b. Medical treatments
   c. Mechanism of injury
   d. Multiple trauma victim
3. Once a patient arrives in the trauma bay, the room should:
   a. Be cool
   b. Be quiet
   c. Be dimly lit
   d. Have music playing

References

American Association of Critical Care Nurses. *Board certification.* https://www.aacn.org/certification?tab=First-Time%20Certification

American Colleges of Surgeons: The Committee on Trauma. (2018). *ATLS: Advanced trauma life support student course manual* (10th ed.). American College of Surgeons.

Board Certification for Emergency Nursing. *About the TCRN exam.* https://bcen.org/tcrn/about-the-exam/

Board Certification for Emergency Nursing. *Reach your full potential with specialty nursing certification.* https://bcen.org

Criddle, L. M. (2022). *Trauma care after resuscitation course manual.* Visionem, Inc.

Emergency Nurses Association. *Emergency Nurses Association University.* https://www.ena.org/enau/educational-offerings

Newgard, C. D., Fischer, P. E., Gestring, M., Michaels, H. N., Jurkovich, G. J., Lerner, E. B., Fallat, M. E., Delbridge, T. R., Brown, J. B., & Bulger, E. M. (2022). The Writing Group for the 2021 National Expert Panel on Field Triage. National guideline for the field triage of injured patients: Recommendations of the National Expert Panel on Field Triage, 2021. *Journal of Trauma and Acute Care Surgery, 93*(2), e49–e60. https://doi.org/10.1097/TA.0000000000003627

Society of Trauma Nurses. *Advanced trauma care for nurses.* https://www.atcnnurses.org

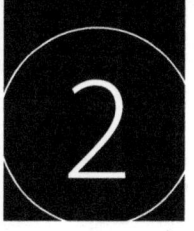

Risk Factors for Trauma
Dawn Carpenter

> Individual characteristics and circumstances can predict who is at most risk for traumatic injury. Additionally, family constructs and social circumstances can predispose individuals and families to become victims of trauma. Social determinants of health and adverse childhood events are risk factors for traumatic events throughout their lives. True "accidents" are rare, as most trauma is preventable. If it's predictable, it's preventable. Thus, most traumatic injuries and deaths are easily preventable.

In this chapter, you will learn to:
1. Identify risk factors for trauma.
2. Recognize how trauma is predictable.
3. Acknowledge how social determinants of health affect trauma patients.
4. Identify how adverse childhood experiences (ACEs) lead to trauma and polyvictimization.

INTRODUCTION

Annually in the United States, more than 23 million individuals are injured, with 36 million people requiring hospitalization. Trauma is the leading cause of death in ages 1 to 44 years and is the third leading cause of death for all age groups. The costs associated with these injuries, including medical expenses and lost productivity, exceeds $4.2 trillion annually. The most common etiologies of trauma include falls, motor vehicle crashes, firearms, and burn injuries. The most common mechanism of injury is blunt force trauma, followed by penetrating, crush, burn, and blast injuries. Trauma can be prevented and the extent of injuries reduced by common safety features such as seat belts, air bags, bike helmets, gun safes and locks, speed limits, and so forth (see Chapter 24).

FATALITIES

Fatal traumatic injuries have a trimodal distribution. The first peak occurs within seconds to minutes of the trauma and is commonly a result of severe brain injury, high spinal cord injury leading to apnea, or rupture of the heart or great vessels causing exsanguination or cardiac tamponade. The great vessels, including the aorta, can tear due to the stress on the tissues because they have fixed points of attachment. These types of injuries are normally lethal even with immediate advanced trauma care.

The second peak occurs within the first 4 hours post injury. These patients typically die from hemorrhagic shock, hemothorax, pelvic or long bone fractures, or splenic and/or hepatic lacerations. The concept of the "golden hour" was designed to improve outcomes for this specific population. The *golden hour* refers to the first 60 minutes after injury, when stabilization of the airway, breathing, and circulation/control of bleeding; disability assessment (i.e., neurologic status); and exposure/environmental (temperature control), commonly referred to as the ABCDEs. Immediate transport to a trauma center with definitive surgical intervention can prevent death and decrease medical sequelae from the injuries.

The third peak occurs several days to weeks after the injury and is related to sequelae of the trauma and resuscitation efforts. These deaths are commonly related to multiple organ dysfunction syndrome (MODS) from respiratory failure such as acute respiratory distress syndrome, renal failure, hepatic failure, cardiac failure, or hospital-acquired infections leading to septic shock. The development of septic shock can also lead to MODS.

Despite the development of Advanced Trauma Life Support courses and improvement in survival, there remains a large population of injured patients needing care. Hundreds of state laws have been implemented to reduce injuries and death, including seat belt requirements, vehicle safety devices, speed limits, drunk driving penalties, enhanced gun safety requirements, and so forth. However, human and social factors remain significant contributors to injuries and deaths. Humans continually find new and creative ways to injure themselves. Children used to ride scooters, bicycles, and skateboards; now we have motorized scooters, electric bicycles, and battery-operated hoverboards. Thus, as our society changes, so do the mechanisms of injury, causing new patterns of injury to emerge.

SOCIAL FACTORS

Trauma is a social disease. Many trauma patients are affected by the social determinants of health and/or ACEs, exposing them to traumatic situations and thus making them more prone to additional traumatic injuries. Additionally, social habits of alcohol, cannabinoids (legal or not), and illicit drugs are common factors altering individuals' judgment, making them prone to traumatic injuries.

Trauma is predictable, including who is most likely to get injured and what injuries are likely to occur. The mechanism of injury is important as it

> **FAST FACTS**
>
> Increased alcohol and drug abuse leads to increased risk for trauma and premature death.

can foretell a pattern of injury that may occur (see Chapter 3). Additionally, the outcome of patients is predictable in that trauma patients with a lower socioeconomic status tend to have worse outcomes. Additional patient-specific risk factors include gender, age, risk-taking behaviors, and social/environmental/lifestyle factors.

Patient factors predisposing to trauma include male gender. Two thirds of trauma patients are male, with the majority being between 15 and 40 years old. Risk-taking behaviors are most common in this age group. The term *young male syndrome'* is the tendency for these men, especially those who are not married or employed, to engage in risky behaviors, such as criminal acts, violence, drug use, driving at high speeds, and undertaking other physical feats to "save face." These young men are more focused on the short-term gains rather than on the longer term consequences of their actions.

At the other end of the age spectrum, older adult trauma patients, especially the frail elders, have the highest risk of mortality and have increased mortality in the setting of less severe injuries. The older adult strives to maintain independence for as long as possible. In rural areas, family may not live in the area to assist them; healthcare and other resources are farther apart; and public transportation is lacking, requiring them to drive beyond what is safe. Additionally, medical conditions and medical events contribute to injuries and deaths. For example, did the patient fall or did they experience syncope from cardiac arrhythmia or hypotension? Did the patient crash the car or have a hypoglycemic event or seizure causing them to go off the road? Medical events should always be suspected as the cause of trauma in a patient older than 50 years. Additionally, older adults do not want to give up their independence, which can also lead to an unsafe environment.

> **FAST FACTS**
>
> Older adult patients have a higher mortality than younger patients who have the same injuries. Even one rib fracture can precipitate the death of an older adult patient.

Social, environmental, and lifestyle factors play a large role in predicting who becomes injured. Social factors predisposing individuals to trauma include whom the person associates with, personal or family exposure to previous traumatic events, and the neighborhood where the individual lives. A person's associates include their intimate partners, which can lead to intimate partner violence (IPV), especially if either or both were exposed to IPV as a child. Nearly 41% of women and 26% of men experience IPV, which can include one or more of the following types: physical violence, sexual violence, stalking, and/or psychological aggression. Additionally, child and elder abuse, alcohol use, and illicit substance use are a few of the other social factors that continue to plague society, creating situations where trauma becomes the norm for many families.

SOCIAL DETERMINANTS OF HEALTH

Trauma disproportionately affects minorities, uninsured persons, and those who are economically disadvantaged. Health disparities exist in the trauma population. *Health disparities* are defined as differences in health outcomes that are closely related to both social and economic disadvantages. These disparities are affected by geographic location of birth and upbringing, as well as the geographic location where the injury occurred and where treatment was obtained.

The place a person is born, raised, injured, and treated shapes their overall health. The neighborhood, social and physical environment, exposure to ACEs, and access to quality healthcare affect outcomes. Crime is considered a social phenomenon and most commonly occurs between people who know each other. Violence and trauma are socially contagious, meaning the nature of trauma and violence includes exposure to various forms of abuse commonly referred to as polyvictimization. Specifically, violence is concentrated in high-risk populations in major cities, where unemployment is higher and people have lower education and income. Fifty percent of firearm fatalities occur in Black persons, 19% in Hispanic persons, and 18% in white persons, with 13% occurring in other ethnic groups. In the early 2000s, overall homicide rates were decreasing; however, Black-on-Black homicide increased 31%, with juvenile offenders increasing to 43%. Black victims have an age-adjusted murder rate 27% greater than white persons.

Trauma patients who have a lower socioeconomic status have worse clinical outcomes. Lower levels of education and income are associated with increased high-risk behavior, increased complication and death rates, and less access to quality healthcare. Additionally, those who are uninsured or underinsured have an increased likelihood of death regardless of their race or mechanism of injury.

ADVERSE CHILDHOOD EXPERIENCES

ACEs may be an isolated event or ongoing circumstances that a child identifies with in a negative way, which may have potentially harmful effects on their long-term health. ACEs include child abuse or neglect, household dysfunction (including domestic violence, substance use, criminal activity, mental illness, and parental absence), being poor, bullying, peer rejection/ lack of friends, school or community violence, serious accidents, traumatic loss of a loved one, sudden or frequent relocations, life-threatening childhood illness or injury, and exposure to or participation in prostitution/sex trafficking. Additionally, kidnapping, natural disasters, torture, war, and refugee camps and terrorism are included within ACEs.

Children who experience chronic traumatic toxic stressors (TTS) have their "flight-or-fight" response triggered. The flight-or-fight response activates the hypothalamic-pituitary-adrenal (HPA) axis and stimulates the sympathetic nervous system. HPA hormones trigger the release of cortisol and norepinephrine/epinephrine, which stimulate the heart (increase heart rate and blood pressure), lungs (dilate bronchioles), and liver (gluconeogenesis). Repeated or persistent stimulation of the flight-or-fight response can result in negative long-term health outcomes, such as hypertension, obesity, cardiovascular disease, and autoimmune diseases. Additionally, and important to the trauma population, the overstimulation of the HPA axis causes epigenetic modifications of the brain, specifically the hippocampus, prefrontal cortex, and amygdala. Remodeling of the amygdala can cause impulsive behaviors. TTS cause the prefrontal cortex, which regulates impulse control, to become underdeveloped, leading to decreased impulse control. Lastly, the response to TTS can alter social and behavioral coping abilities, which may lead to maladaptive behaviors such as alcohol or drug use.

FAST FACTS

Higher number of ACEs increases the risk of traumatic toxic stress, which leads to physiologic changes to the brain, increased impulsivity, and reduced impulse control and leads to maladaptive coping.

Four or more ACEs increase the rate of alcohol abuse (7.4 times), substance abuse (4.2 times), IV illicit substance abuse (11.3 times), and sex with 50 or more partners (3.2 times). Thus, impulsive behaviors, combined with reduced impulse control, and maladaptive behaviors referred to as *trauma organized lifestyle* predispose these children to increased risk for physical and psychological illnesses and trauma throughout their life. Higher numbers of ACEs are also found to be associated with increased rates of unemployment, leading to less access to medical and psychological care and premature death by up to 20 years sooner.

Additionally, trauma centers have been found to have outcome variability, with centers serving higher percentages of people of color having worse outcomes. Trauma centers that treat greater numbers of low-income or uninsured patients tend to have higher mortality rates. Further research into patient factors, staff and provider experience and expertise, as well as facility resources needs further exploration to explain these differences.

FAST FACTS

Nurses should assess for the social determinants of health and ACEs. Any positive findings warrant specific communication to the social work department to further assess the situation and connect the patient to available community services.

SUMMARY

Most trauma is preventable. Exposure to trauma and social environment are common factors contributing to injury. Social determinants of health and ACEs contribute to individuals experiencing trauma. More work must be done to alleviate health disparities for trauma patients.

REVIEW QUESTIONS

1. The nature of trauma and violence includes exposure to multiple forms of abuse, which is commonly referred to as:
   a. Mass casualty
   b. Polyvictimization
   c. Multisystem trauma patient
   d. Multiple partner violence
2. Trauma is:
   a. Exciting
   b. Inevitable
   c. Preventable
   d. Unavoidable
3. Which of the following is a risk factor for trauma?
   a. Having a job with benefits and reliable transportation
   b. Growing up in an urban area in a single-parent home
   c. Living in the suburbs with extended family nearby
   d. Having a college education and steady income

Additional Resources

Bell, T. M., & Zarzaur, B. L. (2013, October). Insurance status is a predictor of failure to rescue in trauma patients at both safety net and non-safety net hospitals. *Journal of Trauma and Acute Care Surgery, 75*(4), 728–733. https://doi.org/10.1097/TA.0b013e3182a53aaa

Brodal, P. (2004). *The central nervous system: Structure and function* (3rd ed.). Oxford University Press.

Brown, D. W., Anda, R. F., Tiemeier, H., Felitti, V. J., Edwards, V. J., Croft, J. B., & Giles, W. H. (2009). Adverse childhood experiences and the risk of premature mortality. *American Journal of Preventive Medicine, 37*, 389–396.

Burke, N. J., Hellman, J. L., Scott, B. G., Weems, C. F., & Carrion, V. G. (2011). The impact of adverse childhood experiences on an urban pediatric population. *Child Abuse & Neglect, 35,* 408–413.

Centers for Disease Control and Prevention. (2010). Adverse childhood experiences reported by adults—Five states, 2009. *Morbidity and Mortality Weekly Report, 59,* 1609–1613.

Centers for Disease Control and Prevention. (2011). CDC health disparities and inequalities report United States, 2011. *Morbidity and Mortality Weekly Report, 60*(Suppl.), 1–109.

Centers for Disease Control and Prevention. (2013). CDC health disparities and inequalities report United States 2013. *Morbidity and Mortality Weekly Report, 62*(3), 1–184.

Cudnik, M. T., Sayre, M. R., Hiestand, B., & Steinberg, S. M. (2010). Are all trauma centers created equally? A statewide analysis. *Academic Emergency Medicine, 17*(7), 701–708.

Dong, M., Giles, W. H., Felitti, V. J., Dube, S. R., Williams, J. E., Chapman, D. P., & Anda, R. F. (2004). Insights into causal pathways for ischemic heart disease: Adverse childhood experiences study. *Circulation, 110,* 1761–1766.

Dube, S. R., Cook, M. L., & Edwards, V. J. (2010). Health-related outcomes of adverse childhood experiences in Texas, 2002. *Preventing Chronic Disease, 7,* 1–9.

Elenkov, I. J., & Chrousos, G. P. (2006). Stress system—organization, physiology and immunoregulation. *Neuroimmunomodulation, 13,* 257–267.

Felitti, V. J., Anda, R. F., Nordenberg, D., Williamson, D. F., Spitz, A. M., Edwards, V., & Marks, J. S. (1998). Relationship of childhood abuse and household dysfunction to many of the leading causes of death in adults: The Adverse Childhood Experiences Study. *American Journal of Preventive Medicine, 14,* 245–258.

Garner, A. S., Shonkoff, J. P., & Committee on Psychosocial Aspects of Child and Family Health; Committee on Early Childhood, Adoption, and Dependent Care; Section on Developmental and Behavioral Pediatrics. (2012). Early childhood adversity, toxic stress, and the role of the pediatrician: Translating developmental science into lifelong health. *Pediatrics, 129,* e224–e231.

Greene, J., & Hibbard, J. H. (2012). Why does patient activation matter? An examination of the relationships between patient activation and health-related outcomes. *Journal of General Internal Medicine, 27*(5), 520–526. https://doi.org/10.1007/s11606-011-1931-2

Haider, A. H., Ong'uti, S., Efron, D. T., Oyetunji, T. A., Crandall, M. L., Scott, V. K., Haut, E. R., Schneider, E. B., Powe, N. R., Cooper, L. A., & Cornwell, E. E. (2012). Association between hospitals caring for a disproportionately high percentage of minority trauma patients and increased mortality: A nationwide analysis of 434 hospitals. *Archives of Surgery, 147*(1), 63–70. https://doi.org/10.1001/archsurg.2011.254

Institute of Medicine & National Research Council. (2013). *Contagion of violence: Workshop summary.* The National Academies Press.

Kochanek, K. D., Xu, J., Murphy, S. L., Minino, A. M., & Kung, H. C. (2011). Deaths: Final data for 2009. *National Vital Statistics Reports, 60,* 1–166.

Mc Elroy, S., & Hevey, D. (2014). Relationship between adverse early experiences, stressors, psychosocial resources and wellbeing. *Child Abuse & Neglect, 38,* 65–75.

National Scientific Council on the Developing Child. (2015). *Excessive stress disrupts the architecture of the developing brain: Working Paper 3.* Updated Edition. https://developingchild.harvard.edu/resources/reports_and_working_papers/working_papers/wp3/

Shonkoff, J. P., Boyce, W. T., & McEwen, B. S. (2009). Neuroscience, molecular biology, and the childhood roots of health disparities: Building a new framework for health promotion and disease prevention. *JAMA, 301,* 2252–2259.

Shonkoff, J. P., Garner, A. S., Committee on Psychosocial Aspects of Child and Family Health; Committee on Early Childhood, Adoption, and Dependent Care; Section on Developmental and Behavioral Pediatrics. (2012). The lifelong effects of early childhood adversity and toxic stress. *Pediatrics, 129,* 232–246.

Sleet, D. A., Dahlberg, L. L., Basavaraju, S. V., Mercy, J. A., McGuire, L. C., & Greenspan, A. (2011). Injury prevention, violence prevention, and trauma care: Building the scientific base. *Morbidity and Mortality Weekly Report, 60*(4), 78–85. www.cdc.gov/mmwr/pdf/other/su6004.pdf

Turner, H. A., Finkelhor, D., & Ormrod, R. (2010). Poly-victimization in a national sample of children and youth. *American Journal of Preventive Medicine, 38*(3), 323–330. https://doi.org/10.1016/j.amepre.2009.11.012

Wilson, M., & Daly, M. (1985). Competitiveness, risk taking, and violence: The young male syndrome. *Ethology and Sociobiology, 6,* 59–73.

References

Criddle, L. M. (2022). *Trauma care after resuscitation course manual.* Visionem, Inc.

Mikhail, J. N., Nemeth, L. S., Mueller, M., Pope, C., & NeSmith, E. G. (2018, September/October). The social determinants of trauma: A trauma disparities scoping review and framework. *Journal of Trauma Nursing, 25*(5), 266–281. https://doi.org/10.1097/JTN.0000000000000388

Oral, R., Ramirez, M., Coohey, C., Nakada, S., Walz, A., Kuntz, A., Benoit, J., & Peek-Asa, C. (2016). Adverse childhood experiences and trauma informed care: The future of health care. *Pediatric Research, 79*(1), 227–233.

Tamás, V., Kocsor, F., Gyuris, P., Kovács, N., Czeiter, E., & Büki, A. (2019, April 12). The young male syndrome: An analysis of sex, age, risk taking and mortality in patients with severe traumatic brain injuries. *Frontiers in Neurology, 10,* 366. https://doi.org/10.3389/fneur.2019.00366

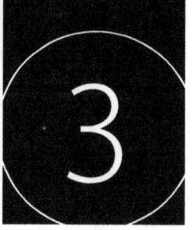

Mechanism of Injury
Alexander Menard

> *The mechanism of injury can provide crucial information in determining the extent and type of damage that results from a trauma. The resulting damage can be* anatomic and/or physiologic. Anatomic *refers to broken structures, like bones, while* physiologic *refers to complex systems, like the nervous system. The mechanism of injury informs responders and caregivers to anticipate injuries, guides assessments, interventions, and management.*

In this chapter, you will learn to:
1. Define mechanism of injury.
2. Differentiate between blunt and penetrating trauma.
3. Understand how mechanism of injury influences injury patterns.

INTRODUCTION

The first information that is conveyed after a trauma occurs is the mechanism of injury. How an injury happened, the types of forces involved, and the organs and tissues suspected of being injured are all part of mechanism of injury. The mechanism of injury is a key factor that first responders utilize to determine where a trauma patient should be transported. The mechanism of injury can inform what services a patient may require, thus directing first responders to transport the patient to a facility with appropriate resources. Injury patterns offer an index of suspicion and direction for care teams to investigate and treat. The mechanism of injury is categorized into two broad areas: blunt trauma and penetrating trauma.

FAST FACTS

Mechanism of injury is a key component for first responders and the trauma care team to decide the level of care (facility capabilities) and diagnostic workup and interventions that are warranted.

BLUNT TRAUMA

The most common type of trauma is blunt force trauma. This includes motor vehicle crashes (MVCs), falls, assaults/physical violence, blast injury (without penetrating projectiles), pedestrian versus vehicle, and contact sports. Blunt force trauma is a result of transferred energy from an object to a person and the resultant displacement and damage to the body (tissues, organs, and bones) and body systems.

FAST FACTS

Blunt trauma is force/s applied to tissue/s resulting in injury(ies). It can be caused by a single force or combination of forces: acceleration, deceleration, shearing, crushing, rotational, or compression.

Motor Vehicle Crashes

MVCs are responsible for nearly 50% of blunt trauma. MVCs result in extensive damage to the body structure and tissues. MVCs can cause blunt trauma to the body by all forces listed above. Distinguishing characteristics of the crash informs the specific body parts and/or systems that need focused evaluation. The mechanism of injury has direct correlation with a pattern of injury (see Table 3.1). Four types of impact occur during a single MVC:
1. The vehicle impacts another object.
2. The occupant (driver or passenger) collides with the interior of the vehicle or other object.
3. Internal tissues collide with ridged structures of the body.
4. Secondary impacts (passengers within a car collide with each other).

Additionally, if a person is ejected, they may also collide with other objects outside the vehicle.

Falls

More than 800,000 patients a year are hospitalized secondary to injuries sustained due to a fall. Fall injuries are a result of vertical deceleration. Given the nature of this mechanism of injury, there is an associated injury pattern that accompanies this type of injury (see Table 3.2). Falls most often result in head injury and/or hip fractures. There are several modifiable and nonmodifiable risk factors for falls (see Table 3.3).

FAST FACTS

Blunt trauma can result in multiple injuries, making this form of trauma more life-threatening than penetrating trauma injuries. Blunt injuries can be less obvious, potentially delaying diagnosis.

TABLE 3.1

Injury Patterns With MVC

Mechanism of Injury	Possible Injury Pattern
Frontal impact	- Cervical spine fracture/s - Anterior flail chest - Pneumothorax - Traumatic aortic disruption - Spleen or liver injury - Fracture or dislocation of the knee and/or hip - Head injury (TBI, skull fracture, laceration, etc.) - Facial fractures
Side impact	- Cervical spine fracture/s - Lateral flail chest - Pneumothorax - Traumatic aortic disruption - Spleen, liver, or kidney injury - Head injury (TBI, skull fracture, laceration, etc.) - Fractured pelvis or acetabulum
Rear impact	- Cervical spine injury - Head injury (TBI, skull fracture, laceration, etc.) - Soft tissue injury to the neck
Ejection	- Difficult to predict injury pattern, but increases risk and severity for all possible injuries
Motor vehicle versus pedestrian	- Head injury (TBI, skull fracture, laceration, etc.) - Traumatic aortic disruption - Abdominal visceral injuries - Fractured lower extremities and pelvis

MVC, motor vehicle crash; TBI, traumatic brain injury.

PENETRATING TRAUMA

Penetrating trauma is defined by a foreign object that penetrates body tissue. Most commonly this is from bullets, knives, industrial equipment, power tools, and/or other projectiles. The severity of the injury is directly related to the tissues and structures that are directly impacted. The amount of damage is also closely related to the force by which the object was thrust. Higher velocity penetrating objects will transfer more energy to the tissues when impacting the body compared with low-velocity objects; thus, high-velocity projectiles cause more tissue damage. The extent of tissue damage is not readily apparent upon presentation and may take hours to days to become apparent.

FAST FACTS

Penetrating trauma is an injury in which the body has been pierced by a foreign body.

TABLE 3.2
Injury Patterns With Falls

Falls	Possible Injury Pattern

From height, standing, or stairs	■ Axial spine injury*
	■ Abdominal visceral injuries
	■ Fractured pelvis or acetabulum
	■ Head injury (TBI, skull fracture, laceration, etc.)
	■ Lower extremity fractures
	  ● Calcaneal fracture with fall from height*
	■ Rib fractures
	  ● Hemothorax or pneumothorax
	  ● Hemopneumothorax

Fall/jump and land on feet	■ Calcaneal fractures ■ Hip and pelvis fractures ■ Axial spinal injury
Fall, land on head/diving	■ Axial spinal injury, cervical spine most common ■ Head injury ■ Near drowning

*Associated with falls from height.

TBI, traumatic brain injury.

TABLE 3.3
Risk Factors for Falls

Modifiable	Nonmodifiable

■ Vision problems
■ Difficulty with ambulation or balance
■ Lower body weakness
■ Vitamin D deficiency
■ Medications (polypharmacy), particularly sedatives, opioids, and antihypertensive agents
■ Home hazards, throw rugs, uneven flooring, or steps
	■ Age
	■ Sex
	■ History of prior falls
	■ Chronic conditions
	  ● Prior stroke
	  ● Parkinson disease
	  ● Dementia
	  ● Sensory loss

High-Velocity Penetrating Trauma

Penetrating trauma is often related to projectiles; missiles; or, more often, gunshot wounds. This mechanism of injury also corresponds to patterns of injury that should be suspected (see Table 3.4). Most commonly, this missile or projectile comes from a firearm. The extent of tissue damage is determined by the caliber and characteristics of the bullet and the velocity of

TABLE 3.4

Injury Pattern: High-Velocity Penetrating Trauma

Gunshot Wounds	Possible Injuries
Truncal	■ Trajectory from the projectile helps predict injured tissues or organ/s. ■ With any penetrating injury to the chest or abdomen, the team should suspect and assess for an injury to the other cavity. ■ Pneumothorax ■ Hemothorax
Extremity/ies	■ Fractured bones ■ Vascular injury ■ Nerve injury ■ Extensive muscle loss ■ Complications: Compartment syndrome can be present on initial presentation or develop hours to a day or two later.

the bullet, which is determined by the amount of propellant in the casing. In general, rifles tend to have a higher velocity than handguns and result in increased tissue damage. Shotguns, on the other hand, usually have more projectiles within the shell, which can cause significant damage at a short range. Pellets spread out as distance from the firearm increases, thus making them less lethal at longer distances.

Muzzle blast is a mechanism of injury of penetrating trauma that describes the cloud of hot gases emitted from the barrel that result after a firearm is discharged against tissues. If the proximity to the body is close, these gases can enter the cavity and cause localized damage. As a bullet enters the body, it may strike a bone, causing the bone to shatter and become additional projectiles that damage tissue. A bullet that strikes a bone may change direction within the body, making it difficult to predict internal injuries.

Low-Velocity Penetrating Trauma

Penetrating trauma includes stab wounds and other impalements. These wounds are typically more obvious but require thorough inspection to identify other penetration sites (see Table 3.5). Low-velocity penetrating trauma often affects only tissues and structures in the immediate area of the injury. The size and shape of the penetrating object and direction of penetration are also important, to understand which tissues and to what extent those tissues may be damaged. Stabbing or impalement injuries can involve intrusion into more than one body cavity. For example, a stab wound to the upper abdomen can traverse the diaphragm and enter the chest cavity as well.

TABLE 3.5

Injury Patterns: Low-Velocity Penetrating Trauma

Stab Wound Location	Common Injury Pattern (Any tissue or organ within direct path of the object must be suspected of injury)
Anterior chest	■ Cardiac tamponade ■ Hemothorax and/or pneumothorax
Posterior chest	■ Hemothorax and/or pneumothorax ■ Spinal cord injury
Left thoracoabdominal	■ Left diaphragmatic injury ■ Splenic injury ■ Hemopneumothorax
Abdomen	■ Abdominal visceral injury ■ Pelvic injuries, including bladder ■ Diaphragm injury

FAST FACTS

Never remove an object that is still embedded in the patient without the ability to explore the injured site because the object may be tamponading the bleeding. Ensure options for surgical control and stabilization are immediately available prior to removal of any penetrating object.

BURN INJURY

Burn injuries may be isolated or occur in conjunction with other traumatic injuries. Gathering information regarding the mechanism of burn injury can differentiate the classification of the burn. Types of burns include thermal, electrical, radiation, and chemical (see Table 3.6). Depending on the type of burn, initial management and treatment vary. For instance, a patient who presents with a chemical burn requires decontamination, whereas a patient who presents with an inhalation injury may need an advanced airway.

SUMMARY

The mechanism of injury is an important part of the initial triage of a trauma patient to ensure transport from the scene to an appropriate facility equipped to manage their potential injuries. The mechanism of injury can also inform hospital caregivers on potential diagnoses and management. Understanding the mechanism of injury can inform the trauma team of

TABLE 3.6

Types of Burn Injuries

Burn	Description
Thermal	Burn secondary to an external heat source that raises the temperature of the skin and tissues and causes tissue cell damage or death.
Electrical	Burn from electrical current. AC or DC.
Radiation	Burn due to prolonged exposure to ultraviolet rays of the sun, or to other sources of radiation.
Chemical	Burns due to strong acids, alkalis, detergents, or solvents to the skin and/or eyes.

AC, alternating current; DC, direct current.

suspected injuries. Several factors can affect patterns of injury for a trauma patient. For example, a patient involved in an MVC might have blunt trauma secondary to hitting the steering wheel and have a penetrating trauma from a tree branch that impaled the neck, as well as thermal injuries to the lower extremities from the fire that ignited in the engine. The mechanism of injury will provide crucial information on what patterns of injury to expect in informing care of the patient.

REVIEW QUESTIONS

1. It is possible to have a patient with both blunt and penetrating trauma. True or false
2. Motor vehicle crash results in this many impact/s:
   a. One
   b. Two
   c. Three
   d. Four
3. This type of burn can result from prolonged exposure to sunlight.
   a. Chemical
   b. Radiation
   c. Thermal
   d. Electrical
4. _____ is an important factor when deciding where a trauma patient should be transported.
   a. Mechanism of injury
   b. Patient preference
   c. Family preference
   d. Alcohol level

References

American College of Surgeons: The Committee on Trauma. (2018). *ATLS: Advanced Trauma Life Support student course manual* (10th ed.). American College of Surgeons.

Centers for Disease Control and Prevention, & National Center for Injury Prevention and Control. (2023, November). *Web-based injury statistics query and reporting system (WISQARS)*. https://www.cdc.gov/injury/wisqars/index.html

Evans, D., Pester, J., Vera, L., Jeanmonod, D., & Jeanmonod, R. (2015). Elderly fall patients triaged to the trauma bay: Age, injury patterns, and mortality risk. *The American Journal of Emergency Medicine*, *33*(11), 1635–1638. https://doi.org/10.1016/j.ajem.2015.07.044

Florence, C. S., Bergen, G., Atherly, A., Burns, E. R., Stevens, J. A., & Drake, C. (2018, March). Medical costs of fatal and nonfatal falls in older adults. *Journal of the American Geriatrics Society*, *66*(4), 693–698. https://doi.org/10.1111/jgs.15304

Lupton, J. R., Davis-O'Reilly, C., Jungbauer, R. M., Newgard, C. D., Fallat, M. E., Brown, J. B., Mann, N. C., Jurkovich, G. J., Bulger, E., Gestring, M. L., Lerner, E. B., Chou, R., & Totten, A. M. (2022). Mechanism of injury and special considerations as predictive of serious injury: A systematic review. *Academic Emergency Medicine*, *29*(9), 1106–1117. https://doi.org/10.1111/acem.14489

McQuillan, K. A., & Flynn-Makic, M. B. (2020). *Trauma nursing: From resuscitation through rehabilitation* (5th ed.). Elsevier.

Toney-Butler, T. J., & Varacallo, M. (2022, January). *Motor vehicle collisions*. StatPearls Publishing. https://www.ncbi.nlm.nih.gov/books/NBK441955/

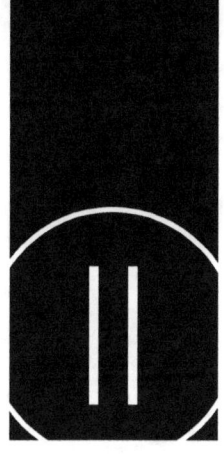

RESUSCITATIVE PHASE OF CARE

Primary Survey
Alexander Menard

> The primary survey is focused on rapid assessment of the patient's vital functions. The primary survey must include the Airway, with restriction of cervical spine motion, Breathing, Circulation, Disability, and Exposure (ABCDEs). Alterations in each of these elements must be addressed before moving on through the rest of the exam. The purpose of the primary exam is to treat any instability to prevent life-threatening deterioration.

In this chapter, you will learn to:
1. Distinguish between the components of the primary survey.
2. State the goal of a primary survey.
3. Recognize different types of shock.

INTRODUCTION

The assessment of a trauma patient is divided into three main phases: primary, secondary, and tertiary surveys. This framework for evaluation is specific to the trauma population and is structured to identify life-threatening injuries first, prioritize interventions and care needs, and identify other injuries when the patient is more stable. This chapter describes the primary survey in detail.

The focus of the primary survey is identification of life-threatening injuries, intervening on those injuries deemed critical and prioritizing the plan of care for the patient. This is done by assessing airway, breathing, circulation, disability, and exposure, more commonly known as the ABCDEs (Table 4.1). The ABCDEs can be assessed within seconds of the initial encounter with a clinician. The clinician can assess ABC and D by simply introducing themselves and asking the patient to state their name and to describe what happened. Thus, the examiner can simultaneously determine that the patient has a patent airway and intact cognition.

Restriction of cervical spine motion is considered the second part of the airway evaluation. Cervical collars are routinely placed by emergency medical services (EMS) prehospital. For patients who present in personal vehicles, a cervical collar should be placed immediately until assessment can be performed. Cervical spine precautions should be maintained throughout

TABLE 4.1

Primary Survey of the ABCDEs

ABCDE	Assessment
A = Airway (with restriction of c-spine motion)	Assess patency: can the patient talk? Inspect for blood or edema obstructing the airway Ability to maintain a patent airway Place cervical collar and maintain c-spine precautions
B = Breathing and ventilation	Assess oxygen saturation Assess ability to take deep breaths
C = Circulation with hemorrhage control	Assess skin perfusion Assess for decreased level of consciousness Observe heart rate for tachycardia Inspect for overt bleeding
D = Disability	Assess neurologic status: GSC, movement, and sensation
E = Exposure	Completely undress the patient to ensure a complete evaluation of all surfaces Obtain temperature to identify any hypo- or hyperthermia

ABCDE, airway, with restriction of c-spine motion, breathing, circulation, disability, and exposure; c-spine, cervical spine; GSC, Glasgow Coma Scale.

the primary and secondary surveys and diagnostic treatments. Avoid head rotation, extension, and flexion. Nursing should educate the awake patient not to move their head and remain still until a formal assessment of the cervical spine can be done. Patients with midline spinal tenderness require CT scan of the neck to assess for bony fractures. Midline spinal tenderness is not the sole indication for spinal imaging; the mechanism of injury alone can warrant radiographic investigation. Caregivers must always be aware of the possibility of a distracting injury, an injury that overshadows another injury, otherwise stated as an injury with significant pain that may prevent accurate assessment and patient report of pain, thus preventing identification of other serious injuries.

FAST FACTS

Airway is the first and foremost assessment during the primary survey. If the patient can verbally communicate and has no hoarseness or stridor, they are less likely to have an airway that is in immediate jeopardy. If the patient does not have a patent airway, or the ability to maintain their airway, the team must first secure the airway, regardless of the underlying issue(s) causing the compromised airway.

AIRWAY (A)

Evaluation of airway patency is the highest priority and the first assessment completed when a trauma patient arrives to a hospital. Rapidly assessing airway patency can be done by asking them their name. If the patient is unable to speak, look for bleeding, edema, injuries, and foreign objects obstructing the airway. Identify fractures in the surrounding area (face, mandibular) or other obvious injuries of the neck that may impede the airway. Focus on restricting the cervical spine movement during this assessment and until the cervical spine can be cleared.

Airway adjuncts can be used to assist in maintaining patent airways. The jaw-thrust maneuver is an initial measure to open the airway but is often only a temporizing measure to optimize airway patency. Nasal trumpet and/or oral bite block are also commonly used. The nasal trumpet can be used in patients who are lethargic but breathing and can be used to nasotracheal suction the trachea. Nursing should never insert a nasogastric tube to any patient with a traumatic brain injury or facial fractures until appropriate imaging and specialist consultation have occurred. Oral bite blocks are used temporarily in unconscious patients to lift the tongue and open the airway to allow for Ambu bagging. At any point, if there is concern that the patient does not have a patent airway or is unable to maintain their airway, a definitive airway (oral or nasal endotracheal tube or tracheostomy) should be considered. Most commonly, patients are intubated orally, but nasotracheal intubation is an option. If patients are unable to be intubated, a tracheostomy or cricothyroidotomy may be placed emergently by surgeons.

FAST FACTS

Frequent reassessment of the airway is needed because a patient's condition can change rapidly, causing loss of patency or ability to maintain an airway, and can occur at any moment (even when a definitive airway is in place). End-tidal carbon dioxide monitoring may be used to ensure that the endotracheal tube is in the correct position.

Restriction of Cervical Spine Motion

Careful attention must be paid to minimize movement of the cervical spine to prevent development or worsening of a neurologic deficit from trauma to the cervical spine. A cervical collar is the standard method for cervical spine immobilization. The cervical collar will remain in place until it can be clinically and/or radiologically cleared. It is important to note that during the primary or secondary surveys is not the time to "clear" the cervical collar; this should be done once the patient is stabilized.

BREATHING AND VENTILATION (B)

Having an airway that is patent does not equate to adequate breathing and ventilation. Careful assessment is needed to ensure patients are adequately ventilated. *Ventilation* refers to adequate exchange of gasses, primarily oxygen and carbon dioxide. Several factors affect the ability to ventilate a patient, including neurologic status, shock, and respiratory mechanics. The condition of the lungs, chest wall, and diaphragm affect ventilation. Impairment of any of these factors can affect the patient's ability to adequately breathe and ventilate. If a patient has inadequate breathing or ventilation, an advanced airway is needed.

FAST FACTS

A patent airway does not ensure adequate respiration or ventilation. Assessment should include rate and depth of respirations. Patients in shock or with severe pain, especially from rib fractures, will breathe rapidly and shallowly. Patients with respiratory rates over 22 breaths per minute should be carefully monitored for impending respiratory failure.

CIRCULATION WITH HEMORRHAGE CONTROL (C)

The statement "it is hemorrhage until proven otherwise" is often verbalized when discussing critically ill trauma patients. Most circulation issues result from bleeding, which causes low circulating blood volume, resulting in a low cardiac output. Compensatory mechanisms include increased heart rate and contractility. Failure of the compensatory mechanisms results in hypotension and shock. Recognizing bleeding, quickly controlling it, and rapidly starting resuscitation are crucial components of this part of the primary survey. Hemorrhagic shock is the leading type of shock affecting trauma patients. Trauma patients may concurrently experience other types of shock, including hypovolemic, cardiogenic, distributive, and obstructive shock (Table 4.2). The cause of the shock must be determined to properly treat the patient. An important concept is that trauma patients can have more than one type of shock at a time, such as hemorrhagic and neurogenic shock. For example, a patient with a urinary tract infection who has a fall may have both septic and hemorrhagic shock.

Hemorrhagic shock is the most common type of shock in the trauma patient. A hemorrhage is the result of rapid acute loss of blood from the vascular system. The average adult's volume of circulating blood is estimated to be 5 liters of blood, which is approximately 7% of body weight. Hemorrhagic shock can be further classified by signs and symptoms.

TABLE 4.2

Types of Shock

Type of Shock	Description
Hypovolemic—Nonhemorrhagic	Inadequate circulating volume related to nonbleeding sources (vomiting, diarrhea, diaphoresis, third spacing, etc.)
Hypovolemic—Hemorrhagic	Inadequate circulating blood secondary to bleeding
Cardiogenic	Pump impairment/failure
Distributive—Septic	Peripheral vasodilation—due to infection
Distributive—Neurogenic	Impaired/disrupted sympathetic tone
Distributive—Anaphylactic	Peripheral vasodilation—due to allergic reaction
Obstructive—Pulmonary embolism	Decreased cardiac output due to impaired blood flow through the pulmonary vessels
Obstructive—Cardiac tamponade	Decreased cardiac output secondary to pericardial fluid accumulation, preventing adequate filling of the ventricles
Obstructive—Tension pneumothorax	Decreased cardiac output secondary to displacement and compression of the great vessels
Adrenal insufficiency	Deficiency in circulating cortisol

Hemorrhage can occur into five areas, including the surrounding environment (outside the body), chest, abdomen/pelvis, retroperitoneum, and long bones. Internal bleeding can be identified by physical examination and imaging with a focused assessment with sonography for trauma (FAST) exam; radiographic images (chest x-ray, pelvic x-ray, etc.); and less commonly, diagnostic peritoneal lavage.

External bleeding is initially managed by direct pressure; if direct pressure is not sufficient and life or limb is threatened, a tourniquet can be applied. Scalp lacerations can bleed profusely; thus, closure with staples or sutures during the primary survey is imperative. The most common spaces for internal bleeding are the chest, abdomen, pelvis, long bone compartments, and retroperitoneum. Interventional radiology may be consulted to achieve intra-arterial control of bleeding from the spleen or other vessels. Surgical exploration may be required to control abdominal or thoracic hemorrhage. A pelvic binder can be applied to control tamponade bleeding from pelvic fractures.

Early and continued resuscitation is the mainstay of treatment, along with control of bleeding. Resuscitation is covered in more detail later in this chapter. Reversal of anticoagulants plays a key role in controlling bleeding.

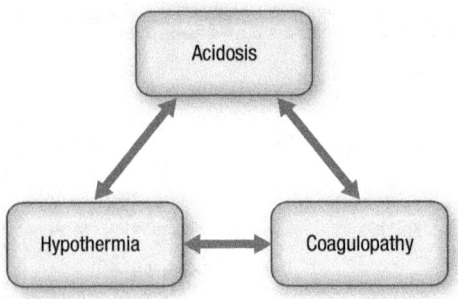

Figure 4.1 The lethal triad.

Resuscitation

Resuscitation is a critical component of managing circulation. The goal of resuscitation is to reverse shock, restore perfusion and tissue oxygenation, and avoid organ damage. Intravenous fluids may be used initially as they are readily available; however, ideally blood products are the best intervention for hemorrhagic shock. A ratio of blood product transfusion of 1:1:1 (red blood cells:plasma:platelets) restores patients' blood loss as closely as possible. Whole blood transfusions are emerging again to avoid the development of coagulopathies.

A systolic blood pressure goal of 90 mmHg is acceptable in the setting of resuscitation and traumatic hemorrhage. This is referred to as permissive hypotension. A blood pressure that is too high will promote ongoing bleeding. Thus, permissive hypotension reduces ongoing bleeding until hemostasis is achieved. Resuscitation should always be performed with warmed fluids and blood products to avoid hypothermia. Hypothermia is one of the tenets of the "lethal triad," which includes acidosis, hypothermia, and coagulopathy (Figure 4.1). Patients who are acidotic, hypothermic, and coagulopathic are at a much greater risk of death.

Recognizing when to slow or stop resuscitation can be challenging. Trauma teams follow a variety of end points of resuscitation. The priority is to stabilize vital signs in order to complete the primary and secondary surveys and obtain necessary diagnostic testing to further identify additional serious injuries. The focus on end points of resuscitation during the primary survey should focus on dynamic measures that assess perfusion and oxygenation.

DISABILITY (D)

Once hemodynamic stability is achieved, a brief neurologic assessment is then completed. Assessment includes level of consciousness, pupillary size and reaction, peripheral motor sensation, and any localized deficits. The Glasgow Coma Scale (GSC) (Table 4.3) is a quick approach to determine a

TABLE 4.3

Glasgow Coma Scale

Evaluation	Documented Response	Points
Best response—Eye opening	■ Spontaneous ■ To voice ■ To pain ■ No response	4 3 2 1
Best response—Verbal	■ Oriented to person, place, and time ■ Confused ■ Inappropriate words ■ Incomprehensible sounds ■ No response	5 4 3 2 1
Best response—Motor	■ Obeys commands ■ Localizes pain ■ Withdraws from pain ■ Flexion to pain (decorticate) ■ Extension to pain (decerebrate) ■ No response	6 5 4 3 2 1
	TOTAL POINTS =	3 to 15
Interpretation	Mild TBI = Moderate TBI = Severe TBI =	13 to 15 9 to 12 <9

TBI, traumatic brain injury.

patient's level of consciousness. A high index of suspicion for an injury to the central nervous system must always be present with any alteration in level of consciousness in a trauma patient. Additionally, recurrent shock; hypoglycemia; or intoxication with alcohol, narcotics, or other drugs can decrease the level of consciousness of a patient.

FAST FACTS

A GCS less than 8 requires intubation. Trauma patients require ongoing reassessment to monitor for changes in GCS.

EXPOSURE/ENVIRONMENTAL CONTROL (E)

The last part of the primary survey includes exposure and environmental control. All surfaces of the patient must be exposed to ensure thorough evaluation. This includes removal of all garments the patient may be wearing. The patient is then at high risk for hypothermia given the removal of clothing, as well as resuscitation with fluids and/or blood products that may be at room temperature. *Hypothermia* is defined as a core temperature below 35°C (95.5°F). Hypothermia is a complication that can lead to coagulopathy and death. Once all surfaces of the patient have been assessed, ensure the patient regains and maintains a normal body temperature. This can be achieved by increasing the temperature in the room, applying warm blankets or warming devices, and warming fluids (blood products or crystalloid).

A patient who is hypothermic cannot be declared dead. Resuscitation and rewarming must continue until the patient returns to a normal body temperature. Only when the patient is normothermic, and a determination has been made to cease resuscitation, can a patient be declared deceased. Severe cases may require advanced therapies such as extracorporeal blood warming.

FAST FACTS

Hypothermia is defined as a core temperature below 35°C or 95.5°F. Nurses should ensure the trauma bay is warm during the primary and secondary surveys. This can be achieved by increasing the room temperature, warm blankets, warm fluids, and other topical warming methods.

SUMMARY

The primary survey is designed to identify and intervene on immediate injuries that lead to imminent patient death. In other words, the primary survey is designed to identify injuries in the order by which death or disability occurs first. Ongoing resuscitation will happen concurrently with the primary survey. At any point, the primary survey can be reinitiated if any component of the ABCDEs requires reevaluation. Adhering to the ABCDEs of trauma care is essential.

REVIEW QUESTIONS

1. The focus of the primary survey is to:
   a. Determine the reason for the trauma
   b. Perform a rapid assessment of the patient's vital functions
   c. Consult specialty services
   d. Clear cervical collar
2. The most common type of shock seen in trauma patients is:
   a. Hemorrhagic shock
   b. Cardiogenic shock
   c. Adrenal insufficiency
   d. Anaphylactic shock

3. The lethal triad includes:
   a. Acidosis, hypothermia, and coagulopathy
   b. Hypotension, hyperthermia, and acidosis
   c. Acidosis, anemia, and hypotension
   d. Hemorrhage, hypotension, and hypothermia

References

American College of Surgeons: The Committee on Trauma. (2018). *ATLS: Advanced Trauma Life Support student course manual* (10th ed.). American College of Surgeons.

Gondek, S., Schroeder, M. E., & Sarani, B. (2017). Assessment and resuscitation in trauma management. *Surgical Clinics of North America*, *97*(5), 985–998. https://doi.org/10.1016/j.suc.2017.06.001

McQuillan, K. A., & Flynn-Makic, M. B. (2020). *Trauma nursing: From resuscitation through rehabilitation* (5th ed.). Elsevier.

Secondary Survey
Dawn Carpenter

> Once the primary survey is completed and ABCDEs have been stabilized with resuscitation, the team proceeds directly into the secondary survey. The secondary survey, completed in the trauma bay, is a comprehensive head-to-toe assessment that seeks to identify other injuries that require urgent intervention. Pertinent medical history in the mnemonic AMPLE is collected. Adjunctive diagnostic testing ensues. Continuous monitoring and reassessment are essential during this phase. As injuries are diagnosed, decisions to transfer or treat are made. If the patient will stay, consultation with specialty services begins and comprehensive treatment plans are implemented.

In this chapter, you will learn:
1. The components of a secondary survey.
2. What an AMPLE history is and why it's needed.
3. What adjunctive diagnostic testing is part of the secondary survey.
4. To identify pertinent reassessment and monitoring.
5. Articulate specialty consultations commonly needed to care for trauma patients.

INTRODUCTION

During the secondary exam, the survey begins with assessment of the head, eyes, ears, nose, and throat (HEENT) and proceeds down the neck, through the chest, abdomen/pelvis, and musculoskeletal systems. Upon completion of inspection and palpation of the anterior body, be sure to maintain spinal precautions and log roll the patient to assess the spine, back, rectum/vagina.

HEAD-TO-TOE EXAM

Head-to-toe examination and assessment are designed to identify any areas of tenderness, open wounds, ecchymosis, edema, and deformities, along with any sensory or motor deficits (Table 5.1). Any abnormal findings warrant additional diagnostic testing. Also see the section "Diagnostic Testing" later in this chapter.

TABLE 5.1

Secondary Survey Assessment by System

System	Assessment
HEENT	*Head* ■ Inspect scalp, face for lacerations, bleeding, and ecchymosis. ■ The scalp is highly vascular and can result in significant blood loss and if severe enough, may require transfusion. Closure of the scalp laceration is urgent to stop ongoing blood loss. ■ Palpate skull and facial bones for deformities, tenderness, and hematoma. *Eyes* ■ Evaluate pupil size, reactivity, and hemorrhage of conjunctiva. ■ Inspect for periorbital ecchymosis, referred to as raccoon eyes and which signifies a skull fracture. ■ Inspect and remove contact lenses. ■ Assess EOM. EOMs that are not intact represent ocular entrapment, an ocular emergency, and requires a stat ophthalmology, plastic surgery, HEENT, or OMF consult (institution specific). *Ears* ■ Inspect for laceration to external ear. ■ Inspect behind ear for ecchymosis over mastoid bone, that is, "battle sign," which is common with basal skull fractures. ■ Inspect the inner ear for bleeding into the ear canal and for ruptured tympanic membrane. *Nose* ■ Inspect for deformity, blood in nasal cavity. *Mouth* ■ Ask the patient to open and close the mouth to identify any malocclusion. ■ Inspect the teeth for missing or broken teeth, tongue for lacerations, active bleeding, or dry blood. ■ Patients with severe facial injuries may require intubation to protect the airway, preventing aspiration of blood, and to secure the airway as edema develops. *Throat/neck* ■ Inspect airway for edema, soot, and blood. ■ Inspect external neck for hematoma, edema, and lacerations.

(continued)

TABLE 5.1 (continued)

Secondary Survey Assessment by System

System	Assessment
	▪ The cervical collar may impede assessment and needs to be opened to thoroughly inspect and palpate.
	▪ Penetrating injuries to the neck commonly require surgical exploration and intubation because hematomas may form.
	General considerations
	▪ Any indication of burn injury to the head, the nurse must suspect airway involvement/inhalation injury and actively inspect for singed nasal hairs or eyebrows, soot in nose or mouth, and erythema or blistering of the skin.
Chest	▪ Inspect for open wounds, abrasions, bleeding, and deformities.
	▪ Ecchymosis across the chest from shoulder to hip likely represents a seatbelt sign, which should heighten the suspicion for blunt cardiac injury.
	▪ Inspect and palpate for paradoxical chest wall respirations, which may indicate flail sections.
	▪ Palpate clavicles and sternum.
	▪ Palpate anterior and lateral chest walls to elicit tenderness, subcutaneous emphysema, and identify any instability.
	▪ Auscultation of breath sounds if not done during the primary survey.
Abdomen and pelvis	▪ Inspect for abrasions, distention, and ecchymosis.
	▪ Auscultate for bowel sounds.
	▪ Palpate abdomen for tenderness.
	▪ Press on iliac wings to assess pelvic tenderness and stability. If unstable and patient is not stable, a pelvic fracture is highly likely; obtain a pelvic x-ray if not already done, and apply a pelvic binder.
	▪ Perform an E-FAST exam to assess for fluid in the pericardial, perihepatic, perisplenic, and pelvic areas and thoracic cavities.
	▪ Unstable patients with a positive FAST with fluid in the abdomen/pelvis need emergent operative exploration.
Extremities	▪ Inspect for deformities, edema, ecchymosis, and hematoma lacerations.
	▪ Assess CSM.
	▪ Palpate for edema, tenderness.
	▪ Lacerations over bony deformities are highly suspicious for open fractures, which require surgical decontamination and IV antibiotics.

(continued)

TABLE 5.1 (continued)

Secondary Survey Assessment by System

System	Assessment
Genitals	■ Inspect for blood at the meatus. Presence of blood at the meatus precludes Foley placement by nursing. ■ Inspect for blood from the vagina or penile lacerations. ■ Bleeding from the vagina requires a speculum exam to further assess for injuries. ■ Consider sexual assault if a rape kit is needed and consult SANE nurse for evidence collection.
Back	■ Log roll while maintaining cervical spine precautions. ■ Inspect the back for ecchymosis, wounds, hematoma, and abrasions. ■ Palpate spine for tenderness, step-offs.
Buttocks and rectum	■ Inspect buttocks and rectum for bleeding, hematoma, abrasions, and wounds. ■ Either perform a digital rectal exam or ask the patient to squeeze their buttocks together to assess for rectal tone.

Neurologic	■ Assess sensation, motor function, and strength of each extremity, and determine if equal bilaterally.
	■ Repeat palpation of pulses in extremities with deformities after turns or movement.
	■ Assess for changes to the patient's neurologic status.
	   ■ Combativeness may indicate a head injury or illicit substances in the patient's system.
	   ■ Patients who are hypoxic may become restless, fidgety, or agitated. Inability to follow directions or repeatedly removing oxygen or cervical collar warrants further investigation.
	   ■ Patients who are lethargic, withdrawn, or not interactive unless stimulated may be in shock or have a concussion or other head injury.

Psychological	■ Assess psychological response to traumatic event (anxiety is common).
	   ■ Anxiety can be a sign the patient is in shock.
	   ■ Providing information on the status of other people involved in the trauma can alleviate anxiety.
	   ■ Trauma patients may be worried about a family member or pet at home alone. Requesting social work to locate next of kin to address these concerns can help calm the patient.

CSM, circulation, sensory, motor; E-FAST, extended focused assessment with sonography in trauma; EOM, extra ocular movements; HEENT, head, eyes, ears, nose, and throat; OMF, oral and maxillofacial; SANE, sexual assault nurse examiner.

FAST FACTS

Unstable patients with a positive extended focused assessment with sonography for trauma (E-FAST) with fluid in the abdomen/pelvis need blood transfusion and emergent operative exploration. Additional diagnostic testing should be delayed until the patient is hemodynamically stable.

Any abnormal finding should be called out loudly so the documenting nurse can record the finding and the team leader can hear the findings. The trauma team leader needs to be aware of all abnormal findings because these findings guide additional diagnostic testing and the treatment plan of care.

If at any time during the secondary survey, the patient becomes unstable, stop the secondary survey, and repeat the primary survey. Upon completion of the secondary survey, obtain a brief history in the AMPLE format (see "AMPLE History"). Data from the secondary survey aids decision-making to determine adjunctive diagnostic testing.

Nurses play a key role during the secondary survey. Nurses listening to the key findings being called out can anticipate additional diagnostic testing to ensure all injuries are diagnosed. Nurses can expect specific interventions to treat these injuries and thus can prepare essential equipment. This ability to foresee necessary treatment can expedite patient care.

Not all injuries are diagnosed during the secondary survey or diagnostic testing. Within hours to a day or so, after initial injuries are treated, pain is controlled, and the patient is mobilized, new pain, edema, and ecchymosis may develop, leading the nurse to recognize that additional injuries may be present and need further testing. Hand and foot or ankle fractures, sprains, strains, and ligamentous injuries are often identified during subsequent assessments throughout the hospital stay. A tertiary survey is completed before discharge to specifically assess for additional injuries (see Chapter 6).

FAST FACTS

If at any time during the secondary survey the patient becomes unstable, stop the secondary survey and repeat the primary survey.

AMPLE HISTORY

The AMPLE history is a succinct assessment of pertinent history that is needed to immediately care for the individual (Table 5.2). The AMPLE history does not preclude a comprehensive medical history, rather it allows rapid identification of factors that require immediate consideration for potential interventions.

TABLE 5.2
Mnemonic for AMPLE and rationale

Mnemonic	Rationale
A = Allergies and reactions	Allergies are required to guide treatment.
	IV contrast may be needed during CT scans. Antibiotics may be required to treat open fractures or contaminated wounds.
M = Medications	Patients taking anticoagulants require reversal agents in the event of serious or life-threatening bleeding. Beta-blockers and calcium channel blockers may blunt or inhibit a patient's tachycardic response to injury.
P = Past illnesses, pregnancy status	Past medical history including neurologic deficits, cardiac history, and pulmonary diagnoses is especially important. For example, a patient with a history of uncontrolled hypertension may be in shock with a normal blood pressure.
L = Last meal	Knowing the last meal is important because trauma patients may need operative interventions, and knowing this status can help anesthesiologists gauge the risk of vomiting upon intubation and induction of anesthesia.
E = Events/Environment related to injury	Pertinent events prior to or pertaining to the crash are helpful in making diagnoses. Example: A patient who felt light-headed or dizzy before falling may have had a medical event such as syncope or an arrhythmia precipitating a fall. The environment, such as how long the patient was at the scene and temperature, help with early identification of hypo- or hyperthermia.

Family, if present, can often provide AMPLE history if known. Family members are usually highly anxious during the initial evaluation. Nursing may be responsible for initial communication with family. This task can be delegated to others, such as clergy, social work, or nursing supervisors, to allow the bedside nurse to maintain focus on the patient.

FAST FACTS

AMPLE history provides critical information needed for the immediate management of the patient.

DIAGNOSTIC TESTING

Laboratory
The acuity and circumstances of the patient determine what laboratory testing is needed. Those who are acutely and critically ill require a panel of labs

(Table 5.3). In some institutions, nurses draw lab work, whereas at other hospitals, it may be the laboratory technician or ED patient care technician who performs this task. Labs can be drawn during insertion of an IV line. However, do not draw labs off an IV that already has IV fluids infusing or has IV fluid infusing distally. The IV fluid is highly likely to affect the testing results and commonly dilutes the samples, leading to erroneous results. Treating these erroneous results can adversely affect patient outcomes.

TABLE 5.3

Initial Laboratory Testing for Acutely and Critically Ill Trauma Patients

Test	Considerations
Required	
Type and crossmatch	■ Required for all trauma patients, when type-specific blood is needed.
	■ Identifies any antibodies in the patient's blood and matches with compatible blood products.
CBC	■ Provides a baseline hemoglobin and hematocrit. Note: Normal values do not preclude transfusion if the patient is unstable or in shock.
	■ Leukocytosis is expected due to the trauma but may also indicate an infection because patient may have fallen due to sepsis and associated hypovolemia.
	■ Platelet count is important to ascertain whether the patient has sufficient platelets to form clots. Thrombocytopenia may be evident in a patient with cirrhosis.
CMP	■ Severe hyponatremia may cause seizures as an etiology for fall or head injury. Hyponatremia in elders may be a result of medications such as HCTZ. Investigate medical history for hypertension or heart failure.
	■ Initial elevated potassium can indicate severe tissue damage, acute kidney injury. Hypokalemia can cause arrhythmias that may have caused syncope and the patient to fall.
	■ Hyperchloremia can represent administration of normal saline and cause hyperchloremic metabolic acidosis.
	■ Low bicarbonate represents metabolic acidosis indicative of shock. Elevated bicarbonate represents metabolic alkalosis, which can occur in severe COPD with chronic hypercarbia. Explore medical history for COPD or OSA.
	■ Elevated BUN and creatinine can reveal either acute kidney injury or CKD.
	■ AST, ALT, and bilirubin can indicate presence of liver injury or shock liver from hypotension.

(continued)

TABLE 5.3 (continued)
Initial Laboratory Testing for Acutely and Critically Ill Trauma Patients

Test	Considerations
INR, PTT	■ An elevated INR can indicate the patient is on warfarin and should be reversed with PCC, vitamin K, or FFP.
Alcohol level	■ Used for medical purposes. Elevated levels indicate alcohol may have been a contributing factor to the patient being injured and requires an SBIRT intervention.
Urine drug screen	■ Used for medical purposes. Positive results indicate substances may be due to (1) medications taken at home, (2) medications given prehospital or in the ED, (3) or have been a contributing factor to the patient being injured and requires an SBIRT intervention.
Patient Specific	
HCG	■ Should be done in all females of childbearing age.
Troponin	■ Should be done for any patient who has sternal, manubrium, or first or second rib fractures or complaints of anterior chest pain.
CPK	■ Assesses for tissue damage that can lead to rhabdomyolysis.
Lipase	■ Assesses for pancreatic injury.
Kleihauer–Betke	■ Required for all pregnant women. Assesses for presence of fetal blood in the maternal circulation; if present, indicates fetal trauma. This is common with high-energy blunt force trauma, abdominal trauma, and when a placenta is located anteriorly in the uterus.
ABG	■ Assesses acid/base, oxygenation, ventilation, and base excess. Severe respiratory and/or metabolic acidosis requires intubation and indicates the need for ventilator adjustments and ongoing resuscitation.
Lactic acid	■ Is a measure of shock from cellular hypoxia.
ROTEM, TEG	■ Identifies deficits in the coagulation cascade and guides transfusion/treatments of hemorrhagic shock.

ABG, arterial blood gases; ALT, alanine transaminase; AST, aspartate transaminase; BUN, blood urea nitrogen; CBC, complete blood count; CKD, chronic kidney disease; CMP, comprehensive metabolic panel; COPD, chronic obstructive pulmonary disease; CPK, creatinine phosphokinase; FFP, fresh frozen plasma; HCG, human chorionic gonadotropin; HCTZ, hydrochlorothiazide; INR, international normalized ratio; OSA, obstructive sleep apnea; PCC, prothrombin complex concentrate; PTT, prothrombin time test; ROTEM, rotational thromboelastometry; SBIRT, screening, brief intervention, referral to treatment; TEG, thromboelastogram.

Serial laboratory testing may be needed to reassess the status of the patient. These decisions are made at the time of admission or subsequently thereafter based on the patient's clinical condition. Serial complete blood count, basic metabolic panel, creatinine phosphokinase, and repeat international normalized ratio testing may be needed to monitor for ongoing bleeding, renal impairment, development of rhabdomyolysis, and rebound coagulopathy, respectively. Lactic acid should be retested if elevated over 2 mmol/L to assess for ongoing tissue hypoxia from shock.

Radiologic Studies

The team leader will decide which diagnostic imaging is needed. Commonly, CT scans of the head, chest, abdomen, and pelvis are needed to diagnose acute injuries. When indicated, patients may need CT scans of the face to assess for fractures and ocular entrapment, which is an ocular emergency. CT angiograms of the neck are commonly needed to assess for vascular injuries, especially if cervical or first or second rib fractures are present. Orthopedic teams may request CT of joints or fractures for surgical planning of fractures. Patients who are suspected of having bladder or rectal injuries may need CT cystogram or rectal contrast to identify these respective injuries. Nurses should be conscientious of how much IV contrast a patient receives and can suggest a bolus of IV fluid to prevent contrast-induced nephropathy, which may lead to renal failure.

After additional potentially life-threatening injuries are identified via CT scans, treatment can then be determined. If urgent or emergent surgery is not required, then other x-rays may be done to identify other, nonlife-threatening injuries. X-rays of extremities are commonly required when edema, ecchymosis, or pain is identified. These can also be done hours later, once surgical intervention has been completed. Nursing should perform regular neurovascular checks to the affected extremity. Any decrease in sensation, escalating pain, or reduced pulses should be reported to the trauma team leader.

FAST FACTS

Normal saline bolus is indicated for patients receiving IV contrast to prevent contrast-induced nephropathy, acute kidney injury, and acute renal failure.

Nursing care of the patient who is undergoing diagnostic testing requires frequent monitoring of heart rate, blood pressure, oxygen saturation, and respiratory rate. Patients can become unstable with ongoing bleeding or become hypotensive when pain medication is administered. Hypoxia can worsen, requiring increased oxygen, noninvasive ventilation, or intubation. Any changes to the patient's vital signs should be reported to the trauma team leader. Aborting studies and returning to the trauma bay to repeat the primary survey may be needed to regain stability.

Decision to Transfer

Any patient at a level III or IV trauma center who becomes unstable at any point should be immediately transferred to a higher level of care. Do not perform CT scans on any patient who is unstable. Rapid transfer for definitive care is essential. If the team leader is busy performing life-saving procedures, nurses should suggest and assist in facilitating the transfer. The decision to transfer can occur at any point, even before the patient arrives.

Level II trauma centers may need to transfer a select few patients who need specialized services. Critically ill pediatric patients may need to be transferred to a children's hospital. Patients with severe burns require specialized care at a burn center. Patients with severe adult respiratory distress syndrome in whom advanced ventilator management, proning, and paralytic agents have failed may need extracorporeal membrane oxygenation (ECMO) and require transport to an ECMO center if this service is not available at the level II center. Patient needs, distance, and weather influence the mode of transport to higher levels of care.

> **FAST FACTS**
>
> Level III or IV trauma centers should focus on stabilizing the patient and prepare for transport for definitive treatment. Do not delay transfer to obtain lab or other diagnostic testing.

REASSESSMENT AND MONITORING

Trauma patients' hemodynamic status can change unexpectedly. Patients should have hemodynamic monitoring with frequent blood pressure checks. Constant reassessment and early interventions are needed to maintain hemodynamic stability. Patients should not leave the trauma bay until they are stable. To be considered stable, the patient should have a minimum of three systolic blood pressures over 100 mmHg. If they are unstable, they should go directly to an operating room. The patient's nurse should remain with the patient through the diagnostic testing period and ensure the patient remains hemodynamically stable.

Children can compensate for longer periods of time, until they suddenly become unstable. Patients who are verging on hypovolemia may be very sensitive to opioid analgesics and become hypotensive with even a small dose. Avoid morphine in patients with renal dysfunction. Patients with renal dysfunction at baseline should receive a bolus of IV fluids prior to contrast to prevent contrast-induced nephropathy and acute kidney injury. Remember, start low, go slow. It's easier to give additional doses of analgesics than to have to rescue a patient from too much.

> **FAST FACTS**
>
> Frail elderly and medically complex patients are also susceptible to opioids and easily become oversedated, leading to hypercarbia and hypoxia. Reduce doses of opioids in the elderly.

Acutely and critically ill trauma patients should be on a cardiac monitor. Continuous monitoring of blood pressures may be necessary and can be done with the insertion of an arterial line. Patients with any chest trauma should have continuous pulse oximetry. Apply oxygen only for those patients who are hypoxic. Providing too much oxygen, when not needed, can displace nitrogen from the alveoli, thus inducing atelectasis.

SPECIALTY CONSULTATION

Consultation with specialty teams is commonly needed to treat traumatic injuries. Orthopedics, neurosurgery, otolaryngology, plastic and reconstructive surgery, and vascular surgery are among the most frequently consulted teams. The urgency of these consultations depends on the type of injuries. Life-threatening injuries are managed first. Limb-threatening injuries may occur concomitantly with multiple teams operating simultaneously to salvage the limb, because revascularization is a high priority.

A period of stabilization may be required before further surgical interventions are undertaken. Ongoing resuscitation, warming body temperature, and correcting coagulopathies and acidosis are critical during this period. Assessment of neurologic function and management of elevated intracranial pressures may be needed prior to additional surgical interventions.

Some traumatic injuries may require fixation in multiple stages. The trauma team will determine when the patient is ready for additional procedures. Temporizing interventions, such as traction for fractures, may be needed to allow for more urgent injuries, such as hemorrhagic shock or severe head injuries, to be stabilized. Facial fracture may be repaired several days later once edema has begun to resolve. Not all fractures require repair during the initial hospitalization. Some facial and orthopedic fractures can be repaired a few days to a week later, on an outpatient basis, while some fractures can be managed nonoperatively.

Additionally, specialty nurses may be integrated into the care of trauma patients, including wound, ostomy, continence nurses and IV nurses, depending on individualneeds. Pregnant patients require collaboration with obstetric nurses, nurse midwives, and obstetricians. Pediatric patients require nurses with pediatric experience and child life specialists. Patients with burns benefit from nurses who have specific burn care expertise.

> **FAST FACTS**
>
> Teamwork is critical to the survival and outcomes of trauma patients. Every team member, regardless of role, institution, department, and so forth, plays an integral role in patient outcomes. Never underestimate your contribution to the care of the patient.

In short, it takes an entire team to care for acutely and critically ill trauma patients. The trauma team coordinates care among the variety of service lines and specialties that are required for each patient. Teams who are skilled communicators improve patient outcomes.

DECISION TO ADMIT

Once all testing is done and injuries are identified, a decision can be made whether the patient requires admission or can be discharged. If the patient is to be admitted, then the decision on appropriate level of care must be made. The team leader will determine, in collaboration with nursing, whether the patient is stable for the floor or requires intermediate or intensive care (see Chapter 13). A patient's medical comorbidities are factors that require consideration in this decision-making process. Patients with complex cardiac and pulmonary problems require more aggressive monitoring. Patients on anticoagulants require reversal and close monitoring for ongoing bleeding and development of thromboses if anticoagulation is reversed.

SUMMARY

In summary, the secondary survey includes a thorough head- to- toe exam, AMPLE history, and diagnostic testing. Ongoing reassessment and monitoring are essential because trauma patients can become unstable, requiring urgent or emergent interventions. Decision to transfer the patient to a higher level of care can be made at any time a team member feels the patient is too ill to keep at the hospital.

REVIEW QUESTIONS

1. Which is a component of the secondary survey?
    a. Assess airway patency
    b. Auscultation of breath sounds
    c. Palpate the chest wall for tenderness
    d. Palpate femoral pulses
2. In an AMPLE history, the A represents:
    a. Airway
    b. Allergies
    c. Atrial fibrillation
    d. Adjunctive testing

3. The most important element a patient who is combative in the trauma bay should receive is:
   a. Sedation
   b. Pain medication
   c. Urine drug screen
   d. A CT scan of the brain

References

American College of Surgeons: The Committee on Trauma. (2018). *ATLS: Advanced Trauma Life Support student course manual* (10th ed.). American College of Surgeons.

McQuillan, K. A., & Flynn-Makic, M. B. (2020). *Trauma nursing: From resuscitation through rehabilitation* (5th ed.). Elsevier.

Zemaitis, M. R., Planas, J. H., & Waseem, M. (2022, January). *Trauma secondary survey*. StatPearls Publishing. https://www.ncbi.nlm.nih.gov/books/NBK441902/

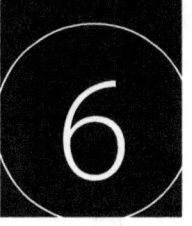

Tertiary Survey
Alexander Menard

> *The tertiary survey is an established standard of trauma care that takes place after initial resuscitation and stabilization. The focus of the tertiary survey is to detect any additional injuries that were not identified in the primary and secondary surveys.*

In this chapter, you will learn:
1. The importance of the tertiary survey.
2. The essential components of the tertiary survey.

INTRODUCTION

Subtle injuries can be overlooked due to more pressing injuries that require immediate lifesaving interventions. Undiagnosed injuries can have a significant impact on a patient's length of stay, course of treatment, rehabilitation, morbidity, and mortality. The tertiary survey was developed to address any occult or less obvious injuries. The tertiary survey was first described in 1990, when a reduction of missed injuries was achieved through an implementation of a trauma tertiary survey. The tertiary survey acts as a formal layer of assessment to identify these injuries in trauma patients. This survey consists of a structured and comprehensive reexamination of the patient and includes a review of every diagnostic study/test performed. Members of the trauma team perform this formal exam; however, nurses play a key role in assessing and identifying potential injuries during their exam and reporting patient complaints to the team. It is imperative that nursing shares any discoveries or concerns about occult injuries with the trauma team during the tertiary exam and at any point during the hospitalization.

FAST FACTS

The goal of the tertiary survey is to identify any missed or occult injuries.

TERTIARY SURVEY

The tertiary survey has become standard of care with the trauma population. This survey is completed by the providers after the primary and secondary surveys and after the patient has been resuscitated and stabilized. The focus is on identifying any missed or occult injuries. The nurse plays a crucial role in identifying potentially missed or occult injuries. Nurses spend large amounts of time with the patient and may notice new swelling or ecchymosis over a particular area and/or may report/document new tenderness. This can lead to further diagnostic testing and detection of an occult injury. Once patients are mobile, it is possible that new symptoms present, and identification of new injuries can occur. This information can be reported from physical and occupational therapists during their assessments and/or therapy sessions. The key to finding these injuries is through documentation and communication with the trauma team. It is not uncommon to find injuries after the primary and secondary surveys as the atmosphere has typically calmed and attention can be drawn to different aspects of care.

The tertiary survey will act as a comprehensive review of diagnostics as well as a reassessment of the patient. Additionally, this will act as a summary that includes review of services that are consulted, identification of incidental findings, review of all imaging, and assurance that best practices have been followed.

While the tertiary survey has become common practice in the care of the trauma patient, the operational procedure and documentation can vary from institution to institution to meet specific needs.

FAST FACTS

The tertiary survey is designed to identify occult injuries.

SUMMARY

The tertiary survey is designed to identify injuries that were not identified during the initial evaluation and resuscitation (primary and secondary surveys), both of which previously focused on prevention of immediate death or loss of limb. The tertiary survey has become a standard of practice across trauma centers and has been proven to improve care of the trauma patient. Everyone involved in patient care can help identify occult injuries, including nurses, physicians, physical therapists, occupational therapists, and speech and language pathologists. Most importantly, any new findings are shared with the trauma service and documented so that appropriate actions can be taken.

REVIEW QUESTIONS

1. The focus of the tertiary survey is to:
   a. Manage emergent airways compromise
   b. Perform a rapid assessment of the patient's vital functions
   c. Identify occult injuries
   d. Clear for discharge
2. The tertiary survey includes:
   a. Reevaluation of the patient and all testing
   b. Ensuring the airway is secure
   c. Ensuring oxygenation and ventilation are adequate
   d. Immediate intervention for active bleeding

References

Enderson, B. L., Reath, D. B., Meadors, J., Dallas, W., DeBoo, J. M., & Maull, K. I. (1990, June). The tertiary trauma survey: A prospective study of missed injury. *Journal of Trauma and Acute Care Surgery, 30*(6), 666–670.

Hajibandeh, S., Hajibandeh, S., & Idehen, N. (2015). Meta-analysis of the effect of tertiary survey on missed injury rate in trauma patients. *Injury, 46*(12), 2474–2482. https://doi.org/10.1016/j.injury.2015.09.019

Keijzers, G. B., Giannakopoulos, G. F., Del Mar, C., Bakker, F. C., & Geeraedts, L. M., Jr. (2012). The effect of tertiary surveys on missed injuries in trauma: A systematic review. *Scandinavian Journal of Trauma, Resuscitation and Emergency Medicine, 20*, 77. https://doi.org/10.1186/1757-7241-20-77

Williamson, F., Grant, K., Warren, J., & Handy, M. (2021). Trauma tertiary survey: Trauma service medical officers and trauma nurses detect similar rates of missed injuries. *Journal of Trauma Nursing, 28*(3), 166–172. https://doi.org/10.1097/jtn.0000000000000578

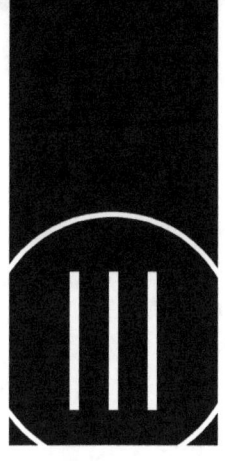

NURSING CARE BY SYSTEM/INJURIES

Neurologic Injuries and Care
Dawn Carpenter

> Trauma patients require detailed nursing assessment to identify neurological deficits. Changes in mental status, weakness, paresthesia, or paralysis are key findings that warrant further investigation. Injuries can range from mild to life-threatening and can subtly or dramatically change. Astute nurses recognize subtle changes and report to the trauma team for their reassessment and treatment. Concurrent neurologic exams during handoff between nurses can identify changes and enhance consistency of documentation.

In this chapter, you will learn:
1. To identify key elements of a detailed neurological exam
2. Articulate nursing interventions for patients with traumatic brain injuries (TBI)
3. Recognize herniation syndrome
4. Distinguish between types of spinal cord injuries
5. Discuss nursing care of patients with spinal cord injuries

INTRODUCTION

All patients with traumatic injuries should receive a thorough neurological exam. The Glasgow Coma Scale (GCS) (see Chapter 4) is used in patients with TBI. A GCS of less than or equal to 8 requires intubation. Nurses must be able to perform detailed neuro exam that includes the cranial nerves (see Figure 7.1 and Table 7.1), pupil exam, motor, and sensation. Spinal cord injuries also require assessment of dermatome levels (see Figure 7.2). The pupil exam can be aided with the use of a bedside pupillometer to quantify change in pupils. This device is specific for indicating neurologic worsening, including increased intracranial pressure (ICP) with severe and moderate to severe TBI.

Types of Neurological Assessment
Motor testing: Observe body position during exam. Ensure patient can move all four extremities and grade strength. Test and grade each extremity for strength (see Chapter 13, Table 13.2). Any changes in strength need to be reported to the trauma providers.

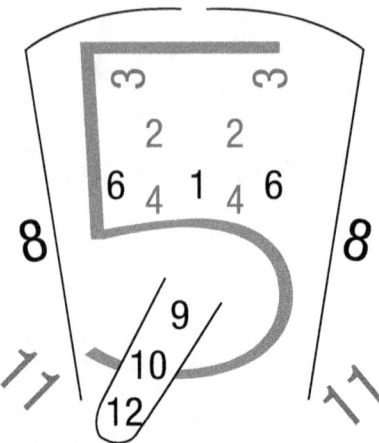

Figure 7.1 Cranial nerve diagram.

Source: Dr.nkumar98, CC BY-SA 4.0 <https://creativecommons.org/licenses/by-sa/4.0>, via Wikimedia Commons. https://commons.wikimedia.org/wiki/File:Nishant_cranial.jpg

TABLE 7.1

Cranial Nerve Function and Testing

Nerve	Name (Type)	Function	How to Test
I	Olfactory (sensory)	Smell	Identify familiar odors with eyes closed, occluding one nostril at a time (not usually tested in hospital)
II	Optic (sensory)	Sight	Visual acuity
III	Oculomotor (motor)	Eye movement	Opens eyelids, eye movement upward/medial, upward lateral, medial, downward lateral Inspect eyelid for droop, and PERRLA
IV	Trochlear (motor)	Eye movement	Eye movement downward and medial
V	Trigeminal (both)	Facial sensation and movement	Identify light touch to forehead, cheek, jaw, and chewing movements
VI	Abducens (motor)	Eye movement	Assess lateral eye movement
VII	Facial (both)	Face: expression and sensory	Facial symmetry: smile, frown, and wrinkle forehead; chewing
VIII	Vestibulocochlear (sensory)	Hearing and balance	Hearing; Whisper and Rinne tests

(continued)

TABLE 7.1 (*continued*)
Cranial Nerve Function and Testing

Nerve	Name (Type)	Function	How to Test
IX	Glossopharyngeal (both)	Tongue and throat	Test gag reflex, ability to swallow
X	Vagus (both)	Parasympathetic	Uvula rises when saying "ah," quality of speech sounds
XI	Spinal accessory (motor)	Head, neck, and shoulder movement and swallow	Shrugs shoulders, moves head against resistance
XII	Hypoglossal (motor)	Speech, chewing and swallowing	Test tongue movement

PERRLA, pupils are equal, round and reactive to light and accommodation.

Sensation testing: Test with both sharp and dull instruments: Test both sides of face with patient's eyes closed, continue from head to toe, assessing each arm, leg, and torso dermatomes. In patients with diabetes and other neuropathies may have altered peripheral sensation at baseline. Report any deficit to the provider for reassessment. Do not assume an individual has a neuropathy unless the patient explicitly reports this finding is normally present.

National Institutes of Health Stroke Scale

Medical events commonly lead to injuries. An example is a trauma patient has a spontaneous hemorrhagic or ischemic stroke that leads to a fall or crashes the vehicle. Nurses must be able to perform the National Institutes of Health Stroke Scale (NIHSS) in the event of a stroke.

FAST FACTS

A thorough and accurate neurological exam is the highest priority to ensure best neurological outcome for the patient. The neuro exam is the window into how the brain and spinal cord is functioning. Always perform a neuro exam during each hand off between shifts and when transferring between units.

TRAUMATIC BRAIN INJURIES

TBI are a broad category of multiple specific and different types of injuries occurring in isolation or concurrently with other TBIs. TBIs are defined as an alteration in brain function, due to an external force (see Table 7.2). TBIs can range from concussion to a devasting brain injury, resulting in death.

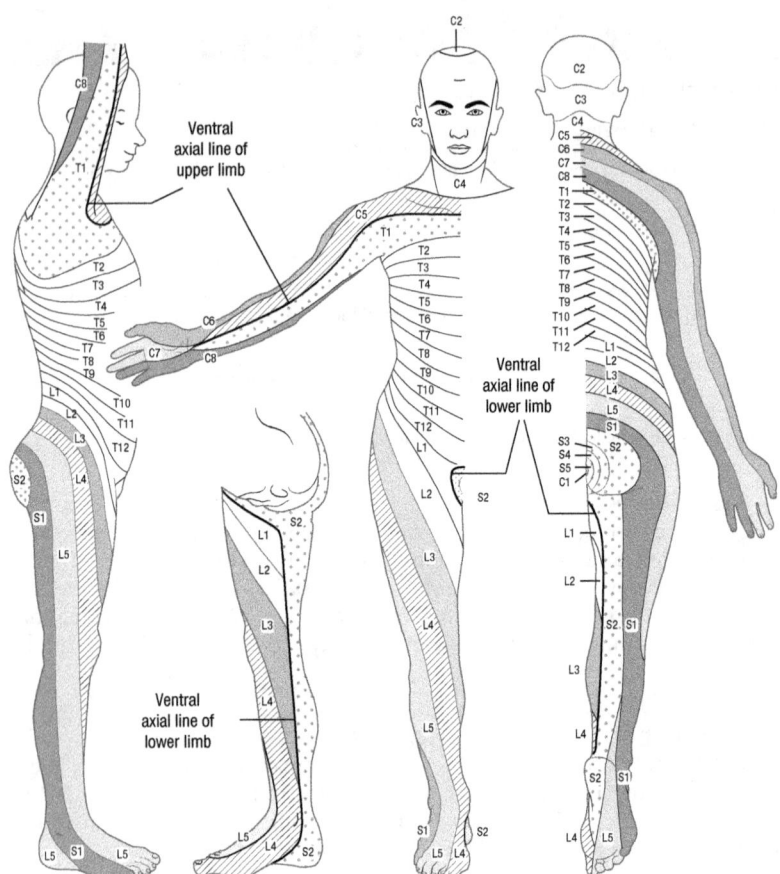

Figure 7.2 Dermatomes.

Source: https://commons.wikimedia.org/wiki/File:Grant_1962_663.png

TBI is the most common cause of trauma related deaths and has a bimodal frequency distribution, with greater risk of TBI in the younger and older populations. Motor vehicle crashes (MVC) are the most common cause of TBIs in the younger people, while falls are the dominate etiology in older populations.

TBIs are diagnosed with both physical exam and radiological findings. TBI is classified by severity, ranging from mild, to moderate, to severe (see Table 7.3). The GCS is used to classify severity (see Chapter 4). The diagnostic test of choice for trauma patients is the CT scan of the brain. CTs are quick and specific for acute blood in the brain.

TABLE 7.2

Types of TBI

Type of Injury	Description
Concussion	Traumatically induced, transient disturbance of brain function.
Hematoma: Subdural	SDH is a collection between the dura mater and the arachnoid layer. ■ Onset more gradual hours, to days to weeks. ■ Subtypes: acute, subacute or chronic SDH. ■ May be traumatic or atraumatic due to anticoagulants. ■ May require surgical evacuation urgently or nonemergently depending on subtype and symptoms.
Hematoma: Epidural	EDH is a collection between the dura mater and the inside of the skull. ■ Classic presentation/sign of EDH = loss on consciousness followed by a brief lucid interval followed by rapid decline in mental status, unresponsiveness. ■ Requires emergent surgical evacuation.
Contusion	Bruising of brain tissue.
Subarachnoid hemorrhage	Bleeding between the arachnoid and pia mater.
Diffuse injuries	Diffuse axonal injury. ■ Impaired function of axons. ■ Ischemia—results from insufficient blood supply from hypotension or lack of oxygen.

EDH, epidural hematoma; SDH, subdural hematoma.

Initial Management of Traumatic Brain Injuries

Management of TBIs requires early recognition and diagnosis. For severe TBIs, securing the patients airway is the initial priority. Patients should be intubated for a GCS <8. Breathing and adjusting ventilator settings is important to achieve and maintain a $PaO_2 > 95$ mmHg and a $PaCO_2$ 35 to 40 mmHg. Circulation needs to maintain adequate blood pressure to perfuse the brain. Lastly, rapid correction of any coagulopathy limits ongoing bleeding. Reversal of anticoagulation is a top priority to stop intracerebral bleeding.

Elevate Head of Bed

Two items are critical to the initial management of all TBIs which includes keeping the head of bed elevated <30 degrees and avoiding all hypotonic intravenous (IV) solutions. Elevate the head of the bed (HOB) once the thoracic and lumbar spine is cleared by the team. If unable to clear the spine immediately, place the patient in reverse Trendelenburg to elevate the head as much as possible.

TABLE 7.3
Severity of TBI

Classification	Criteria
Mild	- Loss/alteration of consciousness: <30 minutes - GCS: 15 - Posttraumatic amnesia: a moment to <24 hours - Radiological changes: No
Moderate	- Loss/alteration of consciousness: >30 minutes, <24 hours - GCS: 9 to 12 - Posttraumatic amnesia: >24 hours, <7 days - Radiological changes: Transient changes
Severe	- Loss/alteration of consciousness: >24 hours - GCS: <8 - Posttraumatic amnesia: >7 days - Radiological changes: Positive, lasting abnormalities

GCS, Glasgow Coma Scale.

Source: Modified from: Brasure, M., Lamberty, G. J., Sayer, N. A., Nelson, N. W., MacDonald, R., Ouellette, J., Tacklind, J., Grove, M., Rutks, I. R., Butler, M. E., & Kane, R. L. (2012, June). *Multidisciplinary postacute rehabilitation for moderate to severe traumatic brain injury in adults* [Internet]. Agency for Healthcare Research and Quality (US); (Comparative Effectiveness Reviews, No. 72.) Table 7.1, Criteria used to classify TBI severity. www.ncbi.nlm.nih.gov/books/NBK98986/table/introduction.t1/

Avoid Hypnotic Fluids

Normal saline (NS) is the initial IV solution of choice. NS has 154 mEq of sodium in each liter, whereas lactated ringers (LR), which is also considered isotonic fluid, has 135 mEq of sodium per liter, thus LR is relatively hypotonic. Patients with severe brain injuries that develop cerebral edema should have all infusions and medications mixed in NS rather than D5W. Pharmacies may need to mix these special for these patients. Large volumes of medication infusions, especially medications such as vancomycin, which commonly require large volumes of 500 mL per dose, can adversely decrease the serum sodium, resulting in worsening cerebral edema. The nutritionist should recommend concentrated tube feedings to 1.5 or 2.0 calories per mL of tube feeding can reduce enteral free water. Additionally, any medications that are to be given enterally should be mixed in NS rather than sterile or tap water.

FAST FACTS

NS should be the in vitro fertilization (IVF) of choice in any patient with a TBI. Avoid all hypotonic IVF, including LR. Mix all infusions and medications in NS rather than D5W when able. Pharmacy may need to custom mix these.

Environment

A dark quiet environment is best for all head injuries, including concussions. A dark quiet room allows the brain to rest. Nurses need to advocate for their patients and ask family to minimize stimulation, reduce number of visitors, and allow the patient to rest. It's acceptable to ask the family not to stimulate the patient. A private room, if available, is best so as not to have additional stimulation by the roommate and their family.

INCREASED INTRACRANIAL PRESSURE

Severe TBI are commonly complicated by cerebral edema which can cause increased ICP. An important concept in the management of ICPs is the Monro-Kellie doctrine which states the cranium is a rigid/fixed container. Intracranial components consist of brain parenchyma (80%), cerebrospinal fluid (10%), and intracranial blood (10%). To maintain equilibrium, the total volume in the skull (brain tissue, cerebral spinal fluid (CSF), and blood) need to remain constant. Increase in the volume of any components within the skull or an addition of a pathologic process can result in increased pressure within the skull. A certain degree of compensation can occur; however, compensation is limited. Sustained increased ICP can result in further brain injury, referred to as a secondary brain injury.

Nurses need to monitor for clinical signs of increased ICP which include focal neurological deficits, nausea, vomiting, vision changes, and pupillary changes. As cerebral edema increases and is not adequately treated or fails to respond to treatment, then the patient's neurological exam may continue to deteriorate until abnormal posturing is noted, including decorticate or decerebrate posturing. These abnormal postures are precursors to brainstem herniation.

ICP monitoring is indicated in all potentially salvageable patients with a TBI and GCS 3 to 8 after resuscitation, and an abnormal head CT scan. Intracranial hypertension is defined as ICP >22 mmHg sustained for >5 minutes. ICP >22 mmHg sustained for >5 minutes requires treatment. ICPs sustained >22 mmHg are associated with an increase in mortality.

FAST FACTS

Intracranial hypertension is defined as ICP >22 mmHg for sustained for >5 minutes.

Any elevation in ICP increases the risk of subsequent injury from brainstem compression or from decreased cerebral blood flow. Decreased cerebral blood flow causes worsening oxygenation, thus causing cellular hypoxia which worsens cerebral edema. Blood flow can be indirectly monitored by calculating cerebral perfusion pressures (CPP). CPP is calculated as mean arterial pressure (MAP) minus ICP.

$$\text{MAP} - \text{ICP} = \text{CPP}$$

Normal CPP is 50 to 70 mmHg. A CPP of <50 mmHg can lead to secondary brain injury, herniation, and brain death. CPP should be maintained between 60 and 70 mmHg for survival and favorable outcomes. Nurses need to document both the ICP and CPP in the medical record and report decreases in CPP below 60 mmHg to providers. When awaiting placement of an ICP monitor, keeping systolic blood pressure (SBP) ≥100 mmHg for patients aged 50 to 69 years old or SBP ≥110 mmHg for patients aged 15 to 49 or >70 years old may decrease mortality and improve outcomes.

Vital signs may change as pressures increases. Tachycardia and severe hypertension are commonly noted if ICPs are not controlled, or interventions fail to reverse the rising ICPs. As pressure builds, "Cushing's Triad" occurs with brainstem herniation. Cushing's Triad includes bradycardia, widened pulse pressure, and agonal respirations that leads to apnea as herniation occurs.

FAST FACTS

Cushing's Triad includes bradycardia, widened pulse pressure, and agonal respirations that leads to apnea.

Types of ICP Monitors

External Ventricular Drains (EVD) are placed by neurosurgeons, neurosurgical residents and/or advanced practice providers at the bedside. The benefit of these devices is their ability to monitor ICP more centrally making them more accurate, drain excess CSF or blood, sample CSF to evaluate for infections and administer intrathecal medications such as antibiotics for ventriculitis.

Parenchymal monitors are inserted in cases of midline shift or malignant brain swelling. However, parenchymal monitors cannot be recalibrated once inserted into the patient. Parenchymal monitors only measure the area local to the tip and can drift with long-term usage. Other parenchymal monitors can measure low brain tissue oxygen ($P_{bt}O_2$). $P_{bt}O_2$ <20 mmHg is indicative of decreased tissue oxygenation and requires provider notification and intervention.

Nursing Care of ICP Monitors

Nursing care of ICP monitors is especially important. Pay particular attention to ensure the team maintains sterility during insertion and throughout every aspect of the circuit to prevents infections. Keep dressings intact and change when soiled or if dressing loosens as hair grows back or if patients become diaphoretic. Transducers and tubing should be flushed with normal saline but NEVER connect to a pressure bag. Transducers should be calibrated prior to insertion. Transducers on EVDs need to be maintained at the level of the Foramen of Monro, which correlates with the tragus of the ear. Use a level to ensure accuracy. Relevel after each time the patient is repositioned.

Nursing care of the ICP monitor includes being present during the insertion process to prime the tubing with normal saline via syringe and cap, then zero and calibrate prior to insertion. Provide analgesics and sedation if needed during the procedure and observes the process to assist in maintaining sterility during insertion. Be sure to wear appropriate personal protective equipment while the catheter is being inserted. Maintain an intact dressing and sterility for the duration of the catheter being in the patient. Level the EVD transducer with the Foramen of Monroe, which corresponds with the tragus of the ear. Zero the transducer per hospital policy, typically Q shift. Relevel the 0 point with any change in position.

Lowering below 0 will facilitate increased drainage, whereas raising the 0 mark to positive centimeters will allow for reduced drainage and allow for weaning of the device. The providers will write orders indicating where the device should be leveled. Always close the EVD when changing the patient's position (i.e.: putting the head of bed down or flat to reposition or obtain CT scan or getting out of bed to chair). Then relevel after each position change. Use an actual level or laser level to ensure the level is correct.

Nursing is responsible for continuous monitoring of the ICP pressures, CPP, ICP waveforms, and output are essential functions of the ICU nurses. Normal CSF is clear yellow/straw colored. Report changes in output color and quantity. CSF can be serosanguineous if a small volume of blood is present in the ventricles. Sanguineous bloody output can cause the catheter to clot and occlude the catheter, thus preventing further drainage. Record hourly CSF output. Report any cloudy output in conjunction with fevers as the patient can develop ventriculitis from an infection. Never flush anything into the EVD and do not connect a pressure bag to the transducer.

FAST FACTS

Flush EVD tubing and transducers with normal saline, but NEVER connect to a pressure bag.

ICP Management

Elevations in ICPs can be caused by any stimulus including patient care, turning, family visitation, and so forth. Ask family to sit quietly and keep lights down and door closed to reduce sounds. Keep the television and music turned off if ICPs are elevated. Coughing, turns, mouthcare can raise ICPs intermittently. Thus, treatment of ICPs is indicated when ICPs remain elevated. If the ICP are sustained over 22 mmHg for more than 5 minutes, this will require additional interventions. Treatment of elevated ICPs is done in a stepwise approach ranging from Tier 0 to Tier 3 (see Table 7.4).

TABLE 7.4

ICP Tiered Management Strategies

Tier	Management Strategies
Tier 0	- Head of bed 30 degrees/or reverse Trendelenburg - Maintain neck in midline position - Cervical collar not too tight - Control environment—Decrease stimuli - Maintain normothermia (avoid fevers) - PRN analgesics and sedatives - Avoid hypotonic fluids, drips, and medications. - Keep PaO_2 >95% - Seizure prophylaxis, when indicated
Tier 1	Tier 0 plus: - Mannitol .5 to 1 g/kg bolus PRN up to Q6 hours (hold for osmolar GAP >20, or serum osmolar gap >320) - The osmolar gap calculates expected serum osmolarity, compared to measured osmolarity to detect any unmeasured compounds, that is, mannitol, in the serum. - Hypertonic saline bolus 30 mL of 23.4% NaCl, bolus PRN up to Q6 hours (hold for Na >160) - Nursing can alternate timing of mannitol and 23% NaCl, such that the patient can receive a dose of either of them every 3 hours if they meet criteria. - Maintain $PaCO_2$ 35 to 38 mmHg
Tier 2	Tier 0 & 1 plus: - Continuous and deeper sedation - Maintain normothermia - May need anti-shivering protocol - Maintain $PaCO_2$ 33 to 35 mmHg
Tier 3	Tier 0, 1, and 2, plus consider: - Decompressive craniectomy (depending on etiology) - Burst suppression (Pentobarbital coma)

PRN, pro re nata.

Positioning: The nurse should ensure the HOB is elevated at or >30 degrees to facilitate venous drainage. Maintain the neck in a midline position to ensure the jugular veins aren't compressed preventing venous drainage. Patients may require turning and repositioning while the HOB is elevated to prevent increased ICPs.

Analgesics: Pain can be difficult to assess in patients with intracranial injuries. Around the clock acetaminophen (if not contraindicated) should be ordered for baseline pain control and concomitantly can prevent hyperthermia/fevers. Intermittent IV analgesics should be attempted first prior to starting an infusion. Analgesic and sedation infusion metabolites can accumulate, making an accurate neuro exam difficult and can falsely depress the mental status.

Sodium management: Allow permissive hypernatremia. The hypernatremia creates an increased osmolality in the vessels to reduce cerebral cellular edema. Additionally, avoid all medications and infusions mixed in hypotonic fluids. All enteral medications should be given in NS. Avoid free water flushes and mixing any enteral medications in free water.

Seizure prophylaxis: Anticonvulsants are recommended to prevent posttraumatic seizures within 7 days of injury. Levetiracetam (Keppra) does not seem to interfere with cognitive function, does not require monitoring of therapeutic levels, and has fewer side effects, making it the drug of choice for seizure prophylaxis for patients with moderate to severe head injuries. If seizures occur at any point, Keppra should be continued, and neurology should be consulted.

Venous access: Patients may need central venous catheters (CVC) as part of their care. CVCs ideally should not be inserted into the internal jugular veins to allow unobstructed venous drainage and prevent jugular deep vein thrombosis (DVT), which can increase ICPs. During subclavian (and internal jugular, if absolutely necessary) CVC insertion, keep the HOB elevated until the patient is prepped, draped, and the provider is ready to insert the finder needle into the vein. During the HOB being in Trendelenburg position for the procedure, monitor the ICP for elevations. As soon as the CVC is positioned in the vein, immediately raise the HOB back to 30 degrees. The provider can suture the line in place and apply the dressing in this position. Minimize the HOB being flat or in Trendelenburg during procedures.

Carbon dioxide: Blood gases should be drawn to ensure $PaCO_2$ ~ 35 mmHg and avoid $PaCO_2$ >40 mmHg or hypercarbia. Carbon dioxide is a potent vasodilator, thus any hypercarbia causes vasodilation and increased intracranial volume of blood. Consequently, any significant hypocarbia ($PaCO_2$ <32 mmHg) causes vasoconstriction and thus can restrict blood flow to the brain, causing a secondary brain injury. Adjustments to the ventilator may be required to achieve the goal $PaCO_2$ 35 to 40 mmHg, or conversely if a patient is spontaneously tachypneic and reducing their $PaCO_2$ to <32 mmHg, increased analgesia or sedation may be required.

Osmolar therapy: Hyperosmolar agents such as mannitol and/or hypertonic saline may be given to decrease the ICP. With the administration of mannitol, it is important to note that the osmolality and osmolar gap must be trended. An osmolality of >320 mOsm/kg or an osmolar gap >20 mOsm/kg are unlikely to offer clinical benefit.

Cerebral spinal fluid drainage: EVD's can be opened to allow intermittent or continuous drainage of CSF. When the EVD is open to continual drainage, the nurse needs to close it hourly to obtain the ICP measurement. The neurosurgeon determines how to manage the EVD.

Refractory elevated ICPs: Hyperventilation for a short period of time, typically 2 to 3 hours, may also be considered to decrease cerebral blood flow and thus decreasing ICP. Depending on the underlying etiology, surgical options such as craniotomy and hemicraniectomy must also be considered. For refractory ICP crisis nonresponsive to treatment, therapies including barbiturate induced coma and hypothermia with targeted temperature management must also be considered.

Complications

Complications of increased elevated ICP include secondary brain injuries from hypoxia, hypotension, herniation, and possibly progression to brain death. Complications of EVD's and other brain monitors include ventriculitis, meningitis, and catheter occlusion from blood. Complications from barbiturate coma includes ileus with associated malnutrition, and hypotension.

BRAIN DEATH

Pronouncement of brain death means there is irreversible loss of brain function, including the brainstem. This is defined by complete loss of consciousness (coma), brainstem reflexes, and the independent ability to breathe (apnea), in the absence of any factors that are reversible. Brain death means the patient is legally deceased, despite the patient continuing to have a heartbeat which is due to being on a ventilator. Cessation of brain function, including the brain stem requires:

- an irreversible brain injury
- excludes other confounding medical conditions
- absence of drug intoxication/poisoning
- normothermia (absence of hypothermia)
- a period of observation (commonly 24 hours) without clinical improvement
- a combination of clinical and ancillary testing
    - Clinical testing includes absence of brain stem functions and apnea testing.
    - Ancillary tests for adults can include EEG, nuclear scan, transcranial Doppler, CT angiogram and MRI/MRA, four vessel angiography.

Ancillary testing is not always a requirement for brain death pronouncement. Each hospital should have their own policies and procedures with specific requirements, timeline, and notification of organ procurement centers. Nurses should be sure to notify the organ procurement organization (OPO), early after a patient has a significant brain injury, in accordance with applicable state laws and hospital policy. Hospitals typically designate specific people who are authorized to perform brain death testing and pronounce a patient brain dead. Commonly it must be an attending, including neurocritical care intensivists, neurologists, neurosurgeons, or other intensivists. Brain death testing should not be performed while the patient is in the emergency department.

FAST FACTS

Pronouncement of brain death means there is irreversible loss of brain function, including the brainstem. Brain death means the patient is legally deceased.

Nursing Care

Nurses play a vital role in communicating with the OPO, notifying them early about patients with severe brain injuries and ongoing communications and updates as the patient progresses. An effective partnership between nursing, providers and the OPO team enhances the opportunities for patients to donate. The OPO cannot write orders in a patient's chart until the patient has been declared dead after cardiac death or brain death. If hospital policy allows, lab work can be sent prior to death for screening to determine if a patient has any communicable diseases that could limit or preclude donation. For ethical and financial reasons, any additional testing such as echo, heart catheterization, bronchoscopy, and so forth, which are necessary to evaluate the organs, must be essential to treat the patient if completed prior to brain death pronouncement. Otherwise, these diagnostic tests should wait till the patient has been pronounced, and consent obtained. Note that consent for donation after death may be the legal next of kin rather than the healthcare proxy. Be sure to reference state laws to ensure consent is granted by the proper individual.

SPINAL CORD INJURIES

Spinal cord injuries (SCI) are caused by both blunt and penetrating injuries. Common causes of blunt SCIs include MVC, falls, and diving. Penetrating injuries from knives, or bullets more commonly cause incomplete injuries. Injuries follow a dermatomal pattern. C1 and C2 injuries are commonly fatal at the scene, as the patient will not have any respiratory drive. Whereas C3, C4, and C5 innervate the diaphragm, and can provide some ventilatory support. Injuries below C5 can cause respiratory failure due to ascending edema and de-innervation of the intercostal muscles. Complete cord injuries above the level of T6 can result in neurogenic shock. Patients can experience complete or incomplete injuries. See Table 7.5 for key terminology.

Nurses must maintain a high index of suspicion for any patient who experienced any dangerous mechanism of injury including a fall >5 steps, axial load to the head, MVC with high rate of speed, rollover or ejection, bicycle, or all-terrain vehicles (ATV) crash. Additionally, ages 65 and older with neurological deficits. These patients require a CT scan to diagnose fractures. Patients with ongoing pain with a negative CT should receive an MRI to assess for ligamentous injuries. There are several spinal cord syndromes that have classic etiologies and resultant physical exams (see Table 7.6).

Neurogenic Shock

Patients with injuries at or above T-6 are at risk for neurogenic shock. Neurogenic shock presents with bradycardia, hypotension, warm perfused skin, and spinal shock. Spinal shock may have loss or decreased sensation, motor, and reflexes immediately after the injury or can develop over hours with additional spine movement, bleeding or as edema develops, further compressing the spinal cord.

TABLE 7.5

Key Terminology for SCI

Term	Description
Neurogenic shock	The loss sympathetic innervation to the heart and loss of vasomotor tone results in bradycardia and hypotension.
Spinal shock	Loss of motor tone and function and/or sensation, including reflexes below the level of the lesion immediately after the injury.
Complete cord injury	Total loss of all motor and sensory function below the level of injury.
Partial cord injury	Some sensation and/or function remains below the level of the injury.
Bony level of injury	Refers to the level of vertebral fracture.
Neurological level of injury	Describes the highest segment of the spinal cord that has normal sensory and motor function. Spinal cord edema can cause a bony injury at one level to have a more proximal neurological level of injury.

TABLE 7.6

Spinal Cord Syndromes

Pattern	Deficits	Etiology
Central cord	Loss of motor strength in the upper extremities more so than the lower extremities. (Can dance but can't play the piano)	Hyperextension injury commonly occurs in elderly patients with preexisting cervical canal stenosis. May or may not have a fracture.
Anterior cord	Paraplegia and bilateral loss of pain and temperature sensation	Cord ischemia.
Posterior cord	Loss of proprioception and vibration, motor is preserved	Compression or spinal artery occlusion leading to cord ischemia.
Brown-Sequard	Ipsilateral loss of motor, proprioception, and vibration; with contralateral loss of pain and temperature	Hemi-transection of the spinal cord.
Conus medullaris*	Normal motor function, no pain, saddle anesthesia, symmetric abnormalities, severe bowel, bladder, and sexual dysfunction. Bulbocavernous and anal reflex preserved.	L1-2 injuries, tumors, and vascular injuries.

(continued)

TABLE 7.6 (continued)
Spinal Cord Syndromes

Pattern	Deficits	Etiology
Cauda equina*	Flaccid paralysis of involved lumbar roots, areflexic lower extremities, asymmetric sensory loss in root distribution, pain present, higher lesions spare bowel and bladder, urinary and/or fecal incontinence, bulbocavernous and anal reflex absent.	L2 to sacral neve root injuries such as pelvic ring and sacral fractures.

Note: *No consistent definition exists to distinguish between the conus medullaris syndrome and cauda equina syndrome, due to variability between individuals' anatomy.

Treatment of neurogenic shock includes ensuring that the patient is not also in hypovolemic, hemorrhagic, or obstructive shock. Expect an initial fluid bolus to be ordered. Reassess the patient to identify sources of bleeding in the chest, abdomen, and pelvis. Commonly extended focused abdominal exam for trauma ultrasound is done. Transfusion may be warranted if bleeding is suspected based on other injuries. Once other life-threatening sources of shock are eliminated, then the treatment for neurogenic shock is vasopressor support. A variety of vasopressor infusions can be used to support the patient in neurogenic shock (see Table 7.7). MAP goal for a patient in shock is typically 65 mmHg, however in SCI, evidence exists to drive MAP to >85 mmHg, to enhance perfusion to the injured spinal cord and can be maintained at this level for up to 7 days.

Nursing Care
Nursing care of a patient who presents with traumatic injuries should be presumed to have a spinal cord injury until proven otherwise. Thus, stabilization of the full spine should be maintained until assessment and imaging can be completed. All traumatically injured patients should initially have a hard cervical collar and full spinal alignment, instituted by emergency medical service (EMS) or immediately by the emergency department nurse upon arrival, if the patient arrived by personal vehicle. Failure to adhere to spine precautions can cause additional injuries to the spinal cord. Variations in practice exist on the best protocol to "clear" a cervical spine and remove the collar. Clinical exams must be done by a provider. Imaging (CT scan and/or MRI) may be needed. Nursing should not remove a collar until diagnostic tests are complete and documentation of the spine clearance is in the patient's chart.

TABLE 7.7

Vasopressor Options for Neurogenic Shock

Vasopressor	Mechanism of Action	Dosing	Notes
Phenylephrine (neosynephrine)	Pure alpha agonist to enhance peripheral vasoconstriction	2 to 300 mcg/min or .1 to 1 mcg/kg/min	Can be infused peripherally.
Norepinephrine (Levophed)	alpha and beta-1 adrenergic agonists to produce both inotropic and vasopressor effects	.5 to 30 mcg/min or .01 to .04 mcg/kg/min	Can be infused peripherally at low doses until central access can be obtained (check hospital policy).
Dopamine	alpha and beta 1 adrenergic agonists to produce both inotropic and chronotropic support	.5 to 5 mcg/kg/min	Can be infused peripherally at low does. Useful if the patient has severe bradycardia.
Epinephrine	Alpha and beta 1 and beta 2 agonists to produce both inotropic and vasopressor effects	.01 to .05 mcg/kg/min	Can be infused peripherally at low does until central access can be obtained (check hospital policy). Useful if the patient has severe bradycardia.

FAST FACTS

Nursing should not remove a collar until diagnostic testing is complete and documentation of the spine clearance is in the patient's chart.

Bluntly injured trauma patients have a 3.7% prevalence of spine injuries. Spine injuries are classified as stable or unstable. For stable injuries, a cervical, cervical-thoracic spine orthotic, or thoracic lumbar spine orthotic or lumbar spine orthotic may be needed for 4 to 6 or more weeks. Unstable fractures require surgical fixation to prevent further injury or paralysis. Timing of surgical intervention is determined by the patient's other injuries that may require more immediate interventions, and by neuro or orthopedic spine surgeon. Maintaining spinal precautions, including keeping the patient's spine aligned, log rolling, and prevention of patient movement and their removal of the patient's collar are of utmost importance until the spine is stabilized.

Postoperative Spine Care

Postoperative care of a spinal cord injury focuses on continual reassessment of neuro exam, monitor for bleeding, early mobilization, and discharge planning to spinal cord injury rehab. Monitor for improvement of neuro exam, including improved sensation and movement. Nerve pain can include burning sensation and pins/needles. Treatment of neuropathic pain commonly includes gabapentin (Neurontin), pregabalin (Lyrica), tricyclic antidepressants, and the serotonin and norepinephrine reuptake inhibitors specifically venlafaxine or duloxetine.

Nursing Care
Nursing care of the patient requiring a cervical collar needs to focus on preventing pressure ulcers where the collar presses on skin. The chin and occiput are most often affected; however, the mandible, ears, shoulders, laryngeal prominence, and sternum are all at risk. Foam padding that comes attached to the collar, should extend beyond plastic at all points, such that plastic does not touch the skin. These pads can be washed in mild soap and water and allowed to air dry for reuse. The patient must have a second collar or extra set of padding such that the patient is always maintained in a collar, while the first set is drying. Additional padding can help prevent breakdown.

Complications

Patients, especially the older adult, who require cervical collars are at increased risk for dysphagia and aspiration. Additionally, a collar that is too tight may prevent cerebral venous drainage from pressure on the jugular veins, causing increased ICP. Many nursing interventions are aimed at prevention and treatment of complications of spinal cord injuries, including, but not limited to acute respiratory failure, infections (urinary tract infection, pneumonia), venous thromboembolism, pressure injuries, constipation, and urinary retention.

Atelectasis and pneumonia: Aggressive pulmonary hygiene interventions are crucial to preventing and treating atelectasis, pneumonia, and mucous plugging. Put the head of be up, minimally 30 degrees, as soon as the thoracic and lumbar spine is cleared for bending. Alternatively, the nurse can place the patient in reverse Trendelenburg to keep the head elevated to reduce the chance of aspiration. Use of incentive spirometry, positive expiratory pressure therapy, cough assist devices, percussive vests, tracheal suctioning, and mobility protocols may be utilized to maintain adequate pulmonary status. Continuous positive airway pressure, Bilevel positive airway pressure and ventilators may be required for ventilatory support.

Deep vein thrombosis (DVT): DVT prevention requires nurses follow strict adherence to applying compression stockings, sequential compression devices, chemoprophylaxis such as enoxaparin, or heparin (when able, given other injuries) and early mobility (once the spine is stabilized). For patients who can't be anticoagulated, an inferior vena cava filter should be considered.

Pressure injuries: Many spinal cord patients develop pressure injuries due to lack of sensation and inability to move frequently. Thus, nurses must be diligent to reposition minimally every 2 hours and stay vigilant inspecting for early signs and stages. Specialty mattresses and beds are helpful. Nurses should teach family members to assist with repositioning and range of motion exercises can assist the nursing team and allows the family to feel useful in the patient's recovery.

Urine retention and constipation: Urinary retention and constipation are common in spinal cord injuries. Early removal of foley catheters reduced the incidence of catheter related urinary tract infections (CAUTIs). Nurses play a central role in the bladder training process. Use of bladder scanning with intermittent straight catheterization every 4 to 6 hours can prevent autonomic dysreflexia (AD). Additionally, prevention of constipation is central in preventing AD. Thus, adherence to an aggressive bowel regimen is key. Maintenance of hydration and addition of fiber can help, but often patients require multiple agents to facilitate regular bowel movements. Stimulants are most useful, and enemas and digital disimpaction may be necessary.

Discharge planning: Patients with spinal cord injuries require aggressive rehabilitation to return home and work. Rehabilitation services with physical therapy, occupational therapy, speech and swallow therapies (S&S), and integration of orthotic teams for adaptive devices are all central to the recovery of the patient.

Autonomic dysreflexia (AD): Patients with a spinal cord injury above T6 level are at risk to develop AD. AD is a dysregulated adrenergic response to a noxious stimulus below the level of the spinal cord injury. AD can be associated with a stimulus, even if the patient is unable to feel it. AD occurs three times as often in complete spinal cord injuries. AD is an acute episode of hypertension with a SBP increased >25 mmHg above the patient's baseline. This is considered a type of hypertensive urgency and may lead to hypertensive crisis if the patient has target organ damage such as intracranial hemorrhage, seizures, and can even lead to death. Other symptoms include flushing and diaphoresis of the skin above the level of the spinal cord injury, blurred vision, and nasal congestion. Below the level of the lesion, the sympathetic overdrive causes pale, cool skin, with piloerection. Bowel or bladder distention are common triggers of AD and can easily be resolved. However, infections can also trigger AD, but takes longer to resolve. If is not treated recognized or treated promptly, it has a 22% mortality rate and 300% increased risk of hemorrhagic stroke. Thus, nurses should continually assess for signs and symptoms of AD and remove possible stimuli.

FAST FACTS

Nursing interventions are aimed at preventing complications of spinal cord injured patients.

BLUNT CEREBRAL VASCULAR INJURIES

Blunt cerebral vascular injuries (BCVI) can occur as a result of any form of blunt injury to either the head or neck resulting in injuries to the internal carotid or vertebral arteries. The most common cause of BCVI are MVC. Either carotid or vertebral arteries can be affected. BCVI occur in 1% of all hospitalized trauma patients and up to 9% of all patients with head injuries. BCVI is caused by stretching of the vessels. Hyperflexion, hyperextension and/or rotational forces of the neck stretch the vessels, causing tears to the intimal lining of the vessel. Thrombus formation occurs to repair the tear in the vessel wall and thus a hematoma forms partially or completely occluding the lumen. These intraluminal clots can embolize cerebral arteries, resulting in an ischemic stroke. BCVI is an independent predictor of higher morbidity and mortality in patients with this injury, historically as high as 25% to 50% for those who do suffer a stroke. Patients with severe facial fractures, basilar skull fractures, cervical fractures, and first rib fractures should be screened for BCVI. Screening for and treatment of BCVI has reduced strokes to ~3%.

Medical treatment with aspirin, Plavix, heparin, or warfarin are all useful to prevent stroke. These treatments may be initially contraindicated for patients with severe brain injuries. Additionally endovascular stenting may be required for higher grade injuries.

Nursing Care of BCVI
Maintain a high index of suspicion for any patient who has severe facial fractures, basilar skull fracture, any cervical fractures, and first rib fractures, as these patients are at high risk for ischemic stroke. Be sure to obtain an NIHSS for any patient who has these injuries and exhibits any signs of stroke. Contact the providers with neurological changes in these populations.

SUMMARY

In summary, TBIs can range from mild to severe and may progress to brain death. Nurses who perform detailed neurological exams can identify early neurological changes and institute timely interventions that can impact patient outcomes. Be sure to perform joint neurological exams during hand-offs between shifts and units. Nursing care of patients with SCI is aimed at preventing complications from immobility.

REVIEW QUESTIONS

1. The first nursing intervention when a patient's ICP is sustained over 22 mmHg for >5 minutes is
   a. Start a Fentanyl infusion
   b. 23.4% Saline bolus
   c. Give a 75 gm Mannitol bolus
   d. Ensure the HOB is >30 degrees

2. A patient with a traumatic brain injury needs central venous access. The nurse notes the resident is prepping the jugular vein. What is the nurse's next step?
   a. Suggest a femoral line
   b. Suggest they place a subclavian line
   c. Get the ultrasound machine to the bedside
   d. Immediately place the patient in Trendelenburg position
3. A patient has uncontrolled ICPs despite giving pro re nata (PRN) fentanyl and versed boluses. Mannitol was given 2 hours ago, and the patient's sodium is 170. What should be the nurses next intervention?
   a. Call the family in
   b. Notify the provider
   c. Give another dose of 23% NaCl
   d. Give a second dose of Mannitol stat
4. An attending neurosurgeon is placing an EVD and the nurse notes a monitor cable touched the neurosurgeons sterile glove while they were getting into position. What is the Nurses next step?
   a. Tell the neurosurgeon
   b. Fill out an incident form
   c. Report it to the charge nurse
   d. Set up and zero the transducer
5. A young adult patient who fell and hit the left side of his head on the cement curb arrives. EMS reports the patient had a brief loss of consciousness but is now awake and alert. Glasgow coma score is 15 on arrival to the ED. While in the ED, the patient became more somnolent, and his left pupil is now 5 mm, and the right is still 3 mm. What is the most likely diagnosis?
   a. Concussion
   b. Subdural hematoma
   c. Epidural hematoma
   d. Subarachnoid hemorrhage

References

Bower, M. M., Sweidan, A. J., Xu, J. C., Stern-Nezer, S., Yu, W., & Groysman, L. I. (2021). Quantitative pupillometry in the intensive care unit. *Journal of Intensive Care Medicine*, 36(4), 383–391. https://doi.org/10.1177/0885066619881124

Brommeland, T., Helseth, E., Aarhus, M., Moen, K. G., Dyrskog, S., Bergholt, B., Olivecrona, Z., & Jeppesen, E. (2018). Best practice guidelines for blunt cerebrovascular injury (BCVI). *Scandinavian Journal of Trauma, Resuscitation and Emergency Medicine*, 26, 1–10.

Carpenter, D., & Menard, A. (2023). *Adult gerontology acute care nurse practitioner certification review* (1st ed.). Springer Publishing Company.

Carpenter, D. (2021). *Fast facts for the adult-gerontology acute care nurse practitioner*. Springer Publishing Company.

Chesnut, R., Aguilera, S., Buki, A., Bulger, E., Citerio, G., Cooper, D. J., Arrastia, R. D., Diringer, M., Figaji, A., Gao, G., Geocadin, R., Ghajar, J., Harris, O., Hoffer, A., Hutchinson, P., Joseph, M., Kitagawa, R., Manley, G., Mayer, S., Menon, D. K. et al. (2020, May). A management algorithm for adult patients with both brain oxygen and intracranial pressure monitoring: The Seattle international severe traumatic brain injury consensus conference (SIBICC). *Intensive Care Medicine, 46*(5), 919–929. https://doi.org/10.1007/s00134-019-05900-x. Epub 2020 Jan 21.

Cowan, H., Lakra, C., & Desai, M. (2020). Autonomic dysreflexia in spinal cord injury. *BMJ, 37*, m3596. https://doi.org/10.1136/bmj.m3596

Dellazizzo, L., Demers, S., Charbonney, E., Williams, V., Serri, K., Albert, M., Giguere, J., Laroche, M., Williamson, D., & Bernard, F. (2019). Minimal PaO$_2$ threshold after traumatic brain injury and clinical utility of a novel brain oxygenation ratio. *Journal of Neurosurgery, 131*(5), 1639–1647. https://doi.org/10.3171/2018.5.JNS18651

Ham, H. W., Schoonhoven, L. L., Galer, A. A., & Shortridge-Baggett, L. L. M. (2014). Cervical collar—related pressure ulcers in trauma patients in intensive care unit. *Journal of Trauma Nursing, 21*(3), 94–102.

Menacho, S. T., & Floyd, C. (2021). Current practices and goals for mean arterial pressure and spinal cord perfusion pressure in acute traumatic spinal cord injury: Defining the gaps in knowledge. *The Journal of Spinal Cord Medicine, 44*(3), 350–356. https://doi.org/10.1080/10790268.2019.1660840

Munakomi, S., & Das, J. M. (2023, January). *Intracranial pressure monitoring.* StatPearls Publishing. https://www.ncbi.nlm.nih.gov/books/NBK542298/

Orman, J. A. L., Kraus, J. F., Zaloshnja, E., & Miller, T. (2011). Epidemiology. In J. M. Silver, T. W. McAllister, & S. C. Yudofsky (Eds.). *Textbook of traumatic brain injury* (2nd ed., pp. 3–22). American Psychiatric Publishing.

Russell, J. A., Epstein, L. G., Greer, D. M., Kirschen, M., Rubin, M. A., & Lewis, A. (2019). Brain death, the determination of brain death, and member guidance for brain death accommodation requests: AAN position statement. *Neurology, 92*(5), 228–232.

Trent, T., Vashisht, A., Novakovic, S., Kanter, G., Nairon, E., Lark, A., Tucker, A., Reddy, V., McCreary, M., Stutzman, S. E., & Olson, D. M. (2023, February 1). Pupillary light reflex measured with quantitative pupillometry has low sensitivity and high specificity for predicting neuroworsening after traumatic brain injury. *Journal of the American Association of Nurse Practitioners, 35*(2), 130–134. https://doi.org/10.1097/JXX.0000000000000822

Ziu, E., Khan Suheb, M. Z., & Mesfin, F. B. (2023, January). *Subarachnoid hemorrhage.* StatPearls Publishing. https://www.ncbi.nlm.nih.gov/books/NBK441958/

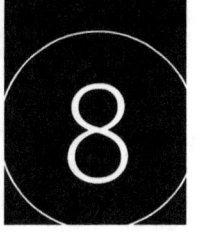

Head, Eyes, Ears, Nose, and Throat Injuries and Care
Alexander Menard

> *Injuries to the head, eyes, ears, nose, and throat, often abbreviated together as HEENT, can occur either in isolation or in conjunction with other multisystem trauma. Visual inspection can lead the nurse to observe injuries to the HEENT. These injuries can affect a patient's ability to see, hear, breathe, manage secretions, impede oral competence, and verbalize self-expression as well as maintain adequate oral intake and nutrition. These injuries can occasionally lead to significant facial deformities, temporary or permanent, that may cause patients to have concerns over their appearance and loss of self-identity and can lead to individuals being ostracized from social groups.*

In this chapter, you will learn to:
1. Recognize signs of trauma to the HEENT.
2. Identify assessments indicated for injuries to the HEENT.
3. Articulate red flags, signs of underlying pathology, and serious injury.

INTRODUCTION

The initial evaluation of the HEENT should start with a visual inspection of visible surfaces. Trauma patients have many reasons to have deformities, lacerations and abrasions, or foreign objects present. Remove helmets, clothing, accessories, or dressings and look under cervical collars during this evaluation. Palpation follows and can be useful in determining pain underlying an otherwise unremarkable exam. Palpation identifies the presence of subcutaneous air in the tissues or other structural pathologies.

HEENT ASSESSMENT

Head
Often injuries to the head will be apparent with blood, cerebrospinal fluid (CSF), or displaced tissues being clearly visible. It may be possible that an injury to the head may manifest with hemotympanum, otorrhea, or

rhinorrhea, which may be blood and/or CSF. The nurse should wash away any dried blood or dirt to properly evaluate an injury to the head. An intact clot should not be disrupted so as not to cause rebleeding; however, the trauma team provider may need to do this to inspect the wound further to determine further interventions.

> **FAST FACTS**
>
> Scalp lacerations can bleed profusely and be hidden in a patient's long, dark hair. They can bleed sufficiently to require transfusion. If left unrecognized, they may lead to hemorrhagic shock and death.

Eyes

Facial injuries, specifically ocular injuries, commonly cause significant periorbital edema and edema of the eyelids, making it difficult to inspect the eye itself. To complete the assessment, the eyelids must be opened. The eye assessment includes a visual inspection and evaluation of visual acuity and extraocular movements. The visual inspection allows the nurse to evaluate the sclera, conjunctiva, and pupillary size. During the eye evaluation, the nurse can determine whether there is a gaze preference, anisocoria, or abnormal eye movements. Further assessment will include evaluation of pupillary responses and accommodation. The nursing assessment will routinely involve the evaluation of visual fields and extraocular movements. The inability of a patient to complete the extraocular movement exam warrants further investigation and might indicate orbital edema or hemorrhage; extraocular muscle entrapment; or cranial nerve III, IV, or VI damage. Abnormalities in the extraocular movement may indicate ocular entrapment, which requires immediate notification to the primary and ears, nose, and throat (ENT) teams. Surgical intervention is required within 60 to 90 minutes to salvage vision in the affected eye.

Anisocoria is the presence of unequal pupils, which can be a normal variation in some individuals. Additionally, patients may have had prior neurologic diagnoses that may affect their eye exam. Other variations may be seen in patients who have had a previous stroke or corneal surgeries and may not have pupillary responses. Abnormal exam findings should be noted, and the patient or family should be asked about their history.

Ears

The external ear evaluation entails visual inspection for deformity, bleeding, lacerations, auricular hematoma, and/or discharge from the ear. In the trauma bay, the tympanic membrane should be inspected for hemotympanum or ruptured membranes. Gross hearing deficits may be noted, but the noise from the trauma bay should be considered and other more serious injuries may take priority. Tinnitus may be the presenting symptom, and hearing loss may not be immediately recognized because of it. Thus, the ICU and floor nurses should be vigilant, with ongoing assessment for tinnitus and hearing deficits. Additional hearing tests can be performed with the use of a tuning fork. The Weber test can detect unilateral conductive or sensorineural hearing loss, and the Rinne test evaluates sound transmission from air and bone conduction. Consultation with otolaryngology or audiology may be needed for persistent hearing deficits. Earrings and any other piercings or jewelry should be removed to prevent artifact on CT scans, which may obscure images.

FAST FACTS

Remove all jewelry, including all piercings, to prevent artifact on CT scans, which may obscure images.

Nose

Assessment of the nose includes determining patency by asking the patient if they can breathe through their nose. Ask the patient to close off one nostril and inhale and then do the same on the other side. Inspect for bleeding, lacerations, and deformity. Septal hematomas may not readily be visible externally. Nasal speculum exams should be performed by the trauma or ENT team if the nares are not patent. Discharge should be noted and characterized. Light palpation for crepitus can aid in the assessment and identification of underlying pathology. Epistaxis may occur with nasal trauma, and a patient may present with nasal packing to control bleeding. Nasal packing should never be removed without expert consultation and confirmation from the primary team.

Mouth/Throat

Visual inspection of the mouth and throat is performed to identify any broken teeth; lip, tongue, or cheek lacerations; or foreign objects, including dentures or piercings, which may cause obstruction. If a patient is emergently intubated and has oral bleeding, inspect the hard palate for lacerations from the laryngoscope. Additionally, it is important to note dentition and or lack thereof. The mouth and throat mucosa can also provide information about the volume status of the patient, for instance, whether the mucosa is moist versus dry and cracked. Evaluation of the neck includes inspection for any tracheal deviation. Auscultation of the neck can identify stridor, which may indicate narrowing of the airway. Stridor indicates impending loss of an airway, and the team must be notified immediately.

FAST FACTS

Stridor indicates impending loss of the airway, and the trauma team must be notified immediately. Patients with stridor may have normal oxygen saturation on room air. This is because the problem is the upper airway, not the lungs. Stridor is an airway emergency.

INJURIES OF THE HEAD

Scalp lacerations may be serious injuries resulting in major blood loss, which can lead to hemorrhagic shock and death. Urgent assessment and control of bleeding scalp lacerations are imperative. This management may include direct pressure, pressure dressings, and surgical closure (suture, staples, and gluing) of the laceration. Before surgical closure of the wound, a thorough inspection for foreign bodies (shards of glass, road debris, etc.) and cleaning must occur.

Maxillofacial fractures include nasal, zygomatic and orbital, and maxillary and mandibular fractures. The most common type of facial fracture is a nasal bone fracture. The zygomatic bone is the bone that gives prominence to the cheek and forms the lateral portion of the orbit. Fractures of this bone are the second most common facial fractures. Maxillary and mandibular fractures follow. These types of fractures are managed in conjunction with the primary trauma team in consultation with the plastic surgery and/or HEENT specialist. Le Fort fractures are transverse fractures of the midface and are divided into three subtypes (Table 8.1). The purpose of classifying

TABLE 8.1

Le Fort Classification of Maxillary Fractures, With Images

Le Forte Fracture

Le Fort I	Le Fort II	Le Fort III
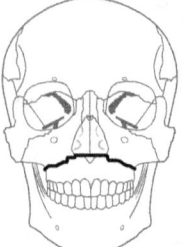	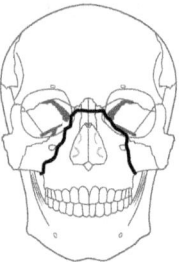	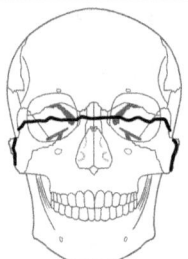
Separation of the hard palate from the upper maxilla secondary to a transverse fracture running through the maxilla and pterygoid plates	Transects the nasal bone, medial-anterior orbital walls, orbital floor, and inferior orbital rims and transversely fractures the posterior maxilla and pterygoid plates	Transverse separation of the nasofrontal suture, medial orbital wall, lateral orbital wall or zygomaticofrontal suture, zygomatic arch, and pterygoid plates (Essentially separation of the maxilla from the skull base)

Source: Le Fort I—https://upload.wikimedia.org/wikipedia/commons/2/2f/LeFort1e.png; Le Fort II—https://upload.wikimedia.org/wikipedia/commons/0/02/LeFort2b.png; Le Fort III—https://upload.wikimedia.org/wikipedia/commons/6/67/LeFort3b.png

facial fractures by the Le Fort system is to determine how stable or unstable the midface is compared with the skull bones.

Nursing Care

The nurse plays a large role in identifying injuries to the head. Cleaning the injury and continued monitoring for ongoing bleeding or signs of infection (warmth, erythematous regions, and or unexpected drainage) are critical tasks for which the nurse may be responsible. Additionally, the nurse can evaluate for drainage that resembles CSF, indicating the cranial vault has been violated and further investigation is warranted to determine the source of the CSF leak. Patients with facial fractures are considered to have open fractures and require prophylactic antibiotics.

Patients with maxillary and mandibular fractures may require maxillary and mandibular fixation, commonly referred to by the slang term *jaw wiring*. These patients cannot open their mouth if they vomit or require intubation. Thus, it is imperative to always keep wire cutters with the patient in case of an emergency, because the wires may need to be cut to open the jaw/mouth. Additionally, the cheeks are sensitive to the metal components and may develop abrasions or become lacerated. Dental wax applied to the hardware can protect the soft tissues from injury.

Nursing interventions include keeping the head of bed (HOB) at 30 degrees or higher (if it is not contraindicated) and applying cold compresses or ice packs. Patients with orbital or nasal fractures should avoid nose blowing and sneezing. Frequent reassessment and pain management are important nursing interventions.

FAST FACTS

Wire cutters must be kept with patients who have maxillary and mandibular fixation at all times and be kept visible and easily accessible. In the event of airway compromise, the wires can be cut to allow access to the airway.

INJURIES OF THE EYES

Eye injuries may be devastating and lead to loss of vision in one or both eyes, depending on the injury. Ocular trauma has two classifications, open-globe injury and closed-globe injury, with subclassifications for each (Table 8.2). Penetrating orbital injuries may result in optic nerve damage and immediate vision loss. Corneal injuries may be painful and result from a foreign body getting into or rubbing against the cornea. Corneal abrasions can be detected by fluorescein staining, penlight, and slit-lamp examination, which can aid in revealing foreign material or injury to the eye.

Foreign bodies that penetrate the eye should not be removed. They should be secured in place. Commonly, a paper cup can be taped over the object and to the patient's face. Removal of the foreign body should occur in the operating room, where bleeding can be controlled.

TABLE 8.2

Ocular Injury Classification

Open-Globe Classification	Closed-Globe Classification
Type: A. Rupture B. Penetrating C. Intraocular foreign body D. Perforating E. Mixed	Type: A. Contusion B. Lamellar laceration C. Superficial foreign body D. Mixed
Visual acuity: A. 20/40 or greater B. 10/50 to 20/100 C. 19/100 to 5/100 D. 4/200—light perception E. No light perception	Visual acuity: A. 20/40 or greater B. 10/50 to 20/100 C. 19/100 to 5/100 D. 4/200—light perception E. No light perception
Pupil: ■ Positive—relative afferent pupillary defect present in affected eye ■ Negative—relative afferent pupillary defect absent in affected eye	Pupil: ■ Positive—relative afferent pupillary defect present in affected eye ■ Negative—relative afferent pupillary defect absent in affected eye
Zone: 1. Isolated to the cornea 2. Corneoscleral limbus to a point 5 mm posterior into the sclera 3. Posterior to the anterior 5 mm of the sclera	Zone: 1. External 2. Anterior segment 3. Posterior segment

Nursing Care

Nurses are instrumental in the care of the patient with ocular trauma. Ongoing assessment of patient-reported symptoms includes loss of vision, blurred vision, double vision, and so forth. Specifically, blurred vision that does not improve with blinking, double vision, loss of a part of the usual visual field (visual field cut or sectorial vision loss), and/or ocular pain are red flags and should trigger a prompt report to the trauma team and evaluation by an ophthalmologist.

FAST FACTS

Vision loss, blurred vision (that does not improve with blinking), sectorial vision loss, and/or ocular pain are all "red flags" and should prompt evaluation by an ophthalmologist.

INJURIES OF THE EARS

The ear is a commonly injured part of the face, given its prominence and delicate structure. Whenever an injury to the ear is present, injury to the middle ear and or temporal bone must be suspected. Sudden hearing loss is a red flag for injury to the inner ear structures. Nurses should also assess the facial nerve by testing the sensation and movement of the forehead, cheek, and chin. Absence of sensation or movement can indicate a facial nerve injury that might be caused by a temporal bone fracture. Further indications of more severe injury include bleeding and CSF leaking from the ear canal. The providers will assess for the presence of foreign bodies within the ear canal, first by external visual inspection and then with an otoscope.

The tympanic membrane and middle ear can be damaged when exposed to blunt or penetrating trauma, blasts, or thermal injuries. Providers assess for this type of injury with the aid of an otoscope. The result of such trauma may be tympanic membrane perforation, middle ear hemorrhage and fracture, damage to the cochlea, or dislocation of the ossicular chain and/or damage to the facial nerve. Lacerations of the ear canal may indicate temporal bone fracture, which would be considered an open fracture, requiring antibiotics. These injuries may result in hearing impairment or loss. Hence, hearing and vestibular function must be assessed.

Nursing Care

Nursing care includes identifying ear injuries as well as monitoring and management. When dealing with an ear injury, it is important to note changes in discharge if any occurs. Blood draining from the internal ear canal is a red flag. Serous or serosanguinous fluid may resemble CSF. Prompt notification to the provider/care team is essential to facilitate diagnostics and treatment.

Ear abrasions and/or lacerations and suture repairs may require bacitracin. The injury should be inspected carefully for signs and symptoms of infection, including erythema, warmth, and/or purulent discharge. Hearing should be continuously assessed throughout each shift through interactions with the patient, and changes should be documented and reported to the trauma providers.

FAST FACTS

Blood draining from the internal ear canal is a red flag and warrants further investigation by the provider.

INJURIES OF THE NOSE

The nose is an important part of the face as it serves as a gateway to the respiratory system and provides structure to the face. The nose is highly vascular, and injuries may result in significant bleeding. Gravity facilitates

TABLE 8.3
Nasal Fracture Patterns by Impact

Impact	Injury Pattern
Anterior impact	Damage to the nasal tip and cartilage
Lateral impact	Depressed displacement of nasal bones, C- or S-shaped nasal dorsum deformities, and medial maxillary wall fractures
Combination anterior and lateral impacts	Septal defects are often associated with fractures of the maxilla, orbit, and septum

drainage into the airway passages, and patients may aspirate and subsequently develop acute respiratory failure. Monitoring the airway is the highest priority. Additionally, patients may swallow this blood and then either vomit blood or develop tarry stools that may resemble an upper gastrointestinal bleed.

Injury to the nose may result in functional and cosmetic defects. Given the position and prominence of the nose, it is the most commonly injured part of the face. Nasal fractures have patterns of injuries depending on the type of impact (Table 8.3). Bruising and tenderness are signs of nasal bone fracture. Additional imaging (CT scan) of the face is the best method to assess for concurrent maxillofacial bony injury. Provider assessment may include palpation for crepitus, anterior rhinoscopy, and endonasal palpation to evaluate for obstruction or narrowing and septal hematoma. Oxymetazoline (Afrin) or phenylephrine nasal sprays can be used to help stop bleeding because they cause vasoconstriction. Alternatively, liquid cocaine, a potent vasoconstrictor, can be sprayed onto the area. Nasal packing or balloon catheters may be useful to tamponade refractory bleeding. Nondisplaced nasal bones do not require surgical intervention. Surgical intervention of displaced fractures is commonly delayed to allow edema to resolve before determining whether fixation is needed.

Nursing Care

Nasal fractures may be painful and associated with significant swelling. Ice packs or cool compresses can be applied and the HOB elevated at least 30 degrees to reduce swelling. Patients should be assessed continually, particularly as swelling decreases, because displaced nasal bone fractures may have been disguised by the swelling. Epistaxis is a concern for the patient with a nasal bone fracture and may result in massive hemorrhage and airway compromise if not managed. Nurses can optimize care for the patient with epistaxis by keeping the HOB elevated, having appropriate suctioning at the bedside, and applying direct pressure until the bleeding stops or more advanced treatments are available. More advanced treatments include nasal tampons, topical vasoconstrictors, cautery, tranexamic acid, and surgical intervention.

In addition to bleeding from the nose, the nurse must be suspicious and inspect for CSF coming from the nose, indicating a fracture into the cranial vault. CSF may be clear, straw colored, or mixed with blood. A halo test can lead providers to determine whether additional testing for CSF is needed. The halo test is performed by placing drainage on a porous material such as filter paper, coffee filter, paper towel, or linen. A double ring will appear if CSF is present. The provider/care team should be notified immediately if there are concerns for CSF discharging from a patient's nose. If a CSF leak is suspected, a sample can be sent for beta-2 transferrin to confirm the diagnosis.

FAST FACTS

CSF coming from the nose indicates a fracture into the cranial vault. The nurse who suspects CSF should notify the provider.

INJURIES OF THE THROAT

Airway trauma may result from head and neck trauma. Laryngeal trauma can be a result of blunt, penetrating, or burn trauma. Suspicion or confirmation of laryngeal trauma requires immediate assessment and intervention to secure the airway. Obvious injuries are addressed in the primary survey. Additional airway discussion is reviewed in Chapter 4. Airway compromise can develop over hours to a day as edema forms. This can be seen with blunt trauma to the neck and/or inhalation injuries, in which swelling in the subsequent hours can result in airway compromise.

Strangulation

Strangulation injuries are a result of a mechanical force being applied to the neck and surrounding structures. This includes manual strangulation as well as suicide attempt by hanging. The result of this type of force is compression of the major vessels in the neck supplying blood and oxygen to the brain, compression of the trachea, and/or fracture of the hyoid bone or cricoid cartilage. Death follows rapidly if the compression is not stopped/relieved. A high level of suspicion for cervical spine injury must be maintained in these patients. Care requires immediate evaluation and intervention by the medical team to secure an airway. Once the airway is secure, additional resources should be mobilized. These additional resources include mental health providers, social work, and law enforcement, depending on the circumstances surrounding the injury.

Nursing Care
For patients with suspected or confirmed injuries to the throat, maintain a high index of suspicion for airway compromise. Continued assessment is needed and should include visual inspection and auscultation with a stethoscope to identify stridor. Other red flag signs of airway compromise include

hoarseness, dysphagia, odynophagia, and drooling due to the inability to manage saliva. Stridor (audible with or without a stethoscope), increased work of breath, accessory muscle use, arrhythmia, and alteration in mental status are late findings. If a patient is exhibiting any of these signs, immediately activate the trauma team, as intubation or emergent trach is imminent. Concurrently, elevate the HOB to 45 degrees and increase oxygen. Bring suction tubing, canister, and Yankauer, as well as intubation tray and trach tray, to the bedside. Anticipate that the patient with airway compromise likely will need a surgical airway and tracheostomy performed. Surgeons prefer these procedures to occur in the operating room, where a more controlled environment exists and they have access to the appropriate equipment. It is important to note that nursing instinct or intuition is also applicable and should not be ignored; if something does not feel or look right, it is appropriate to ask for help.

FAST FACTS

Careful assessment of the airway should be completed with any injuries to the head and face.

SUMMARY

Care of the patient with injuries to the HEENT will often involve consultation with a specialist. The specific specialist team that is consulted depends on the specific injury and each institution's specific resources, which may include plastic and reconstructive surgery, oromaxillofacial surgery, otolaryngology, and/or ophthalmology. Injuries to the HEENT are highly visible and may be associated with patients' emotional and psychological distress over alteration to their body and image. Support should be offered to these patients as early as reasonably and medically possible. Injury to the HEENT can have potential impacts on several of the patient's senses, including hearing, vision, smell, taste, and so forth. Nurses can be instrumental in the healing of these wounds by providing excellent nursing care including but not limited to pain management, dressing changes, continued assessment, encouragement, and education on nutrition and its role in wound healing.

REVIEW QUESTIONS

1. What nursing intervention can be implemented to address a patient with epistaxis?
   a. HOB elevation and cautery
   b. HOB elevation and direct pressure
   c. Application of topical vasoconstrictors and surgical intervention
   d. Application of topical vasoconstrictors and cautery

2. These are considered "red flag" findings related to the eye (select all that apply):
   a. Ocular pain
   b. Sudden loss of sight
   c. Blurred vision that improves with blinking
   d. Sudden sectorial vision changes
3. Stridor is an indication of:
   a. Upper airway narrowing
   b. Increased oxygenation
   c. A cuff leak
   d. Temporal bone fracture

References

Krulewitz, N. A., & Fix, M. L. (2019, February). Epistaxis. *Emergency Medicine Clinics of North America*, *37*(1), 29–39. https://doi.org/10.1016/j.emc.2018.09.005

Landeen, K. C., Kimura, K., & Stephan, S. J. (2022, February). Nasal fractures. *Facial Plastic Surgery Clinics of North America*, *30*(1), 23–30. https://doi.org/10.1016/j.fsc.2021.08.002

McQuillan, K. A., & Flynn-Makic, M. B. (2020). *Trauma nursing: From resuscitation through rehabilitation* (5th ed., pp. 410–453). Elsevier.

Nojoumi, A., & Woo, B. M. (2021, August). Management of ear trauma. *Oral and Maxillofacial Surgery Clinics of North America*, *33*(3), 305–315. https://doi.org/10.1016/j.coms.2021.04.001

Sunder, R., & Tyler, K. (2013). Basal skull fracture and the halo sign. *CMAJ: Canadian Medical Association Journal = Journal de L'Association Medicale Canadienne*, *185*(5), 416. https://doi.org/10.1503/cmaj.120055

Van Hoecke, H., Calus, L., & Dhooge, I. (2016). Middle ear damages. *B-ENT*, *12*(Suppl. 26), 173–183.

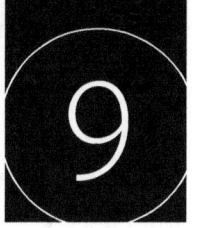

Cardiovascular Injuries and Care
Dawn Carpenter

> *Cardiovascular injuries can range from asymptomatic to precipitously lethal at the scene. For patients who survive and arrive at the hospital, ongoing reassessment and monitoring are essential, because patients can rapidly deteriorate. Nurses must remain vigilant and possess a high index of suspicion for cardiovascular injuries.*

In this chapter, you will learn:
1. Key cardiovascular assessments to identify cardiovascular injuries.
2. To interpret vital signs in trauma patients.
3. To recognize signs and symptoms of specific cardiovascular injuries.
4. To articulate ongoing monitoring of patients with injuries.
5. To prioritize nursing interventions for patients with cardiovascular injuries.

INTRODUCTION

Specific knowledge is needed to quickly identify the rapidly changing signs and symptoms of cardiovascular injuries. The nurse must be able to interpret and critically analyze hemodynamic data. Additionally, nurses must perform detailed assessment of the cardiovascular system and be ready to set up and implement invasive continuous hemodynamic monitoring.

CARDIOVASCULAR ASSESSMENT

Steps for correct assessment of the cardiovascular system are, in order, inspection, palpation, and then auscultation. Inspect the entire anterior chest, looking for abrasions, lacerations, ecchymosis, and deformities. Inspect the arms, hands, feet, legs, and hips for dependent edema. When the cervical collar is removed or changed, inspect the neck for jugular venous distention (JVD).

Palpate the chest for tenderness, crepitus, instability, or paradoxical movement with respirations and for thrills and heaves and to assess point of maximal impulse. Palpate the peripheral pulses, including radial, popliteal, dorsalis pedis, and posterior tibial. Grade the strength of the pulses. If the pulses cannot be palpated, use a Doppler to assess for pulses.

Auscultate heart sounds using both the diaphragm and bell of a quality stethoscope. The disposable stethoscopes used in isolation rooms are usually not sufficient to be able to hear the finer details of a thorough cardiac exam. The diaphragm of the stethoscope is better to hear high-pitched sounds, such as S1 and S2. Muffled heart sounds may indicate cardiac tamponade, an emergency that may require pericardiocentesis or emergent surgery. The bell of the stethoscope is better to hear low-pitched sounds such as S3 and S4. Extra heart sounds, such as S3 and S4, may indicate the presence of ventricular dysfunction, possibly indicating the development of heart failure. Listen in the five locations, including:

- Aortic area at the right sternal border, second intercostal space
- Pulmonic area at the left sternal border, second intercostal space
- Erb's point at the left sternal border, third intercostal space
- Tricuspid area at the left sternal border, fourth intercostal space
- Mitral area (or apex) at the fifth left intercostal space, midclavicular line.

Circulatory, Sensory, and Motor Exam

The circulatory, sensory, and motor exam is especially important in patients with cardiovascular injuries. Changes seen in this exam are as important as vital signs when vessels are injured. Changes in sensation and motor occur prior to pulse loss. Additionally, unequal blood pressures (BPs) can signify aortic injury or dissection.

FAST FACTS

Muffled heart sounds, distended neck veins, and narrowed pulse pressure may indicate cardiac tamponade, an emergency that may require pericardiocentesis or emergent surgery.

HEMODYNAMIC MONITORING

Nurses are primarily responsible for hemodynamic monitoring. Patients with traumatic injuries should initially have continuous telemetry monitoring, continuous respiratory rate, serial BPs, and continuous pulse oximetry. Once the patient is admitted, continuous monitoring should occur in the ICU and intermediate level of care. Providers will need to decide what monitoring is needed for patients admitted to the floor. Nurses can always begin monitoring based on the patient's needs and contact the trauma provider to notify them of the concerns so they can evaluate whether a higher level of care is needed.

Interpretation of Vital Signs

Nurses play a key role in the interpretation and critical appraisal of vital signs in trauma patients. Vital signs are more than just numbers; they are the window into the patient's overall status. Interpretation must occur in conjunction with physical exam findings and laboratory data and must be interpreted in light of expected findings. The nurse should anticipate expected vital signs, and if the patient's findings are not as expected, the nurse needs to ask why. In other words, identify what doesn't fit the rest of the picture. For example, most traumatically injured patients do not present with fever. Thus, if a trauma patient has a fever on arrival, perhaps they have an underlying infection that caused them to become a trauma patient. Several other factors need to be considered that can affect vital signs and alter the expected findings. These variations in vital signs are described in the next few paragraphs. It is important to note that trends in vital signs are important. Evolution of vital signs over time may have significant implications. For example, a progressive increase in oxygen may indicate pulmonary pathology, or decreased BP can indicate a cardiac pathology or infection.

Telemetry Monitoring

Patients need to be monitored for progressive tachycardia or bradycardia. Bradycardia may indicate a reason the patient experienced syncope, which may be the cause of the trauma. Additionally, patients who take beta-blockers, calcium channel blockers, or other antiarrhythmic agents may not become tachycardic. Tachycardia is a compensatory sign of hemorrhagic shock as the patient tries to maintain adequate blood and oxygen supply to the tissues. Any tachycardia in a trauma patient must be reported to the trauma team for reassessment. Hypovolemic or hemorrhagic shock requires aggressive resuscitation. Patients may also develop tachycardia as a result of uncontrolled pain, anxiety, or toxic ingestions such as amphetamines or cocaine. Additionally, tachycardia is one of the signs of systemic inflammatory response syndrome (SIRS). SIRS may be directly related to the trauma itself or result from burns or other medical conditions that precipitated the cause of the trauma (i.e., sepsis causing syncope and a fall). Burn patients may also be tachycardic from SIRS, and they can quickly become hypovolemic from third spacing of fluids and need aggressive fluid resuscitation. Patients may also become tachycardic if a fever develops.

Temperature

Frequent assessment of the patient's temperature initially is important to avoid hypothermia and implement early rewarming. Patients may be exposed to ambient outdoor temperatures for prolonged periods, making them hypothermic or hyperthermic, depending on the local environment. Additionally, trauma patients are stripped of all their clothes in the field to identify injuries. Early rewarming is critical to avoid hypothermia-induced coagulopathy.

> **FAST FACTS**
>
> Hypothermia can induce coagulopathy; thus, early rewarming is critical to avoid and treat hypothermia in a bleeding trauma patient.

A fever is defined as a temperature greater than 38.3°C (>101°F) for most patients, with a lower threshold of greater than 38.0°C (>100.4°F) for elderly and immunocompromised patients. Fevers can arise in trauma patients for a variety of reasons. They can be a direct result of severe trauma, present before admission, or develop during hospitalization. All fevers should be reported to the providers for assessment. Fevers within the first 48 hours of admission are frequently due to atelectasis or preexisting infection that could be the cause of the trauma, commonly a fall resulting in injury. Aggressive pulmonary hygiene with incentive spirometry, positive expiratory pressure, and ambulation is advised.

> **FAST FACTS**
>
> A fever is defined as a temperature greater than 38.3°C (>101°F) for most patients, with a lower threshold of greater than 38.0°C (>100.4°F) for elderly and immunocompromised patients. Not all fevers indicate infection. Antibiotic stewardship is critical to avoid creating resistant organisms.

Fevers may be a sign of infection (e.g., occult traumatic perforated bowel injury, pneumonia, urinary tract infections, cellulitis, catheter-associated bloodstream infections, viral infections). A thorough history of each infectious etiology should be documented and symptoms reported to the team for further evaluation and decisions on whether antibiotics are appropriate. Antibiotic stewardship is a priority to reduce antibiotic resistance; therefore, unless clear evidence for infection is identified, not starting antibiotics is encouraged. Antibiotics are avoided because other sources of noninfectious fever occur in the setting of trauma patients during hospitalization, including blood in the brain tissues, deep vein thrombosis, or pulmonary embolus, among others.

> **FAST FACTS**
>
> Antibiotic stewardship is a top priority to minimize antibiotic resistance.

Respiratory Rate

Reassessment of respiratory rate is critical. Patients should be monitored for increasing respiratory rate because this may indicate the patient is going into early stages of shock. Increased respirations are the body's innate compensatory mechanism to meet its need to supply more oxygen to the tissues. Tachypnea can be a compensatory mechanism for shallow respirations from progressive atelectasis or be a sign of uncontrolled pain. On the contrary, bradypnea can be a sign of excess opioid dose. Patients who are bradypneic may need either naloxone (Narcan) or respiratory support to prevent apnea. Patients with bradypnea should have opioid doses reduced, and other treatment options should be sought. Additionally, many patients have undiagnosed sleep apnea that is observed while the patient is hospitalized. Referral for diagnostic testing after discharge is recommended.

Blood Pressure

Initially in the trauma bay, a manual BP should be obtained and compared with an automated BP reading. Frequent serial BPs are essential to monitor for hypotension from ongoing bleeding, assess resuscitation efforts, and diagnose delayed or occult bleeding as well as to monitor for stability after resuscitation. Arterial lines may be necessary in hemodynamically unstable patients for continuous monitoring. Nurses are responsible for the priming of the tubing, inflation of the pressure bag to the appropriate level, and calibration and leveling of the transducers to ensure accurate readings.

There is no universally accepted definition of hypotension. In the trauma bay, a systolic blood pressure (SBP) less than 100 mmHg is considered hypotensive. In sepsis, generally a mean arterial pressure (MAP) less than 65 mmHg is considered shock. The formula to calculate a MAP is

$$MAP = 2/3 \text{ diastolic pressure} + 1/3 \text{ systolic pressure}$$

MAPs should be recorded in the vital signs along with the SBP and diastolic BP (DBP) readings. What's important for nurses to follow is the trend in BP.

A decreased DBP indicates peripheral vasodilation, such as seen with neurogenic shock or other distributive types of shock, such as sepsis. When a DBP trend decreases over time from 70s and 60s into the 40s and 30s, nurses should suspect a distributive shock. Early in the hospitalization, neurogenic shock should be suspected, but after the first 72 hours, a low DBP can signify sepsis and septic shock.

FAST FACTS

Downtrending DBPs should lead the nurse to suspect vasodilation because they may be leading to a distributive shock such as neurogenic or septic shock.

Permissive Hypotension

In patients with active bleeding, permissive hypotension (SBP 80–90 mmHg or MAP 50–60 mmHg) may be acceptable to minimize excessive bleeding and facilitate clot formation to achieve hemorrhage control. Bleeding control can also be achieved by direct pressure, closure of wounds, and intravascular intervention or surgery. Nurses should not automatically presume permissive hypotension is acceptable. Open discussion with the team is imperative because permissive hypotension has innate risks of hypoperfusion of vital organs, which can lead to organ failure. Thus, permissive hypotension should not be performed for prolonged periods. Additionally, patients with any concomitant brain injuries should not experience any hypotension, to avoid secondary brain injury from hypoperfusion.

BPs need to be assessed in relation to patients' normal BPs that are taken during a healthy state. Ask family members about the patient's baseline BP. Lack of adherence to antihypertensive agents can lead the patient to have uncontrolled hypertension. In this situation, a normal BP may signify relative hypotension and warrant intervention to avoid organ damage from hypoperfusion. Conversely, patients may have relative hypotension based on their medical treatment regimens. For example, in a patient with heart failure, an SBP in the 90s may be normal and not indicate hypotension or require interventions.

Patients should be monitored for trends in BP relative to other vital signs. Are the patient's last few BPs decreasing while the heart rate (HR) and respiratory rate are increasing? If so, this is a worrisome trend and warrants reassessment by the team because the patient's status is deteriorating. Conversely, if the HR is increasing and BP is stable, the patient is stabilizing and reassuring that the patient may not need further resuscitation.

When the patient is initially admitted, antihypertensive agents may be held to monitor for ongoing bleeding and ensure hemodynamic stability; these medications should be resumed once the patient's BP normalizes. Angiotensin-converting enzyme inhibitors or angiotensin receptor blockers may be held for longer periods if the patient experiences acute kidney injury (AKI) or receives multiple doses of IV contrast.

FAST FACTS

Patients' BPs need to be assessed in relation to their normal BPs that are taken during a healthy state. Ask family members about the patient's baseline BP, and monitor for trends in vital signs.

Continuous Pulse Oximetry

Continuous pulse oximetry is essential to monitor for worsening respiratory status from chest trauma such as development of or worsening pneumothorax or hemothorax, blossoming pulmonary contusions, progressive atelectasis, developing pneumonia, aspiration, or pulmonary embolism. Pulse oximetry readings can be altered by other factors, including presence of carbon monoxide and skin tone. Both darker skin tones and presence of carbon monoxide poisoning can lead to artificially high readings, resulting in unrecognized tissue hypoxia. In these situations, an arterial blood gas measurement is useful to obtain more accurate oxygenation.

Identifying normal saturations for patients based on their medical history is important. Normal pulse oximetry in patients breathing room air should be greater than 92%. However, patients with chronic lung diseases such as severe chronic obstructive pulmonary disease, emphysema, or interstitial lung disease can have lower pulse oximetry readings at baseline. Patients with chronic lung disease may have baseline oxygen saturations of 88% to 92%. Concurrently identify whether the patient uses supplemental oxygen, continuous positive airway pressure, or bilateral positive airway pressure at home. These devices should be continued while the patient is hospitalized.

FAST FACTS

When a patient becomes hypoxic, it's imperative to treat the underlying cause. Nurses should not just turn up the oxygen.

SHOCK

Shock is defined as the imbalance between oxygen consumption and oxygen delivery. Thus, if the tissues are not getting enough oxygen, they will become hypoxic and convert from normal aerobic metabolism to anaerobic metabolism, producing lactic acid.

FAST FACTS

Shock is defined as the imbalance between oxygen consumption and oxygen delivery.

Compensatory Mechanisms

The body's innate compensatory mechanisms occur in response to shock (Figure 9.1). The respiratory rate increases to expand the supply of oxygen. Thus, one of the earliest signs of shock is tachypnea. Accurate measurement and recording of respiratory rates are critical to early identification of shock.

Hypotension triggers the adrenal medulla to release epinephrine and norepinephrine. This fight-or-flight response results in increased HR and cardiac contractility to maintain cardiac output and thus BP.

Hypotension also activates the renin-angiotensin-aldosterone system, causing peripheral vasoconstriction and increasing systemic vascular constriction. As vasoconstriction occurs, blood is further shunted away from the peripheral tissues. This enhances preload and thus increases cardiac output. Vasoconstriction facilitates this increased cardiac output toward the vital organs to preserve organ function. Vasoconstriction of the renal arteries causes oliguria and concentration of the urine to preserve fluid in the body. Additionally, as blood is shunted away from peripheral tissues, these tissues may become hypoxic. This hypoxia causes cells to shift from aerobic metabolism to anaerobic metabolism, resulting in production and accumulation of lactic acid.

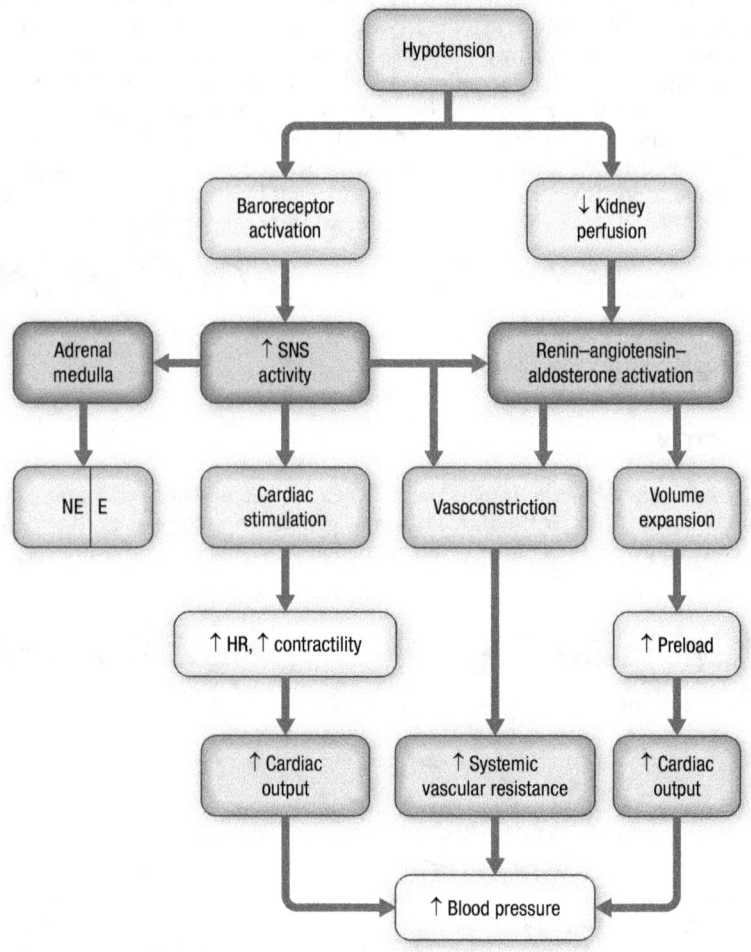

Figure 9.1 Compensatory mechanisms that help maintain perfusion.

Sources: Used with permission from: "Compensatory mechanisms are triggered in shock to help maintain arterial blood pressure despite a fall in cardiac output" from Chapter 20 Shock https://basicmedicalkey.com/shock-2/. authored by Shann Kim; Received permission for use via email on 7/5/23 from Cao Xuan cu <clinicalpub@gmail.com>

Additionally, the hypothalamic-pituitary-adrenal axis activates release of corticotropin-releasing factor to stimulate the release of cortisol, which increases glucose levels in the tissues, leading to hyperglycemia. Severe hyperglycemia is a marker of how critically ill the patient is at the time of admission.

Exam Findings in Shock
Exam findings in shock differ depending on how long a person has been in shock (Table 9.1). Early stages of shock include mild tachycardia, tachypnea, and oliguria. In the late stages of shock, the patient is obtunded, cold and mottled, severely tachycardic, and anuric, and has evidence of other organ damage.

Types of Shock
Trauma patients may present with more than one type of shock concurrently or develop a different type of shock during their hospitalization. For example, a patient who fell off a roof, landing on their feet, and is critically injured presents in hemorrhagic hypovolemic shock due to bleeding from long bone fractures and is concurrently in neurogenic shock from a spinal cord injury. Or perhaps they had a myocardial infarction leading to the fall and present with cardiogenic shock. Another example is an elderly patient who fell and is in hemorrhagic shock from a spleen laceration, but the reason they fell was septic shock from a urinary tract infection. Nurses should never assume that a trauma patient is experiencing only hemorrhagic shock. One needs to keep an open mind and consider other types of shock. Table 9.2 reviews how to differentiate between types of shock.

TABLE 9.1

Physical Assessment as Shock Progresses

System	Exam Findings as Shock Progresses
Neurologic	- Anxiety - Restlessness - Confusion - Lethargy
Respiratory	- Tachypnea - Hypoxia - Respiratory failure
Cardiovascular	- Tachycardia* - Decreased strength of pulses - Hypotension
Renal	- Oliguria - Dark urine output - Anuria
Integumentary	- Pale - Diaphoretic - Mottled - Cold

Note: *Except in neurogenic shock.

TABLE 9.2

Differentiating Among Types of Shock

Type of Shock	Vital Signs	Physical Exam
Hypovolemic:		
■ Hemorrhagic	■ Tachycardia, hypotension	■ Pale, cool skin; weak, thready pulse; and oliguria
■ Nonhemorrhagic	■ Tachycardia, hypotension	■ Pink skin, weak, thready pulse, and oliguria
Neurogenic	■ Bradycardia, hypotension	■ Warm, dry skin; loss of sensation, muscle tone, and reflexes
Septic		
■ Early	■ Fever, tachycardia, tachypnea	■ Warm, pink, flushed skin; full bounding pulse; and decreased UOP
■ Late	■ Hypothermia, tachycardia	■ Cold, mottled, and obtunded
Cardiogenic (i.e., pump failure)	■ Tachycardia, hypotension	■ Cold, mottled skin, oliguria, elevated BNP and troponin, and ischemia on EKG 　■ RV failure: peripheral edema; hepatojugular reflux, ascites 　■ LV failure: S3, hypoxia, crackles, bibasilar crackles, PND, orthopnea, cough, hypoxia, and pink frothy sputum 　■ Biventricular failure: signs of both RV and LV failure
Anaphylactic	■ Tachycardia, hypotension	■ Pruritus, urticaria, facial or tongue/perioral edema, cough, and dyspnea
Obstructive		
■ PE/fat embolism	■ Tachycardia, hypotension	■ Elevated JVD, pulsus paradoxus
■ Cardiac tamponade	■ Tachycardia, hypotension	■ Elevated JVD, muffled or distant heart sounds, narrow pulse pressure
■ Tension pneumothorax	■ Tachycardia, hypotension	■ Elevated JVD, absent breath sounds on ipsilateral side, tracheal deviation to contralateral side

BNP, brain natriuretic peptide; JVD, jugular venous distention; LV, left ventricle; PE, pulmonary embolism; PND, paroxysmal nocturnal dyspnea; RV, right ventricle; UOP, urinary output.

FAST FACTS

Trauma patients may present with more than one type of shock concurrently or develop a different type of shock during hospitalization.

Hypovolemic shock: Most trauma patients experience hemorrhagic hypovolemic shock from bleeding. Common sites of bleeding are at the scene from external loss, especially from scalp lacerations, as the scalp is highly vascular. Other sites are the abdomen from splenic or liver lacerations, chest from hemothorax, and thighs from femur fractures. Patients may need multiple transfusions or even a massive transfusion protocol (MTP) to replace volume quickly. Whole blood is ideal because it replaces all components that are lost from bleeding. The next best option is to replace packed red blood cells (PRBCs), fresh frozen plasma, and platelets at a 1:1:1 ratio. The platelets usually are around 6 units in one "pooled" bag. The amount of IV fluids (IVF) administered should be minimized during resuscitation to reduce postresuscitation complications.

Rapid assessment to determine whether a patient is in hypovolemic shock includes measures such as the shock index (SI) or modified SI. The SI is defined as the HR divided by SBP (HR/SBP):

$$\text{Shock index} = \text{HR/SBP}$$

Example: HR 110, BP 80/60, SI = 110/80 = 1.375. Normal range is .5 to .7 in healthy adults. An SI greater than 1.1 predicts increased risk for morbidity and mortality, including need for MTP activation and/or admission to critical care units.

Alternatively, the modified shock index (MSI) is a better predictor of mortality than SI for patients in the ED, because HR and SBP are often affected by other factors in these patients. The MSI is defined as HR divided by mean MAP:

$$\text{Modified shock index} = \text{HR/MAP}$$

An MSI greater than 1.4 is a predictor of higher morbidity and mortality. For example, a patient with an HR of 110 bpm and a MAP of 50 mmHg has an MSI of 2.2 and is at greater risk of death.

Nonhemorrhagic hypovolemic shock: Trauma patients may present in a dehydrated state or develop nonhemorrhagic hypovolemic shock. Examples include patients with burn injuries or bowel injuries with third space fluids and elderly patients who become dehydrated and fall, injuring themselves. Dehydration may be caused by poor oral intake or exposure to extreme heat, or occur after strenuous exercise such as having just completed a marathon. The inflammatory process stimulates leaky capillaries. Thus, patients with burns may have third space fluids into the interstitium and thus develop hypovolemia. Additionally, patients who have intra-abdominal injuries, especially pancreatic or small bowel injuries, commonly third space large volumes of fluid. Patients who have large nasogastric tube output or are febrile, diaphoretic, or tachypneic may also become hypovolemic. Treatment of nonhemorrhagic hypovolemia includes boluses and maintenance IVF. A passive leg raise can help determine volume responsiveness by increasing venous return to the heart. An improvement in BP indicates that the patient might benefit from additional volume resuscitation.

Distributive shock: Distributive shock encompasses neurogenic, septic, and anaphylactic shock states as each develops vasodilatory effects due to their respective pathophysiology. Distributive shock states have low systemic vascular resistance, which in the absence of a pulmonary artery catheter, can be noted by a low DBP. The low DBP in the setting of a normal SBP can lower the MAP below 60 to 65 mmHg and thus cause hypoperfusion of vital organs.

Neurogenic shock: Patients in neurogenic shock are usually bradycardic and have lost part or all sensation, motor, and reflexes below the level of the injury. Hypotension is common. In trauma patients, assessment for and correction of hemorrhagic or hypovolemic shock should occur first. Vasopressor use is commonly required, and neurosurgeons may desire enhanced MAP to perfuse the tissues surrounding the injury site to prevent additional functional loss of this penumbra. MAP goals may be as high as 85 to 90 mmHg. Phenylephrine causes pure alpha stimulation to enhance peripheral vasoconstriction and can be infused peripherally. Dopamine can also be infused peripherally at low doses and has beta-2 stimulation to increase HR as well. Norepinephrine at low doses can be infused via adequate peripheral IV for a short period but may require a central venous catheter (CVC) for duration infusions.

Septic shock: Trauma patients can occasionally present due to being in septic shock, and the associated hypotension may cause syncope and thus injury. Alternatively, trauma patients who are admitted may develop septic shock if they develop pneumonia or infection due to indwelling devices such as urinary catheters, CVCs, intravenous pressure monitors, or due to the development of intra-abdominal abscesses, and so forth. Treatment in brief includes (1) obtaining cultures, (2) antibiotic administration and source control by removal of lines or drainage of abscesses, (3) administration of IVF boluses, and (4) initiation and titration of vasopressors.

Anaphylactic shock: Anaphylactic shock in trauma patients is rare but can occur if a patient has an allergic reaction to IV contrast or administration of urgent antibiotics in the trauma bay, when allergies may not immediately be known. Antibiotics are required urgently for open fractures and contaminated wounds and just before skin incision if surgery is necessary. Additionally, pain medications are commonly used in the trauma bay and throughout hospitalization; thus, allergic reactions to analgesic agents may occur as well.

Cardiogenic shock: Cardiogenic shock is primarily characterized by a low cardiac output that may result in multisystem organ failure and death. ST-elevation myocardial infarction (STEMI) causes more than 80% of all cases of cardiogenic shock. Coronary arteries may be injured during blunt chest trauma, and these injuries are the most overlooked in patients who die from trauma. Additionally, patients may experience a STEMI or syncope from arrhythmia or hypotension and injure themselves by falling or crashing a vehicle, and so forth. Patients in cardiogenic shock commonly present with hypotension that is refractory to fluid resuscitation. These patients should have an EKG and troponin level testing to identify the presence of myocardial ischemia or infarct. If a STEMI is identified, a STEMI alert should be immediately activated. Commonly, these patients require pharmacologic management and percutaneous intervention. Trauma patients with bleeding or those with traumatic brain injuries require careful consideration when anticoagulation is needed to treat the STEMI. Consultation between the attending cardiologist and traumatologist should occur to prioritize interventions and discuss anticoagulation options.

Obstructive shock: Obstructive shock occurs due to an acute obstruction of blood flow through the heart or pulmonary arteries, causing decreased cardiac output. In trauma, the most common cause of obstructive shock includes tension pneumothorax, cardiac tamponade, and pulmonary embolism. Pressure from a tension pneumothorax shifts the vena cava and other great vessels, obstructing the blood supply returning to the heart, or prevents forward blood flow through the heart. Cardiac tamponade results from fluid buildup in the pericardial space that causes compression of the heart, thus reducing BP. Other causes of obstructive shock include massive pulmonary embolism, venous thromboembolism, fat embolism, and amniotic fluid embolism, and results in an acute obstruction of blood flow from the right ventricle. Shock caused by obstruction quickly progresses to rapid cardiac deterioration, hemodynamic instability, and cardiovascular collapse. Immediate interventions to relieve the obstruction are essential to preserving the patient's life.

Ongoing Monitoring of Shock

Patients in shock require ongoing physical examination, continual reassessment of vital signs, hemodynamic monitoring, and serial laboratory data to identify clinical worsening, stabilization, or resolution of the shock. Shock resolution varies by type and cause of shock. Hemorrhagic shock, with bleeding control mechanisms and appropriate and aggressive resuscitation, resolves in a few hours, whereas septic and neurogenic shock may require a few days to resolve.

Physical exam: Frequent reassessment of physical exam findings can provide clues to whether the shock state persists or is resolving. Nurses need to monitor urine output, cap refill, skin color and temperature, diaphoresis, and neurologic status, as well as BP and vasopressor requirements. Persistent shock states may result in organ damage. The kidney is one of the first organs to be affected by shock.

Vital signs: An arterial line is commonly needed for continuous BP readings, which can provide information on volume status, specifically hypovolemia. The arterial waveform tracing is monitored for pulse pressure variations (PPVs) with respirations. If the waveform increases in amplitude during spontaneous inspiration (patients on positive pressure ventilation are monitored during exhalation), this can indicate the need for further resuscitation. As the intrathoracic pressure decreases, the thorax becomes a negative pressure, thus augmenting venous return, and enhances cardiac output. A variation greater than 10 mmHg is associated with hypovolemia.

Hemodynamic Monitoring Devices and Methods
Hemodynamic monitoring can be either static or dynamic. Static monitoring reflects a single point in time. Examples of static parameters include manual BPs, use of ultrasound to assess inferior cava collapsibility/variability, and pulmonary artery occlusive pressure. Dynamic parameter provides continuous readings during fluid resuscitation, demonstrating real-time changes during interventions. Dynamic parameters include pulse arterial line readings, PPV, stroke volume variation, central venous pressure monitoring, pulmonary artery catheters (PACs), and so forth. Dynamic parameters are superior to static parameters in that interventions can be assessed concurrently during the intervention and adjustments can be made on a real-time basis.

PACs can provide additional hemodynamic data. Classic patterns of hemodynamic data exist for the different types of shock. While PACs have fallen out of favor due to variability of data interpretation, impacts of other factors in producing results, and risk of serious complications, the concepts of the parameters (preload, afterload contractility) are still commonly referred to during bedside discussions (Box 9.1).

Laboratory Findings
Assessment of a patient in shock requires repeated laboratory data to confirm the shock is resolving. The type of testing may vary by type of shock. The results should confirm and correlate with physical exam findings and hemodynamic data. Required testing commonly includes serial complete blood counts (CBCs), arterial blood gas and lactic acid levels, mixed venous oxygen saturation (SVO2), complete metabolic panel (CMP), and coagulation studies.

Complete blood count: Initial transfusions to treat hemorrhagic shock are not dependent on lab value results; thus, one should not wait for anemia

Box 9.1 PARAMETERS DEFINED

1. Preload—The force that stretches the cardiac muscle before contraction, also known as the volume of venous filling on the right side of the heart.
2. Afterload—The pressure the heart must exert to push out blood during ventricular contraction, also known as systolic pressure.
3. Contractility—The innate ability of the heart to contract given varying preloads and afterloads.

to be present on CBC to transfuse. Once bleeding is controlled and initial resuscitation has stabilized the patient, transfusion should occur according to CBC results. In a nonbleeding patient, the transfusion criteria are a hemoglobin of less than 7.0 g/dL or, for patients with cardiac ischemia, greater than 8 g/dL. If the patient is no longer bleeding, each unit of PRBCs should increase the hemoglobin by 1 g and increase the hematocrit by 3%. Patients whose hemoglobin fails to increase with 1 g/unit PRBCs may still be bleeding and may require additional transfusions.

During the initial phase of the coagulation cascade, a platelet plug is formed to facilitate a clot. Thus, in severe trauma, the platelets may be consumed into clots and the platelet count may fall. Ideally, a 1:1:1 transfusion of RBCs to plasma to platelet transfusion is completed. However, patients who have hemorrhaged or continue to have blood loss may require additional platelet transfusions.

FAST FACTS

Initial transfusions to treat hemorrhagic shock are not dependent on lab value results; thus, one should not wait for anemia to be present on CBC to transfuse.

Arterial blood gas: Repeat arterial blood gases are useful to monitor for resolution of metabolic acidosis. Patients in shock may have a metabolic acidosis, commonly from lactic acidosis. With adequate resuscitation, the base excess should begin to normalize (normal range −2 to 0 to +2). The more negative the base excess, the worse the acidosis. Hypercarbia must be corrected to avoid concomitant respiratory acidosis; hypoxia must be corrected to maintain adequate tissue oxygenation. Hyperoxia must be avoided because it worsens atelectasis.

Mixed venous oxygen saturation: SVO2 measures the venous oxygen saturation of the blood returning to the heart. Samples should be taken from the distal port of a PAC. A sample from a CVC distal tip in the superior vena cava (referred to as SCVO2) can be used as a surrogate; however, it does not include venous return from the coronary vessels. Thus, the results are not as accurate as a true SVO2 measurement. Normal SVO2 is approximately 60% to 80%. The lower the SVO2, the more oxygen consumption is occurring at the cellular level. A high SVO2 indicates that the tissues are not extracting oxygen due to microvascular shunting, as is seen in profound shock. Conversely, a low SVO2 can also indicate a low cardiac output failing to meet oxygen demands, low hemoglobin or oxygen saturation levels, or that oxygen consumption has increased without adequate oxygen delivery.

Lactate: Elevated lactic acid levels develop when cells become hypoxic, shifting from aerobic to anaerobic metabolism, resulting in lactic acid production. Serial lactate levels should be checked every 2 to 4 hours to ensure the lactate level has normalized or "cleared" to less than 2.0 mmol/L. If the lactic acid level remains elevated, either the tissues are still in an underperfused state or a new source of lactic acid production has developed. Additionally, a history of liver dysfunction can interfere with lactic acid clearance by the liver.

Comprehensive metabolic panel: The CMP is valuable in assessing several parameters. The bicarbonate level may be low, indicating metabolic acidosis, and as it normalizes, it indicates that shock is resolving. Blood urea nitrogen (BUN) and creatinine levels signify kidney function. Normal BUN/creatinine indicates the kidney has been well perfused. Shock can cause hypoperfusion to the kidney, causing an AKI. Trauma patients commonly experience AKI, because many also receive nephrotoxic agents, including contrast for CT scans and antibiotics, which can worsen AKI. The CMP also provides information regarding the liver. Aspartate and alanine aminotransferase levels increase with both direct liver injury and hypoperfusion. Bilirubin can increase due to breakdown of transfused and extravasated blood. Calcium levels should be monitored during and after resuscitation because of significant reductions in calcium secondary to binding with citrate, which is used in blood products to prevent coagulation during storage.

Coagulation: Coagulation studies are frequently assessed in trauma patients to discern whether a coagulopathy exists. Repeat assessments of the international normalized ratio (INR) and fibrinogen, as well as thromboelastography or rotational thromboelastometry, are needed to ensure all components of the clot formation process have been restored to a normal balance. Liver dysfunction from injury or shock may result in an elevated INR, signifying that the synthetic function of the liver is reduced. Patients with severe traumatic injuries may become coagulopathic due to hypothermia or because they have consumed the available clotting factors and thus may need additional replacement of clotting factors in the form of cryoprecipitate.

Treatment of Shock
Treatment of shock is multifactorial and is determined based on the type of shock (Table 9.3).

END POINTS OF RESUSCITATION

Knowing when the patient has been resuscitated is multifaceted and includes both physical exam and laboratory findings. Physical exam findings are important. Findings include mental status that has returned to baseline, resolution of tachycardia, and warm skin that is not pale or mottled. The patient should ideally be making more than .5 mL/kg urine output per hour unless they have an AKI. Vital signs, including HR, respiratory rate, and BP, should be in the normal range. Additionally, patients with a MAP sustained above 65 mmHg should be weaned off vasopressors. Nurses and providers need to know when the patient has responded to treatment and the shock state is resolved, to prevent harm from the interventions. In other words, too much IVF or blood products may be detrimental and lead to acute lung injury or volume overload. Prolonged and high doses of vasopressors may

TABLE 9.3
Treatment of Shock

Type of Shock	Interventions/Options
Hypovolemic	
■ Hemorrhagic	■ Stop the bleeding/hemorrhage 　■ Surgically 　　● Damage control surgery for the most severe abdominal cases 　　● External fixation of pelvic fractures 　　● Rodding of femur fractures 　■ Intravascularly in interventional radiology with arterial embolization 　■ Suture/staple laceration (especially scalp lacerations) 　■ Direct pressure, pressure dressings ■ Tranexamic acid—bolus and infusion ■ Transfusion of PRBCs, FFP, platelets, and cryoprecipitate ■ Calcium gluconate (1 g for every 4 units PRBCs) ■ Reversal of anticoagulation

Anticoagulant	Reversal Options
Warfarin	■ PCC, Vitamin K, and FFP
Dabigatran (pradaxa)	■ Praxbind (idarucizumab) PCC
Apixaban (eliquis) and rivaroxaban (xarleto)	■ Andexxa (andexanet alfa) PCC
Edoxaban (savaysa)	PCC

Type of Shock	Interventions/Options
■ Nonhemorrhagic	■ IVF with lactated Ringer or normal saline
Neurogenic	■ Ensure patient is not in hemorrhagic shock ■ IVF bolus initially ■ Vasopressors
Obstructive	
■ Tension pneumothorax	■ Needle decompression ■ Follow with chest tube insertion
■ Cardiac tamponade	■ Pericardiocentesis ■ To OR for pericardial window
■ Pulmonary embolism/fat embolism	■ Anticoagulation if not contraindicated ■ Consider percutaneous thrombectomy ■ Consider open thrombectomy
Septic	■ Obtain cultures and lactic acid level ■ Start antibiotics ■ IVF bolus 30 mL/kg ■ If needed, start vasopressors (norepinephrine first line)

(continued)

TABLE 9.3 (continued)
Treatment of Shock

Type of Shock	Interventions/Options
Cardiogenic	<ul><li>Ensure patient is not having a STEMI</li><li>Bolus for RV failure, diuresis for LV failure</li><li>Vasopressors (norepinephrine first line)</li><li>Inotropic agent</li></ul>

FFP, fresh frozen plasma; IVF, IV fluids; LV, left ventricle; OR, operating room; PCC, prothrombin complex concentrate; PRBCs, packed red blood cells; RV, right ventricle; STEMI, ST-elevation myocardial infarction.

lead to organ ischemia and failure; thus, active weaning of vasopressors is an essential function of the nurse.

Laboratory markers are also important to demonstrate the resolution of shock. Stabilized hemoglobin, hematocrit, and platelet counts are important findings but must be checked to ensure they remain stable. Lactate clearance and normalized base deficit on an arterial blood gas evaluation are markers used to identify the resolution of shock. Lactate clearance may be delayed due to underlying liver dysfunction such as cirrhosis or acute liver injury, as in shock liver from hypoperfusion.

Ongoing reassessment is critical to ensure that recurrent shock does not develop. Trauma patients may have ongoing or recurrent bleeding, requiring additional transfusions or repeated doses of reversal agents, especially for patients receiving warfarin. Patients who have third spacing of fluids into tissues from the SIRS response may require repeated IVF boluses.

CARDIAC INJURIES

Blunt Cardiac Injury

Blunt cardiac injury (BCI) refers to blunt traumatic injury to the heart. Blunt trauma to the chest can cause a range of injuries, including a cardiac contusion of the myocardial muscle, disruption of a heart valve, rupture of a cardiac chamber, or coronary artery dissection. In 75% of cases, these injuries are accompanied by a sternal fracture. The most common mechanism of injury is motor vehicle crashes involving speeds over 30 miles per hour with sudden deceleration. Other mechanisms include falls, assaults, explosions, and direct force injury to the chest wall. BCI can manifest as arrhythmias and cardiac wall motion abnormalities.

Commotio cordis occurs as a significant direct impact to the anterior chest wall. It can precipitate ventricular fibrillation cardiac arrest in patients without any known structural heart problems. Commotio cordis is a rare condition but is commonly observed in young athletes struck in the anterior chest with a hard object, such as a baseball, lacrosse ball, or hockey puck.

Survival after cardiac arrest from commotio cordis is about 60%. Prompt and continuous CPR with immediate defibrillation at the scene improves survival outcomes for these patients.

Cardiac contusions are usually the result of direct blunt force trauma to the anterior chest, including the sternum and/or manubrium. Cardiac contusions are the most common type of BCI, with some patients being asymptomatic. Signs and symptoms include arrhythmia (most common), chest pain, and shortness of breath. Sinus tachycardia is the most prevalent arrhythmia, although patients may experience premature atrial contractions, premature ventricular contractions, atrial fibrillation, or right bundle branch block. Diagnostics include EKG and echocardiography. A 12-lead EKG should be done to rule out myocardial ischemia or infarction as source of chest pain. Transthoracic echocardiography should be done to inspect for valvular damage, pericardial effusion, or hypokinesis of wall motion. Cardiac enzymes, including creatine phosphokinase and troponins, are released after a cardiac injury; thus, interpretation of results is limited.

Cardiac rupture is the most lethal type of BCI. Most patients have ventricular rupture, as the atria are more compliant. Patients with atrial rupture are more likely to survive to reach the ED, whereas most patients with uncontained ventricular rupture die at the scene. When patients do survive to reach the ED, signs of cardiac rupture are similar to those of pericardial tamponade, including hypotension, distended neck veins, and muffled heart sounds. In patients with concomitant hemorrhagic shock, distended neck veins may not be obvious; thus, bedside cardiac ultrasound may demonstrate the pericardial effusion or injury. In a loud trauma bay, muffled heart sounds may be difficult to appreciate.

Other cardiac injuries include coronary artery laceration, dissection, and/or thrombosis, which may result in a myocardial infarction. The left anterior descending artery is most affected because of its anterior location on the left ventricle.

Nursing Care of Cardiac Contusions
Nurses must maintain a high index of suspicion for BCI in patients with a predisposing mechanism of injury, specifically sternal fractures. Telemetry monitoring for the first 24 hours should be implemented when BCI is suspected. Any tachycardias, arrhythmias, new chest pain, shortness of breath, hypotension, or distended neck veins should be reported to the trauma team. Transthoracic echocardiography should be anticipated. Severe cases may require vasopressor support, antiarrhythmic agents, and consultation with cardiology. The nurse should ensure the potassium level is kept above 4 mEq/L, magnesium at 2 mg/dL, and calcium in the normal range.

Penetrating Cardiac Injury

Penetrating cardiac injuries are uncommon but life-threatening. The mortality rate for penetrating cardiac injuries is approximately 40% but may vary widely depending on the specific injury. The most common mechanisms of injury in penetrating cardiac trauma are stabbings and gunshots. The right ventricle is the most affected chamber of the heart. Multichambered penetrating trauma increases mortality. Penetrating trauma to the "cardiac box," the areas of the anterior thorax bordered superiorly by the clavicles, inferiorly by the xiphoid, and laterally by the nipples, requires a high level of suspicion for penetrating cardiac injury. For the patient with penetrating thoracic trauma who loses vital signs within 10 minutes and still has signs of life (pulseless electrical activity, agonal respirations, and reactive pupils or spontaneous movement), a resuscitative thoracotomy is indicated.

Resuscitative thoracotomy is a high-anxiety, emergent situation and requires the nurses to remain calm and function appropriately. Depending on the institution and situation, it can be done in the trauma bay or operating room. Multiple staff are required and may be asked to perform several tasks, including administering transfusions, initiating the fluid warmer, accessing and opening sterile equipment for the surgical team, setting up suction, focusing operating lamps, opening sutures, setting up chest tube cannisters, and so forth.

Cardiac Tamponade

Cardiac tamponade occurs when blood or air accumulates in the pericardial sac to such an extent it compresses the heart to the point that the heart cannot fill. The effects of blood in the pericardial space impede venous return of blood and prevent ventricular filling, thus reducing cardiac output. This decreased cardiac output can quickly lead to obstructive shock and imminent death if not immediately corrected. Cardiac tamponade is most associated with penetrating chest trauma, although it may occur with severe blunt chest trauma, such as with a sternal fracture. Classically, a stab wound to the anterior left chest at the left sternal border penetrates the cardiac box, causing bleeding into the pericardial sac.

Classic signs of cardiac tamponade include tachycardia, muffled heart sounds, and JVD. Muffled heart sounds may be difficult to appreciate in a noisy trauma bay. Additionally, tamponade physiology demonstrates hypotension with a narrow pulse pressure and is usually refractory to fluid boluses. Pulse pressure is the difference between SBP and DBP.

$$Pulse\ pressure = SBP - DBP$$

The rapidity of a patient's hemodynamic decline depends on the rate of blood accumulation in the pericardial sac. Normally, about 25 mL of fluid is in the pericardial sac; however, even increments of 50 to 100 mL may have a substantial impact on intracardiac pressures, reducing the ventricular filling volume. Diagnosis of cardiac tamponade may be challenging because many critically ill trauma patients may have concomitant injuries causing simultaneous hemorrhagic shock. Thus, distended neck veins may not be visible due to hypovolemic shock. Additionally, the cervical collar must be opened to visually inspect for JVD. Bedside staff must have a high index of suspicion when patients fail to respond to fluid boluses.

> **FAST FACTS**
>
> The Beck triad comprises classic signs of cardiac tamponade: hypotension, muffled heart sounds, and JVD. JVD may be absent if the patient is also in hemorrhagic shock.

Cardiac tamponade may be difficult to differentiate from tension pneumothorax. Both have similar features of tachycardia, hypotension, and distended neck veins; however, tension pneumothorax does not have muffled heart sounds. Tension pneumothorax does have absent breath sounds on the affected side. Bedside ultrasound can easily identify cardiac tamponade and discern between tension pneumothoraces. Chest x-ray provides rapid diagnosis of tension pneumothorax.

Patients with traumatic cardiac tamponade require immediate intervention. Pericardiocentesis is viewed as a temporary intervention because the underlying source of bleeding must be contained. Pericardiocentesis is a viable option for a community hospital that doesn't have cardiothoracic surgeon availability. Surgical intervention with pericardial window or thoracotomy or sternotomy can be performed and allows direct visualization and repair of injured vessels or myocardium. A drain is commonly left in place to avoid reaccumulation of fluid in the pericardial sac.

Nursing Care of Cardiac Tamponade

Patients with cardiac tamponade require continuous assessment and hemodynamic monitoring. Cardiac monitoring, frequent BP measurements, and continuous pulse oximetry are critical. Nurses maintain adequate IV access and initiate fluid, blood, or vasopressors as needed. They also can assist in setting up for procedures such as insertion of arterial lines or central lines, or pericardiocentesis. Prompt transport for definitive surgical intervention with a succinct SBAR handoff is critical to ongoing care.

Postoperative nursing care prioritizes the maintenance of a patent pericardial drain to avoid recurrent tamponade from ongoing oozing or overt bleeding with an obstructed or clotted pericardial drain. The drain output should be recorded at least hourly. Ongoing overt bleeding must be reported to the trauma team.

> **FAST FACTS**
>
> Any injury to the "cardiac box," the areas of the anterior thorax bordered superiorly by the clavicles, inferiorly by the xiphoid, and laterally by the nipples, requires a high level of suspicion for penetrating cardiac injury.

VASCULAR INJURIES

Vascular injuries occur in the setting of blunt or penetrating trauma and may be arterial or venous in origin. These injuries may lead to hemorrhage and, conversely, can also lead to thrombosis. Common symptoms of vascular trauma include pain, visible bleeding, ecchymosis, edema, and induration. These injuries can be identified by direct visualization, palpation, ultrasonography, CT angiography (CTA), or angiography.

Arterial Injuries—Great Vessels

Aortic and pulmonary vessels: Traumatic aortic disruption is a cause of sudden death in the trauma patient. For trauma patients who have traumatic aortic dissections, immediate identification and management are essential for survival. Findings of these injuries include a chest x-ray displaying a widened mediastinum, new and sudden paralysis, BP variation between the right and left arms (under normal circumstances, the SBP should not differ by more than 12 mmHg), and diminished or absent pulses. Traumatic pulmonary artery injury is uncommon yet frequently fatal. The presenting findings may be a large hemothorax or concern for pseudoaneurysm noted on CTA of the chest. Accessing the pulmonary artery is difficult and may require a sternotomy or posterolateral thoracotomy. If there is a proximal injury, bypass may be required and thus not all institutions would be readily able to intervene. Surgical interventions are needed to address traumatic injuries to the great vessels. Endovascular repair, when possible, has become more favorable because it has been shown to improve mortality.

Arterial injury—extremity: Vascular extremity trauma can be a result of blunt, penetrating, or both forms of trauma. Vascular extremity injuries account for a small number of civilian trauma presentations but occurs at a higher frequency in the military population. Interventions that are commonly seen in the hemorrhaging vascular trauma patient include direct pressure to the site of bleeding, direct pressure on the pulse proximal to the injury, and application of a tourniquet proximal to the injury site. Further assessment of the injury will include CTA of the extremity and surgical intervention if deemed necessary by the primary team.

Venous injuries: Injuries to the superior vena cava and inferior vena cava, also known as traumatic venous injuries, are also uncommon but have an exceedingly high mortality rate. These injuries can be seen in the setting of a motor vehicle crash with acceleration-deceleration forces or penetrating trauma in the setting of a stabbing or gunshot wound. These patients may present in hypovolemic shock, and injuries are identified through direct visualization, ultrasonography, CT imaging, or angiography. Given the location of the vena cava, it is difficult to attain hemostasis without surgical repair. In the setting of extremity venous bleeding, direct pressure and tourniquet placement most often control the bleeding. This is in stark contrast to the types of noncompressible venous injuries previously discussed.

Nursing Care
Nursing care for injuries to the great vessels includes close hemodynamic monitoring and is likely to include impulse control. This treatment will include medication to ensure the HR is less than 80 bpm and the MAP is 60 to 70 mmHg. Variations in target BP and HR may vary among institutions. In the case of a patient hemorrhaging from the great vessels, the nurse can expect that blood transfusions will occur but also should note that this may be balanced with allowing permissive hypotension, as described earlier, until definitive repair can occur.

Arterial vascular injuries often require surgical intervention; thus, the nurse will be responsible for monitoring the surgical site or access point for the procedure. Nurses monitor for complications of the procedure, which may include rebleeding, limb ischemia, and/or paralysis in the case of aortic injuries. The patient is evaluated for a developing hematoma and signs of infection such as erythema, warmth, and discharge. In addition, neurologic exams are important to monitor for signs of ischemic stroke and to evaluate lower extremity function to detect spinal cord ischemia. The nurse should note any bowel movements, especially bloody bowel movements, which can indicate intestinal ischemia or an aorto-enteric fistula. Any suspicion of a complication must be reported to the team immediately.

Nursing care of the patient with an extremity arterial injury will include close hemodynamic monitoring as well as extremity monitoring. Nurses can and will hold direct pressure, pressure to pulse locations proximal to the injury, as well as apply a tourniquet at the direction of the trauma team. It is crucial that the exact time a tourniquet is placed is documented and relayed to the team. The pulse and skin exam are crucial to the treatment and management of these patients. Decreased or absentf pulse or a change in extremity color or temperature must be reported to the team immediately because it could indicate pathology and threaten the viability of the extremity.

Peripheral venous injuries are most amenable to direct pressure. However, injury to the superior or inferior vena cava carries a high mortality given the inability to apply direct pressure and is difficult to access based on the anatomic location.

SUMMARY

In summary, cardiovascular injuries may be lethal. The nurse must be prepared to assess and manage traumatic injuries to the cardiovascular system. Trends from vital signs can aid the nurse in determining patient stability, recognizing specific injuries, and predicting patient deterioration.

REVIEW QUESTIONS

1. Muffled heart sounds, JVD, and hypotension are cardinal signs of what?
   a. Hemothorax
   b. Cardiac tamponade

    c. Aortic dissection
    d. Pneumothorax
2. Auscultating at the left sternal border, fourth intercostal space, will allow the nurse to evaluate which heart valve?
    a. Mitral
    b. Tricuspid
    c. Aortic
    d. Pulmonic
3. Commotio cordis consists of
    a. Ventricular fibrillation cardiac arrest
    b. Cardiac rupture
    c. Cardiac contusion
    d. Myocardial infarction

References

American College of Surgeons: The Committee on Trauma. (2018). *ATLS: Advanced Trauma Life Support student course manual* (10th ed.). American College of Surgeons.

Criddle, L. M. (2017). *TCAR, trauma care after resuscitation: A course for nurses across the trauma spectrum*. Laurelwood Group, TCAR Education Programs.

Das, J. M., Anosike, K., & Waseem, M. (2023, January). *Permissive hypotension*. [Updated August 7, 2022]. StatPearls Publishing. https://www.ncbi.nlm.nih.gov/books/NBK558915/

Drummond, K. E., & Murphy, E. (2011). Minimally invasive cardiac output monitors. *Continuing Education in Anaesthesia Critical Care & Pain*, *12*(1), 5–10.

Haberal, M., Sakallioglu Abali, A. E., & Karakayali, H. (2010, September). Fluid management in major burn injuries. *Indian Journal of Plastic Surgery*, *43*(Suppl.), S29–S36. https://doi.org/10.4103/0970-0358.70715

Lee, R. N., Rodrigues, T. S., Gan, J. T., Han, H. C., Mansour, R., Sanders, P., Farouque, O., & Lim, H. S. (2023). Commotio cordis in non-sport-related events: A systematic review. *JACC: Clinical Electrophysiology*, *2023*, 1321–1329.

Maron, B. J., Haas, T. S., Ahluwalia, A., Garberich, R. F., Estes, N. M., III., & Link, M. S. (2013). Increasing survival rate from commotio cordis. *Heart Rhythm*, *10*(2), 219–223.

McQuillan, K. A., & Flynn-Makic, M. B. (2020). *Trauma nursing: From resuscitation through rehabilitation* (5th ed.). Elsevier.

Murphy, P. B., Severance, S., Holler, E., Menard, L., Savage, S., & Zarzaur, B. L. (2021). Treatment of asymptomatic blunt cerebrovascular injury (BCVI): A systematic review. *Trauma Surgery and Acute Care Open*, *6*, e000668. https://doi.org/10.1136/tsaco-2020-000668

Nair, L., Winkle, B., & Senanayake, E. (2023). Managing blunt cardiac injury. *Journal of Cardiothoracic Surgery*, *18*(1), 71.

Nasser, K., Matsuura, J., & Diep, J. (2021, February). Blunt chest trauma causing a displaced sternal fracture and ST-elevation myocardial infarction: A case report. *Clinical Practice and Cases in Emergency Medicine*, *5*(1), 85–88. https://doi.org/10.5811/cpcem.2020.12.49875

Nguyen, L. S., & Squara, P. (2017, November 20). Non-invasive monitoring of cardiac output in critical care medicine. *Frontiers in Medicine (Lausanne)*, *4*, 200. https://doi.org/10.3389/fmed.2017.00200

Okorare, O., Alugba, G., Olusiji, S., Evbayekha, E. O., Antia, A. U., Daniel, E., Ubokudum, D., Adabale, O. K., & Ariaga, A. C. (2023). Sudden cardiac death: An update on commotio cordis. *Cureus, 15*(4), e38087.

Pendleton, A. C., & Leichtle, S. W. (2022). Cardiac tamponade from blunt trauma. *The American Surgeon, 88*(6), 1319–1321. https://doi.org/10.1177/0003134820942170

Rooke, D. A., Burke, C. R., Bulger, E. M., Van Eaton, E., & Nandate, K. (2021, September 10). Traumatic suprahepatic inferior vena cava injury survival of a rare case. *Trauma Case Reports, 36*, 100535. https://doi.org/10.1016/j.tcr.2021.100535. Erratum in: Trauma Case Rep. 2023 February 17; 45: 100799.

Vahdatpour, C., Collins, D., & Goldberg, S. (2019). Cardiogenic shock. *Journal of the American Heart Association, 8*(8), e011991.

10

Pulmonary Injuries and Care
Alexander Menard

> The pulmonary system is complex and requires nurses to possess refined assessment skills to suspect traumatic injuries to the pulmonary system and recognize the need for early interventions. Nurses must be familiar with key concepts of airway management and strategies to support and ensure adequate ventilation.

In this chapter, you will learn to:
1. Identify key elements of a pulmonary exam.
2. Recognize injuries to the pulmonary system.
3. Articulate nursing interventions to manage pulmonary injuries.
4. Discuss nursing care of the patient with a chest tube.
5. Discuss complications of traumatic pulmonary injuries.

INTRODUCTION

All trauma nurses must be familiar with common pulmonary and chest injuries and their associated treatments as well as monitoring for complications. Nurses need to have the ability to recognize normal and abnormal findings in order to care for trauma patients who have injuries to the pulmonary system. The highest priority in caring for trauma patients is to continually assess airway patency and ensure adequate oxygenation and ventilation. This requires the nurse to possess astute assessment skills.

PULMONARY EXAM

The most important part of the initial evaluation of a trauma patient is an assessment of the airway. The first question that must be asked is, Does the patient have a secure airway? Additionally, the patient must be able to protect their airway. Altered mental status, secretions, blood, and vomiting can impair the airway. The nurse must be able to recognize signs of impending airway compromise and respiratory failure. Stridor and hoarseness are signs of critical airway narrowing that require immediate treatment. Signs of impending respiratory failure include stridor, tachypnea, accessory muscle use, nasal flaring, retractions of the sternocleidomastoid muscles, inability to lie flat, and tripod positioning. Shallow respirations and decreased level of consciousness can occur in hypercarbia or late in hypoxia. Cyanosis is a late finding. These signs require the nurse to report these findings to the primary team while simultaneously implementing nurse-led interventions to manage the impeding airway compromise. Examples of nurse-led intervention include oral suctioning, elevating the head of bed (if the spine is stable), encouraging incentive spirometer (IS) use or positive expiratory pressure (PEP) therapy, and initiating bag mask ventilation if there is no contraindication, such as facial fractures. When the thoracic or lumbar spine is injured and the patient must lie flat, the patient should be placed in reverse Trendelenburg position. The physical exam of the pulmonary system follows the standard approach of inspection, auscultation, and palpation.

Inspect

Observe the patient's general appearance, including color of the face and lips, noting if they are pale or flushed or diaphoretic. Assess respiration rate and depth and look for any use of accessory muscles as well as the ability to speak in full sentences. These signs can indicate increased work of breathing and/or respiratory distress or failure. Observe for paradoxical chest wall movements that can indicate a flail section. With paradoxical respirations, the abdomen moves paradoxically to the chest wall, indicating respiratory distress. Stand at the foot of the bed if you are able. Does the patient have equal chest rise and fall? If not, it could indicate an emergent pathology that needs intervention, such as a pneumothorax or flail section.

Assess the pulse oximeter reading and waveform. Ensure an adequate waveform to ensure the monitor reading is accurate. Is the patient on supplemental oxygen (nasal canula, noninvasive or invasive ventilation)? Once the spine is cleared and the patient can sit upright, observe the position of the patient. Is the patient able to sit upright versus the tripod position? Tripod positioning often indicates dyspnea.

Auscultate

First, listen to the patient's breathing without a stethoscope. Determine whether there is an audible wheeze, stridor, or other adventitious sounds before applying the stethoscope. Then, auscultate using the stethoscope to the upper airway (neck) followed by the anterior and posterior chest for adventitious breath sounds (Table 10.1). Using the diaphragm, auscultate the lungs starting in the apices, moving downward, comparing each lung level to each other. Avoid auscultating over the scapula.

Palpate

Palpation provides critical information to the nurse and trauma team. Tenderness with palpation can indicate underlying injury, such as a fractured rib or chest wall contusion. Subcutaneous emphysema (crepitus) is an indication of air in the subcutaneous space, which may be present with a pneumothorax. Paradoxical movement of the chest wall represents a flail chest.

TABLE 10.1

Types of Breath Sounds and What They Might Represent

Type	Findings	Possibly Representing
Breath Sounds		
Vesicular	Normal breath sounds	Normal
Wheezes	High-pitched, continuous sounds	Asthma, COPD
Rhonchi	Low-pitched, continuous musical sounds within the large and medium airways	Bronchitis, pneumonia
Crackles (rales)	Faint popping sounds caused by air passing through accumulated fluid within small and medium airways	CHF, infection
Stridor	Loud, high-pitched sound on inspiration produced by upper respiratory tract	Upper airway obstruction from edema or foreign body
Absent	No noise appreciated	Pneumothorax, right stem intubation
Other Chest Sounds		
Pleural rub	Described as "grating" or "creaky"	Pneumonia, pulmonary embolism, pleurisy (pleuritis)

CHF, congestive heart failure; COPD, chronic obstructive pulmonary disease.

Percussion

Percuss following the same areas as auscultation, avoiding ribs and other bony structures. Percussion can determine the size and borders of organs as well as the presence or absence of air, fluid, or solid structure. See Table 10.2 for a description of common sounds.

FAST FACTS

Stridor indicates airway narrowing and is a sign of an impending airway emergency. Stridor requires the nurse to immediately notify the trauma providers and respiratory therapists for urgent interventions. Racemic epinephrine nebulizer is commonly a first step. Intubation may be required.

TRAUMATIC PULMONARY INJURIES

Pulmonary system injuries can include specific injuries to the lung parenchyma or to the thoracic cage, which includes ribs, sternum, and scapula.

TABLE 10.2
Percussion Sounds

Sound	Description	Findings
Dullness	A quiet thug	Represents presence of fluid, such as a hemothorax or pleural effusion, in the chest cavity
Resonance (normal)	Low-pitched sound, hollow in terms of sound quality with moderate duration	Represents air-filled lungs
Tympany	High-pitched sound, longer in duration compared with resonance	Represents extra air, such as occurs with a pneumothorax or over the stomach or bowels

Trauma patients may experience specific pathology within the lungs, such as aspiration, lung contusion and/or laceration, pneumothorax, or hemothorax. Injuries to the thoracic cage include fractures such as rib fractures and can impair chest wall stability, as in the setting of flail segment. Other injuries that can occur to other structures within the chest include injury to the bronchus, esophagus, or diaphragm. Additionally, severely injured patients can experience sequelae from their injuries, including hemodynamic instability and pneumonia or acute respiratory distress syndrome.

FAST FACTS

Flail segment is defined as two or more contiguous ribs that are fractured in two or more places.

Pulmonary Parenchymal Injuries

Pneumothorax: A pneumothorax is a collection of air outside the lung but still within the pleural cavity and may result in a partial or complete collapse of the lung. A pneumothorax can be identified with radiographic imaging such as a chest x-ray (CXR) or CT scan or by using ultrasound. Several exam findings can indicate a pneumothorax, including diminished or absent breath sounds or unequal breath sounds. Tympany may be identified when percussing over the pneumothorax. Management of the pneumothorax depends on the size and overall condition of the patient. A small pneumothorax may be conservatively managed without intervention and with close monitoring for spontaneous resolution. Repeat CXR should be done in a few hours to monitor for expansion. When intervention is needed, the standard management includes tube thoracostomy, also known as a chest tube placement. A pigtail catheter can be used in the absence of hemothorax.

Open pneumothorax: Open pneumothorax occurs when air accumulates in the pleural cavity as a result of a hole between the pleural space and the external chest wall. With each breath the patient takes, negative pressure is generated and more air will be sucked from the atmosphere into the pleural space. This increases pressure, compressing the lung. Immediate treatment includes an occlusive dressing taped closed on three sides to prevent air from entering the chest with inhalation while permitting air to leave the chest with exhalation. Ultimate treatment requires a tube thoracostomy and surgical repair of the chest wall defect.

Tension pneumothorax: A tension pneumothorax has all the features of a pneumothorax with the effect of the trapped air compressing surrounding structures and shifting the heart and great vessel to the contralateral side. This compression can cause reduced blood return to the heart, resulting in tachycardia and hypotension. Without quick identification and intervention, tension pneumothorax can lead to obstructive shock. Findings consistent with a tension pneumothorax include chest dissymmetry, respiratory distress, agitation, hypoxia, tachycardia, and hypotension. Tracheal deviation and jugular venous distention can be seen, but these are late findings. Tension pneumothorax is a medical emergency and requires prompt intervention to relieve the pressure in the pleural space. Decompression of the tension pneumothorax can be achieved by either needle decompression or tube thoracotomy.

Hemothorax: A hemothorax is the accumulation of blood in the pleural space. It is the result of damage to intercostal vessels, lung parenchyma, mammary arteries, and great vessels of the heart. Clinical findings of a hemothorax are broad and have overlap with those of a pneumothorax, including decreased breath sounds on the affected side. Dullness will be noted with percussion. Additionally, a hemothorax can be detected with the use of CXR, CT scan, and/or ultrasound. Management of the hemothorax is also dependent on size. A chest tube will drain the blood from the pleural space.

Chest tubes: Chest tubes are commonly required in trauma patients who have thoracic injuries. In this setting, chest tubes are placed to remove air or fluid (blood) from the pleural space to allow the lung to reexpand. The nurse must have a good understanding of how chest tubes work. The main goal of a chest tube is to facilitate the lung expansion to its full capacity. A chest tube allows this to occur by draining air or fluid from the pleural space. Initially when a chest tube is placed, it will be placed to suction. See Figure 10.1 for a review of dry suction chest tube components. Chest tube assessment and management are discussed in the nursing care section below.

Nursing Care
Care of the patient with a chest tube requires astute assessment and attention to detail. The nurse plays a key role in preparing for setup, maintenance of the tube, and prevention of complications.

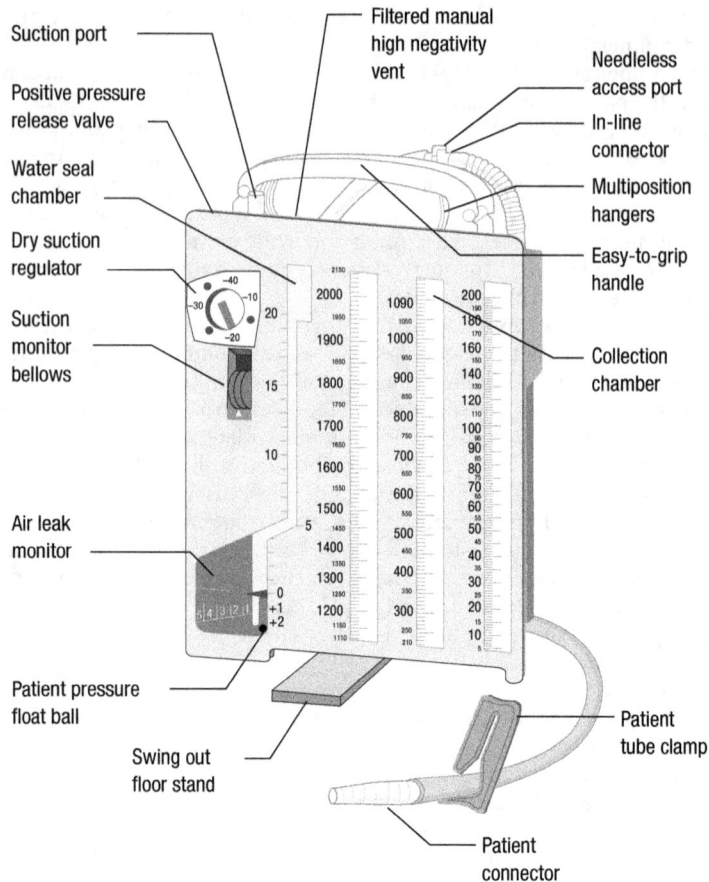

Figure 10.1 Dry suction chest tube system.

Source: https://commons.wikimedia.org/wiki/File:Labelled_chest_tube_drainage_system.png

To prepare for the chest tube setup, the nurse assembles the required equipment. Equipment varies depending on whether a pigtail catheter or tube thoracostomy is being placed. Pigtail catheters typically have a disposable tray with the catheter included, whereas the thoracostomy tube is separate from the chest tube insertion tray. The insertion tray has a variety of sterile supplies, including scalpel, scalpel blades, scissors, clamps, and so forth. Extra supplies, such as sutures and dressings, may be required and if not included in the sterile tray, should be kept close to the tray or attached to the outside. A variety of tube sizes should be available.

The nurse is responsible for setting up the chest tube drainage system and suction canister. When opening the drainage system, the nurse makes sure to keep the connector and tubing sterile when placed on the sterile drapes. Drainage systems vary by type. Typically, they all have a water seal chamber that requires instillation of water to monitor for air leak. Some types require additional water in a separate chamber to establish the centimeters of suction, whereas dry canisters have a dial to set the level of suction. Most commonly −20 cm of suction is used for trauma patients.

The nurse can assist with positioning the patient. For a pigtail catheter insertion, an anterior approach is common. The patient should be positioned on their back with the head of the bed up 30 degrees. For a tube thoracostomy, the patient should be on their back and have their arm raised over their head, if their injuries allow.

The nurse is responsible for accessing and administering prescribed medications (pain, sedative, and anxiolytic) during the placement of the tube; therefore, the nurse should request the providers' preferred medications beforehand. The provider inserting the tube will administer any local analgesic, whereas the nurse will be required to administer any analgesics or sedatives. Conscious sedation monitoring is required during and after the administration of these medications.

Once the chest tube is placed, monitoring the patient and the tube is a high priority for the nurse. Findings with a chest tube that need to be reported to the team include a new air leak and excessive output. An air leak can be identified in the water seal chamber; at the bottom of the chamber is an air leak monitor. An air leak indicates that there is air getting into the system. This air can come through the patient and indicates that the pleural injury has not healed yet. An air leak can also be present when air enters the system at any point from the patient's skin, through the chest tube to the connections or tubing. The nurse can determine if the air leak is coming from the patient or from a part of the system outside the patient's body. This can be determined by momentarily clamping the chest tube at the insertion site. If the air leak stops, the leak originates from the patient, if it does not stop, and then the leak is coming from the system. Nurses should never leave a chest tube clamped unless they have explicit instructions and a written order from the medical team. Unexpected clamping of a chest tube can cause accumulation of air and may lead to tension physiology (hypotension, tachycardia, and hypoxia) which is a medical emergency.

FAST FACTS

Nurses should never leave a chest tube clamped unless they have explicit instructions and a written order from the medical team.

When a chest tube is placed for management of a hemothorax, there are key features that the nurse must assess. These include the color, quantity, and consistency of the fluid being drained. The nurse should alert the medical team when the initial output with placement exceeds 1 to 1.5 L.

After the initial placement, an hourly bloody output of 150 to 200 mL/h for two to four consecutive hours must be reported to the medical team. Both instances indicate significant bleeding that may require surgical intervention for control. Transfusions are likely to be required.

FAST FACTS

An initial chest tube output of 1 to 1.5 L or an hourly output of 150 to 200 mL/h for two consecutive hours must be reported to the medical team.

Pulmonary contusion: A pulmonary contusion, bruising of the lung parenchyma, can impair gas exchange. The impaired gas exchange is due to torn capillaries causing blood in the lung parenchyma and/or alveolar edema, making it difficult for oxygen to move from the alveoli into the capillaries. Pulmonary contusions may exist on presentation but also can evolve over 24 to 72 hours after the initial insult. Exam findings of contusions include decreased breath sounds over the contusion, dullness to percussion, hypoxia, and shortness of breath. Hemoptysis may be noted with severe pulmonary contusions.

Nursing Care

Nursing care for the patient with a pulmonary contusion includes pulmonary hygiene and mobility. Pulmonary hygiene includes use of incentive spirometry, PEP therapy, chest physiotherapy, coughing, and deep breathing. The nurse must be aware that the pulmonary contusion can worsen or "blossom" over the course of 24 to 72 hours after the initial insult. Supplemental oxygen may be required. For severe cases, noninvasive ventilation or intubation and mechanical ventilation may be needed. The nurse should not increase oxygen without first performing pulmonary hygiene measures. If the patient requires increases in oxygen, the trauma providers must be notified to reassess the patient. The nurse must make sure patient has adequate pain control to facilitate pulmonary hygiene measures to be effective.

Pulmonary laceration: Pulmonary lacerations may result from blunt or penetrating injuries, pleural or lung perforation secondary to rib fractures, or inertial decelerations. Pulmonary lacerations result in the disruption of the alveolar walls and the tearing of pulmonary parenchyma. In most cases, pulmonary lacerations heal quickly but do require the use of a chest tube. If this is not the case or if there is ongoing or massive hemorrhage, surgical intervention may be required.

Nursing Care

Care of the patient with a pulmonary laceration is similar to that of a patient with a pneumothorax or hemothorax. Careful monitoring of the chest tube output and vital signs is needed to identify early signs of shock.

> **FAST FACTS**
>
> A chest tube should never be clamped unless an explicit order is written by the medical team. If a chest tube is clamped and the patient develops shortness of breath or respiratory distress, the tube must be immediately unclamped and suction returned.

THORACIC CAGE

Fractures

The thoracic cage is the osseocartilaginous structure that encloses the thorax and includes 12 pairs of ribs, the sternum, manubrium, and scapula. Ribs are the most commonly injured part of the thoracic cage. The sternum and scapula provide an additional layer of protection. A significant amount of force is required to fracture the first or second rib, sternum, or scapula. These injuries prompt the team to be highly suspicious of additional injuries to the head, neck, spinal cord, lungs, and great vessels. Fractures to the ribs, sternum, and scapula can be identified with chest x-ray; however, CT scans provide more detail and specificity.

Rib fractures: Of the 12 pairs of ribs, the first seven are attached anteriorly to the sternum and posteriorly to the spine. Ribs 8 to 10 attach similarly but connect to the costal cartilage of the sternum in the front. Ribs 11 and 12 only attach posteriorly to the spine. The main purpose of the ribs is to protect the organs underneath, including the heart, lungs, kidneys, spleen, and liver. Rib fractures are exquisitely painful. Even one rib fracture can lead to impaired respiration, ventilation, and oxygenation due to acute pain causing reduced lung expansion. Impaired respiration can occur immediately or be delayed over the course of hours to days as atelectasis worsens. Impaired ventilation can be identified by an arterial blood gas (ABG) analysis or monitoring capnography. It can also be qualitativly assessed by looking at respiration rate and depth, as well as the overall work of breathing, including accessory muscle use.

Flail segment: Flail chest is defined as two or more contiguous fractured ribs in two or more places. It is characterized by paradoxical movement of that segment of the chest during inspiration and expiration (Figure 10.2). This commonly leads to impaired ventilation, which usually requires respiratory support with noninvasive ventilation or intubation and mechanical ventilation.

> **FAST FACTS**
>
> Flail chest is defined as two or more adjacent ribs fractured in two or more places.

Sternal fracture: The sternum requires significant force to cause a fracture. Sternal fractures are most commonly a result of blunt, anterior chest

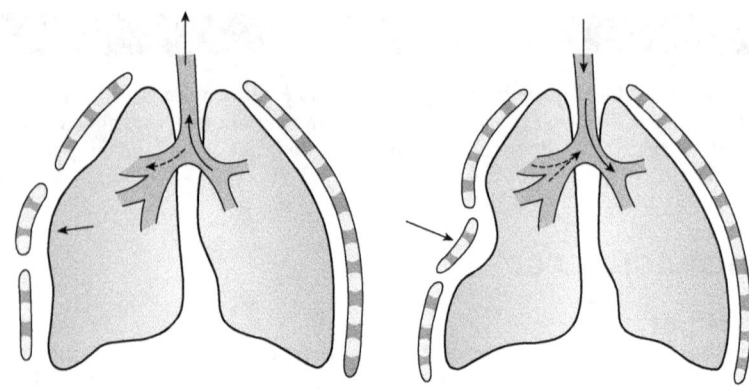

Figure 10.2 Paradoxical breathing.
Source: https://commons.wikimedia.org/wiki/File:Paradoxical-breathing.png

wall trauma and deceleration injuries, such as occurs in high-speed motor vehicle accidents. The sternum overlays and protects the lungs, heart, and great vessels; thus, pulmonary contusions and blunt cardiac injury may result from such an injury. Fractures of the manubrium, the most superior portion of the sternum, are associated with severe concomitant injuries to underlying organs. A 12-lead EKG, troponin test, and echocardiogram are indicated to evaluate for blunt cardiac injury (see Chapter 9) and to rule out cardiac chest pain. Operative repair of sternal fractures is rarely indicated. The most common symptom of sternal fracture is point tenderness at the site of fracture.

Scapula fracture: Scapula fractures are uncommon, but when present, are often associated with high-energy trauma. Most scapula fractures are managed without surgical intervention and with immobilization in a sling and swath.

Nursing Care
Nursing care for the patient with rib fractures includes aggressive pain management to facilitate pulmonary hygiene and early and frequent mobility. Multimodal pain regimens are the standard of care. These regimens commonly include scheduled acetaminophen, lidocaine patches for local pain control, muscle relaxers such as methocarbamol (Robaxin) or cyclobenzaprine (Flexeril), and as-needed opioids such as oxycodone or hydrocodone. Other pain treatment adjuncts include nonsteroidal anti-inflammatory drugs (NSAIDs) such as ketorolac (Toradol) or ibuprofen. NSAIDs are contraindicated in patients with chronic kidney disease or acute kidney injury because they can worsen renal function. NSAIDs can also worsen bleeding and thus have limited use during the initial trauma resuscitation but can be helpful after bleeding has ceased. Gabapentin (Neurontin) is useful to treat

nerve pain. Nerve blocks and epidural catheter infusions play a role when other agents fail. Additionally, ketamine bolus and infusions are useful for treatment of severe pain, although may require a higher level of monitoring in an intermediate care unit or ICU, depending on hospital policy.

The oral route for narcotics is preferred because it provides for longer pain control and should be administered first. Intravenous agents should be second-line agents. If the gastrointestinal tract is not functioning, a patient-controlled analgesic is helpful, so the patient doesn't need to wait for the nurse to bring a dose. Ongoing reassessment of pain is crucial in the management and care of the patient with rib fractures.

The most severe complications that can result from rib fractures are atelectasis and pneumonia, which occur from ineffective ventilation due to lack of pain control. Appropriate pain control, mobility, and pulmonary hygiene have the largest impact on reducing these complications. Pulmonary hygiene can be achieved with the use of an IS. Frequent use of the IS while the patient is hospitalized is imperative. The nurse is responsible for teaching proper use of the IS as well as encouraging patients to use it hourly. Engaging families to encourage the patient to perform IS helps the family feel they are doing something to help the patient's recovery. Documenting how the patient is doing with the IS is important. A downtrend in documented volume indicates poor ventilation or pulmonary mechanics and warrants further intervention. Noninvasive ventilation with continuous positive airway pressure (CPAP) or bilevel positive airway pressure (BiPAP) may be needed to avoid intubation.

Other Thoracic Injuries

Traumatic diaphragmatic injury: Traumatic diaphragmatic injuries can occur with both blunt and penetrating trauma and are often difficult to identify. It is more common to diagnose diaphragmatic injuries on the left side given anatomic structures as the liver spans along the right diaphragm. This type of injury is uncommon, but if the injury is not identified, it carries a significant increase in morbidity and mortality. Diaphragmatic injuries commonly require repair to prevent herniation of abdominal contents into the chest.

Esophageal perforation: Esophageal perforation is a rare injury; however, it is more common with penetrating injuries than blunt force trauma. Perforation results in transmural disruption of the esophagus and allows contents of the esophagus to leak into the mediastinum. This is a surgical emergency. The result of esophageal contents leaking into the mediastinum is local inflammation and if not corrected, can cause systemic inflammation, resulting in sepsis or septic shock. Many esophageal injuries can be detected on CT scan. Esophagram or contrast-enhanced imaging can also be useful in the diagnosis; however, flexible esophagoscopy is nearly 100% sensitive in the setting of penetrating trauma. There are several methods for management, including nonoperative management, which is an option for patients with a contained leak who are hemodynamically stable. Operative interventions range from primary repair, esophageal diversion, and exclusion, to esophagectomy.

Nursing Care
Initial care for the patient with an esophageal perforation includes close monitoring in the ICU to monitor for mediastinitis and sepsis. Patients will be unable to eat, and thus will most likely require parenteral nutrition versus jejunostomy feeding. These patients will maintain strict nothing by mouth (NPO) status. Depending on the management plan, operative versus nonoperative, the patient might have a chest tube in place and possibly a Jackson–Pratt (JP) bulb drain to suction near the surgical repair site as well. Careful monitoring and documentation of the drain output are important in the care of these patients.

Oxygenation and Ventilation

Oxygenation and ventilation are two separate measurements but are interdependent physiologic processes that reveal how the pulmonary system is working. Oxygenation is the physiologic process involving absorption of oxygen across the alveolar capillary membranes into the bloodstream, whereas ventilation is the movement of air in and out of the lungs.

Arterial Blood Gas Interpretation
An ABG test can provide insight into how well a patient is oxygenating and ventilating. The typical sequence of the ABG values is as follows:

$$[pH/PaCO_2/PaO_2/HCO_3/SaO_2/\text{base excess/deficit}]$$

Definitions of these values and normal ranges are listed in Table 10.3.

ABG Interpretation
To assess ventilation, the $PaCO_2$ is evaluated, and to assess oxygenation, the PaO_2 and SaO_2 are evaluated. Carbon dioxide is an acid and affects the pH of blood. Too much CO_2 results in hypercarbia and lower pH, whereas too little CO_2 results in hypocarbia with a high arterial blood pH (alkalosis).

Step 1. Evaluate the pH—Is the patient acidemic (pH <7.38) or alkalotic (pH >7.42)?

TABLE 10.3

AGB Values and Normal Ranges

Value	Representation—In Arterial Blood	Normal Range
pH	Acid-base level in the blood	7.35 to 7.45
$PaCO_2$	Partial pressure of carbon dioxide	35 to 45 mmHg
PaO_2	Partial pressure of oxygen	75 to 100 mmHg
HCO_3	Calculated concentration of bicarbonate	22 to 26 mEq/L
SaO_2	Calculated arterial oxygen saturation	95% to 100%
Base excess/deficit	Calculated relative excess/deficit of base	−2 to +2

AGB, arterial blood gas.

Step 2. Evaluate the PCO_2 and HCO_3

- If the pH is acidemic and the PCO_2 is greater than 45 mmHg, then it is a respiratory acidosis.
- If the pH is acidemic and the HCO_3 is less than 22 mEq/L, then it is a metabolic acidosis.
- If the pH is alkalotic and the PCO_2 is less than 35 mmHg, then it is a respiratory alkalosis.
- If the pH is alkalotic and the HCO_3 is greater than 26 mEq/L, then it is a metabolic alkalosis.

Oxygen Delivery Options

Trauma patients may require supplemental oxygen due to hypoxia from their injuries. Room air is composed of 21% oxygen and 78% nitrogen. The other 1% is composed of carbon dioxide and other gases. Nitrogen keeps the alveoli open and distended and prevents atelectasis. If supplemental oxygen is provided, nitrogen is displaced from the alveoli and can cause worsening atelectasis. Thus, unless the patient is hypoxic (oxygen saturation <92% for healthy individuals), supplemental oxygen should be avoided. For patients with chronic obstructive pulmonary disease, an acceptable oxygen saturation is 88% to 92%. Oxygen should not be increased without first having the patient perform pulmonary hygiene maneuvers (IS, PEP, cough, and deep breaths). Nurses should wean the oxygen down to room air as the patient stabilizes.

When the patient is truly hypoxic, oxygen should be applied. The goal fraction of inspired oxygen (FiO_2) is the minimum required to achieve 92%; for ventilated patients with severe chest injuries, the goal is to achieve ≤50% FiO_2 before weaning off positive end-expiratory pressure (PEEP).

FAST FACTS

Supplemental oxygen displaces nitrogen in the alveoli, thus worsening atelectasis. Aggressively wean oxygen to minimize atelectasis. Encourage the patient to perform pulmonary hygiene measures prior to increasing oxygen. If the patient has persistent hypoxia, requiring increased oxygen, contact the trauma provider to consider noninvasive measures.

Oxygen delivery options range from nasal cannula to a non-rebreather to high-flow nasal cannula (Table 10.4).

Noninvasive Positive Pressure Ventilation

Noninvasive positive pressure ventilation includes CPAP and BiPAP. CPAP provides the same pressure on inspiration and expiration and is used to treat hypoxia. BiPAP provides extra pressure to augment inspiration and thus promotes greater tidal volumes (TVs) and promotes oxygenation. CPAP and BiPAP can be administered via nasal pillows, nasal mask, or

TABLE 10.4

Oxygen Delivery Options

Oxygen Delivery Method	Flow Rate; Percent FiO_2
Nasal cannula	1 L/min; ~24%
	2 L/min; ~28%
	3 L/min; ~32%
	4 L/min; ~36%
	5 L/min; ~40%
	6 L/min; ~44%
Simple face mask	6 to 10 L/min; ~35% to 60%
Non-rebreather	15 L/min; ~65% to 95%
Venturi mask	2 to 4 L/min; ~24%
	4 to 6 L/min; ~28%
	6 to 8 L/min; ~31%
	8 to 10 L/min; ~35%
	10 to 12 L/min; ~40%
	12 to 15 L/min; ~55% to 60%
High-flow nasal cannula	30 to 60 L/min; 21% to 100%

FiO_2, fraction of inspired oxygen.

full-face mask. The basic settings for nurses to document for CPAP are the FiO_2 and pressure. For BiPAP, the three basic settings include the FiO_2, inspiratory positive airway pressure and expiratory positive airway pressure. Contraindications for positive airway pressure in trauma patients include facial fractures, oral or pulmonary secretions or bleeding, inability to remove the mask if the patient vomits, and impaired mentation with inability to protect the airway. Patients with a Glasgow Coma Scale score of 8 or less should be intubated.

Nursing Care

Whenever a patient is on supplemental oxygen or noninvasive positive pressure ventilation (NIPPV), it is crucial that the nurse perform a detailed pulmonary exam, continuously encourage the patient to perform incentive spirometry, and actively mobilize the patient. Patients on NIPPV should not be restrained so that they can remove the mask if they need to vomit. The nurse should ensure that the patient has adequate pain control to perform incentive spirometry. Mobilization should be encouraged and facilitated. There is no need to wait for physical therapists to get patients out of bed.

Patients should be out of bed as much as possible and progress to walking as other injuries allow. Intubated patients in the ICU can be mobilized as well as long as injuries have been stabilized.

Document the IS results and amount of oxygen the patient is receiving. Report declining IS and oxygen saturations as well as need for increased oxygen to the trauma provider team. These patterns are important because these changes represent worsening pathology that needs further interventions. The first assessment that must be made when a patient's oxygen need is increasing is to ensure the pulse oximeter is functioning properly and to determine whether it needs repositioning.

Patients on NIPPV require frequent reassessment to ensure they maintain the ability to remove their mask if they need to vomit. Additionally, nurses need to monitor the nose and face for the development of pressure injuries, which can occur with any form of oxygen delivery system or NIPPV. Protective coverings such as hydrocolloids, transparent film, and silicone should be used on the high-contact pressure areas to prevent skin breakdown and prevent small air leaks.

Airway Management

Airway management is a critical component for all trauma patients. Airway assessment and management are the very first steps during the primary survey. Any change in the patient's condition requires reassessment of the patient's airway. Interventions should be in accordance with the Advanced Trauma Life Support (ATLS) guidelines, which are covered extensively in Chapter 4.

Airway Obstruction

Nurses must be able to identify airway obstruction and/or impending airway obstruction. Airway obstruction must be identified quickly so that an intervention to relieve or bypass the obstruction can be pursued. Airway obstruction can occur suddenly or gradually. Signs of airway obstruction are evidenced by hoarseness; stridor; and an acute inability to manage oral secretions, speak, or ventilate. Patients can compensate until the obstruction becomes severe enough to significantly impair ventilation and, finally, oxygenation. Patients with impending airway obstruction **require immediate intervention**. Treatment options, depending on etiology, may include suction, racemic epinephrine nebulizer, NIPPV, blended helium and oxygen (heliox) via mask, IV steroids, intubation, tracheostomy, or cricothyrotomy.

Intubation

Trauma patients may require intubation for a variety of reasons (Box 10.1). An airway cart should be immediately available in the trauma bay and ICU. This cart should be checked every shift to ensure all equipment is available and functioning.

> **Box 10.1 INDICATIONS FOR INTUBATION**
>
> - Airway injury/compromise
> - Inability to protect the airway against aspiration of oral or pulmonary secretions and vomiting
> - Inability of the patient to maintain a patent airway
> - Reduced level of consciousness (GSC ≤8)
> - Failure to ventilate/severe hypercarbia
> - Failure to oxygenate/severe hypoxia
> - To facilitate a surgical intervention
> - Anticipation of a deteriorating clinical course

Intubation is a high-risk situation, requiring a skilled team, closed-loop communication, and appropriate resources readily available at the bedside. Nursing and respiratory therapy share responsibilities for setting up the room and equipment. Preparedness includes ensuring suction is available and working, including the canister, tubing, and yankauer. It is important to ensure that the Ambu bag is readily available and connected to oxygen. The intubation tray or cart should be checked regularly and include various sizes of direct laryngoscopy blades; tubes; lubricant; and a high-resolution video laryngoscopy system such as a GlideScope, which should be readily available. Other special equipment may be needed for difficult airways, including a fiberoptic bronchoscope, bougie, and tube exchangers. Many institutions include these devices on a high-risk airway cart. Commonly, trach trays and/or percutaneous cricothyrotomy trays are kept in these carts. These are commonly required for patients who cannot be intubated due to severe facial trauma, an injured larynx, or other neck injuries.

Other tasks nurses may need to perform to secure an airway include assisting with proper patient positioning. The nurse may be responsible for administering medications and monitoring oxygen saturations, heart rhythm, and blood pressure during and following the procedure. Anticipate the patient may become hypotensive during or after intubation. Ensure the IV is patent, and have a bolus of IVF and connected to the patient's IV. Vasopressors and tubing should be immediately available at the patient's bedside.

Once the endotracheal tube (ETT) is inserted, confirm placement with end tidal CO_2, bilateral breath sounds, bilateral chest rise and a chest radiograph must be obtained. Listen for absence of air in the epigastric region. Observe for improving and stabilizing oxygenation on saturation. Document tube position at the teeth and initial ventilator settings. Ensure the tube is secured properly. Initiate ongoing analgesics and sedation to ensure the patient doesn't experience cognitive awareness and pain while still paralyzed.

Ventilator Management

Initial ventilator settings are provided by the providers and adjusted based on ABG results. Most trauma patients initially require full support of volume control continuous mandatory ventilation.

Providers select the settings, including TV, respiration rate, FiO_2, and PEEP. TV is calculated according to ideal body weight (IBW). IBW is based on a patient's height; thus, the nurse should obtain an accurate height. Measuring the patient with a tape measure should be routine practice. An accurate height is critical to prevent errors in calculating TV, which if too high, can cause volutrauma to the lungs. Initial TV should be less than 8 mL/kg IBW. The formula for calculating TV is as follows:

- IBW for men: 50 kg + 2.3 kg for each inch over 5 feet tall
  - Example: a man who is 6 feet tall = 50 + (2.3 * 12) = 77.6 mL/kg IBW
  - Initial TV for an average height man should range between about 520 and 600 mL
  - Rarely should TV exceed 600 mL
- IBW for women = 45.5 kg + 2.3 kg for each inch over 5 feet tall
  - Example: a woman who is 5 feet, 7 inches tall = 45.5 + (2.3 * 7) = 61.6/kg IBW
  - Initial TV for an average height woman should range between around 360 and 480 mL
  - Rarely should TV exceed 500 mL

Respiration rates should be set slightly higher than a normal rate to compensate for possible metabolic acidosis and ensure the patient is not hypercarbic, especially for patients with brain injuries. A common rate to set is 16 to 20 breaths per minute. Initially, provide 100% FiO_2 and PEEP of 8 cm water pressure. A higher PEEP will assist in recruiting alveoli that have become atelectatic during intubation or at the scene. Further adjustments are based on results of an ABG. Once the patient is through the ED and operating room and settled in the ICU, rapid weaning of the FiO_2 to at or below 50% is important to prevent worsening atelectasis and oxygen toxicity. Once FiO_2 is below 50%, then wean PEEP by 2 cm, no more frequently than every 4 hours.

Troubleshooting the Ventilator

Nurses spend the most amount of time at the bedside and will routinely respond to ventilator alarms and should have understanding of methods to troubleshoot alarms (Table 10.5). Ventilator management requires an interdisciplinary approach with nurses, providers, and respiratory therapists.

Ventilator Weaning

Every day, patients should have a sedation awakening trial (SAT). The only absolute contraindication to performing an SAT is if the patient requires paralytic agents. Otherwise, nurses should stop all analgesic and sedation agents for a period of time to allow the patient to awaken. Minimizing sedation is known to decrease the risk of post-ICU syndrome. If the patient's

TABLE 10.5

Troubleshooting Ventilator

Alarm	Possible Causes	Diagnostic and Treatment Options
■ High peak inspiratory pressure With normal plateau pressure	■ Occlusion of ETT tube 　■ Patient biting ETT 　■ ETT kinked 　■ Patient coughing against ETT 　■ Gagging on ETT 　■ Secretions in tube	■ Increase sedation ■ Add bite block to ETT ■ Prop tube up ■ Suction ETT ■ Administer antiemetic ■ Suction ETT
	■ Bronchospasms	■ Administer albuterol, consider Atrovent
	■ Condensation in ventilator tubing	■ Evacuate excess fluid from tubing
	■ Patient dyssynchrony with ventilator	■ Increase sedation ■ Change ventilator mode, consider SBT with/without PSV
■ High peak inspiratory pressure with high plateau pressure	■ Mainstem bronchus intubation	■ Obtain CXR and pull ETT back
	■ Pneumothorax	■ CXR 　■ Needle decompression 　■ Pigtail catheter 　■ Tube thoracostomy
	■ ARDS	
	■ Abdominal compartment syndrome	■ Shift to low TV ventilation (4–6 mL/kg IBW)

(continued)

TABLE 10.5 (continued)

Troubleshooting Ventilator

Alarm	Possible Causes	Diagnostic and Treatment Options
		■ Make room in abdomen:
		■ NGT to suction
		■ Rectal tube/enema
		■ Paracentesis
		■ Paralytics
		■ Surgical intervention to open abdomen
■ Breath stacking/ auto PEEP	■ Insufficient expiratory time	■ Decrease RR on vent
	■ RR too fast, preventing full exhalation	■ May need sedation if patient is spontaneously overbreathing
	■ Obstructive lung disease	
		■ Decrease inspiratory time
		■ Albuterol or Atrovent neb
		■ Consider steroids
Low volume	■ Patient disconnected from ventilator	■ Check all connections
	■ ETT is dislodged	■ Evaluate if patient needs ETT or can remain extubated, and if not, requires reintubation
	■ Patient in spontaneous mode and is becoming bradypneic, apneic, or fatigued	■ Return to full vent support to rest
	■ Cuff leak	■ Check ETT cuff pressure—add pressure
		■ Check pilot balloon to ensure it's not blown or patient hasn't bitten through it—if so, change ETT

(continued)

TABLE 10.5 (continued)
Troubleshooting Ventilator

Alarm	Possible Causes	Diagnostic and Treatment Options
■ Hypoxia	■ Progressive underlying disease	■ Ensure proper treatment of disease
	■ Pneumothorax	■ CXR
		■ Needle decompress
	■ Pulmonary edema	■ Pigtail catheter
		■ Tube thoracostomy
	■ Aspiration	
		■ CXR, identify etiology
	■ Patient reposition/alveolar fluid shifts	■ Consider diuresis
	■ Pulmonary embolism	■ Suction ETT
		■ Preoxygenate prior to turns
		■ Sedation/analgesia prior to turns
		■ CT chest PE protocol
		■ Anticoagulation

ARDS, acute respiratory distress syndrome; CT, computed tomography; CXR, chest x-ray; ETT, endotracheal tube; IBW, ideal body weight; NGT, nasogastric tube; PE, pulmonary embolism; PEEP, positive end-expiratory pressure; PSV, pressure support ventilation; RR, respiratory rate; SBT, spontaneous breathing trial; TV, tidal volume.

condition warrants, the nurse can restart analgesia sedation at or below 50% of the previous infusion dose. Additionally, patients should have daily spontaneous breathing trials (SBTs). SATs and SBTs can be protocolized to happen routinely as long as patients meet specific criteria, which may vary by institution. Typically, patients should be hemodynamically stable and weaning off vasopressors. FiO_2 should be at or below 50% and on 8 or less of PEEP through the ventilator to support an SBT.

Extubation Criteria
The next step with an intubated patient is to determine when the patient is ready for liberation from mechanical ventilation. The goal is to extubate all patients

from the ventilator as soon as possible. An SBT should be completed daily for all intubated patients, unless contraindicated. An **absolute contraindication is if the patient is on a paralytic agent**. An SBT includes placing the patient on a spontaneous mode of ventilation, which can include placing the patient on a T-piece, pressure support ventilation, or continuous positive pressure. The goal of an SBT is to determine whether a patient will breathe spontaneously to maintain sufficient oxygenation and ventilation for a period of time. SBT duration ranges from 30 to 120 minutes. Clinicians can allow the patient to stay in this mode for longer periods without extubation, while allowing the patient to meet other extubation criteria, such as improved mental status. Other factors that influence readiness for extubation include reversal of the pathology that forced the intubation, hemodynamic stability, ability to clear secretions, and stable mental status. A scoring system is widely used to predict the success of extubation: the rapid shallow breathing index (RSBI). This RSBI formula is:

[RSBI = Respiratory Rate/TV in liters]

Example: RR 20/TV .4 = 50

A resulting score below 105 is predictive of a likely successful extubation, whereas a score higher than 105 is predictive of an unsuccessful extubation. Ultimately, whether to extubate a patient is a clinical decision that considers a variety of factors and patient characteristics (Box 10.2).

Nursing Care

The nurse plays a crucial role in airway management. The nurse is one of the first team members at a patient's bedside when an airway issue arises. The nurse must be confident in initial interventions to aid a patient with an airway issue. It is within the nurse's scope of practice to increase the percent oxygen being delivered in an acutely decompensating patient. Nurses

---

Box 10.2 EXTUBATION CRITERIA

- Reason for intubation resolved
- Hemodynamically stable MAP 60 to 65 mmHg, with minimal vasopressor requirements
- FiO_2 <50% and PEEP ≤8 cm H_2O
- PaO_2 >60 mmHg; Sat >90%; PaO_2/FiO_2 >150 on PEEP 5 to 8 cm H_2O
- pH >7.25; $PaCO_2$ <60 mmHg
- RSBI <105
- Able to have head of bed up 30 to 45 degrees
- Adequate muscle strength
  - Able to lift head off bed
  - Negative inspiratory force at least −20
- ETT cuff leak present
- Minimal pulmonary secretions

may need to initiate bag mask ventilation or provide maneuvers to open the patient's airway, including the head tilt chin lift (when not contraindicated) or jaw thrust maneuver.

With the mechanically ventilated patient, the nurse is responsible for routine oral care, chest physiotherapy, and endotracheal suctioning. Mechanical ventilation often requires pain and sedation medication titration within the prescribed parameters. The nurse should ensure all patients on mechanical ventilation have a daily sedation interruption and attempt to wean the ventilator settings or an SBT unless contraindicated.

Failure to Wean From Mechanical Ventilation

Patients who fail to wean from mechanical ventilation may require a tracheostomy. Detailed assessment to identify and correct the cause of wean failure is essential to prevent tracheostomy. Common reasons patients fail to wean from the ventilator include active cardiac ischemia, concomitant heart failure or volume overload, neurologic injuries, malnutrition, infection, and fibrotic changes from acute respiratory distress syndrome (ARDS).

Tracheostomy
Tracheostomy is a common procedure performed on the critically ill patient. It is an advanced airway and is indicated for:
1. Prolonged ventilator weaning/dependence.
2. Penetrating laryngeal trauma.
3. Spinal cord injuries or other neuromuscular disease.
4. Severe brain injuries, to provide patent airway and facilitate discharge to rehabilitation center.
5. Prophylactic placement prior to maxillomandibular fixation for jaw fractures.
6. Acute upper airway obstruction with inability for/failed ETT placement.
7. Chronic aspiration.

When a patient has a tracheostomy, the upper airway is bypassed and the functions of the upper airway (warming, filtering, and humidifying inspired air) are lost. Providing humidified air or oxygen, as a trach collar, along with appropriate fluid intake, promotes thinning and mobility of secretions. Early mobility of the patient can aid in mobilizing secretions.

Nursing Care
Caring for a patient with a tracheostomy includes suctioning the patient, routine tracheostomy care, oral hygiene, and assessing for potential complications. Functions of the upper airway include warming, filtering, and humidifying air. A tracheostomy is a foreign object and secretions can form around the tracheostomy tube. The stoma and surrounding tissues must be kept clean and dry to prevent skin breakdown.

> **FAST FACTS**
>
> Monitor tracheostomies for pressure injuries from the tracheostomy flange.

Pulmonary Sequelae

Aspiration
Broadly, aspiration is the act of breathing in something that does not belong in the lungs. This can be a foreign object; particles of food; liquids, including blood; gastric contents; and oropharyngeal secretions. Aspiration does not always result in an infection. Initial aspiration causes a chemical pneumonitis or noninfective irritation of the lungs. Aspiration does not require antibiotics unless the patient develops pneumonia. Aspiration increases morbidity and mortality and is the nidus for ARDS. Risk factors of aspiration include neurologic impairment, mechanical ventilation, poor cough and secretion management, dysphagia, esophageal dysmotility, and gastric distention from ileus or bowel obstruction.

Pneumonia
Pneumonia is an inflammatory process involving the distal airways and alveoli caused by an infectious agent. This can be a complication of thoracic trauma. Pneumonia can also occur after an aspiration event, either during the trauma or at some point throughout the hospitalization, or as a complication of immobility and/or interventions such as intubation with mechanical ventilation.

Mediastinitis
Mediastinitis is inflammation or infection that involves the mediastinum, the space within the thorax that is bordered by the pleural sacs, the thoracic outlet, and the diaphragm. Because the mediastinum houses many vital structures of the body, this pathology can be life-threatening. Mediastinitis occurs when the integrity of mediastinal structures is compromised, which may be traumatic, infectious, or iatrogenic in origin. One of the more common causes of traumatic mediastinitis occurs in the setting of esophageal perforation.

Nursing Care
The most important nursing care related to aspiration is the preventative measures nurses can use to reduce risk of aspiration. These include engaging speech language pathology for formal assessment and therapies, such as upright positioning during meals, small bites, thickened liquids, and so forth. A fiberoptic endoscopic swallow study may be needed to directly observe for aspiration. This is usually completed by the speech therapist. Appropriate oral hygiene is also associated with reduction in aspiration events. Nursing

care to prevent pneumonia includes interventions to improve gas exchange, including weaning oxygen and ensuring proper patient positioning to improve lung expansion and aeration (sitting upright, out of bed to chair, and ambulation if not contraindicated). Incentive spirometry and PEEP therapy should be used with patients.

SUMMARY

In summary, care of the trauma patient with a pulmonary pathology or complication is common. Nurses must have the knowledge and skills to manage a wide range of traumatic pulmonary injuries. Nurses must be proficient in weaning oxygen, understanding ventilation methods and modes of ventilation, and chest tube management. Most important of all, nurses must possess astute physical exam skills to identify early deterioration of patient clinical status.

REVIEW QUESTIONS

1. Tracheal deviation and jugular venous distention are late signs of:
   a. Trauma
   b. Tension pneumothorax
   c. Pneumothorax
   d. Scapula fracture
2. Interpret the arterial blood gas:
   pH7.19/PaCO$_2$ 65 mmHg/PaO$_2$ 90 mmHg/Bicarb 24 mEq/L/O$_2$ Saturation 95%/Base Excess −2
   a. Metabolic acidosis
   b. Respiratory alkalosis
   c. Metabolic alkalosis
   d. Respiratory acidosis
3. Stridor is indicative of
   a. Flail chest
   b. Narrowed airway
   c. Readiness for extubation
   d. Pneumonia

References

Alqahtani, J. S., & AlAhmari, M. D. (2018, May). Evidence based synthesis for prevention of noninvasive ventilation related facial pressure ulcers. *Saudi Medical Journal, 39*(5), 443–452. https://doi.org/10.15537/smj.2018.5.22058

American College of Surgeons: The Committee on Trauma. (2018). *ATLS: Advanced Trauma Life Support student course manual* (10th ed.). American College of Surgeons.

Carboni Bisso, I., Gemelli, N. A., Barrios, C., & Las Heras, M. (2021, February 27). Pulmonary laceration. *Trauma Case Reports, 32*, 100449. https://doi.org/10.1016/j.tcr.2021.100449. Erratum in: Trauma Case Rep. 2023 March 01; 45: 100818.

Castro, D., Patil, S. M., & Keenaghan, M. (2023, January). *Arterial blood gas.* [Updated September 12, 2022]. StatPearls Publishing. https://www.ncbi.nlm.nih.gov/books/NBK536919/

Dogrul, B. N., Kiliccalan, I., Asci, E. S., & Peker, S. C. (2020, January). Blunt trauma related chest wall and pulmonary injuries: An overview. *Chinese Journal of Traumatology, 23*(3), 125–138. https://doi.org/10.1016/j.cjtee.2020.04.003

Hochhegger, B., & Altmayer, S. (2022, July–August). Traumatic sternal fractures. *Radiologia Brasileira, 55*(4), IX. https://doi.org/10.1590/0100-3984.2022.55.4e3

McQuillan, K. A., & Flynn-Makic, M. B. (2020). *Trauma nursing: From resuscitation through rehabilitation* (5th ed.). Elsevier.

Mubang, R. N., Sigmon, D. F., & Stawicki, S. P. (2022, July 26). *Esophageal trauma.* StatPearls Publishing.

Müller, F. (2015, March). Oral hygiene reduces the mortality from aspiration pneumonia in frail elders. *Journal of Dental Research, 94*(3 Suppl.), 14S–16S. https://doi.org/10.1177/0022034514552494

Parker, L. C. (2014, November). Tracheostomy care. *Nursing Critical Care, 9*(6), 38–41. https://doi.org/10.1097/01.CCN.0000453466.57833.dd

Pumarejo Gomez, L., & Tran, V. H. (2023, January). *Hemothorax.* [Updated August 8, 2022]. StatPearls Publishing. https://www.ncbi.nlm.nih.gov/books/NBK538219/

11

Gastrointestinal Injuries and Care
Dawn Carpenter

> *Injuries to the abdominal organs and gastrointestinal tract can range from mild to lethal. Solid organ injuries are readily observed on CT scan, whereas other injuries, such as pancreatic or small bowel, may be more difficult to detect. Ongoing assessment and serial abdominal exams are essential to ensure all diagnoses are recognized and treated promptly. Nurses are integral team members who can communicate changes in patients' conditions, such as ongoing pain and worsening assessment findings.*

In this chapter, you will learn to:
1. Identify key examination findings of the gastrointestinal tract.
2. Detect solid organ injuries.
3. Identify hollow organ injuries.
4. Articulate serious complications of splenectomy.
5. Verbalize key nursing care for patients' intra-abdominal injuries.

INTRODUCTION

Trauma nurses should be familiar with common intra-abdominal injuries, their associated treatments, and monitoring for complications. Nurses need to have the ability to recognize normal and abnormal findings in order to care for the trauma patient who has injuries to the abdominal cavity. The highest priority is to assess for bleeding and detect injuries within the abdominal cavity. Abdominal injuries may not initially be apparent and can manifest hours to days after presentation. The nurse must possess astute assessment skills.

GASTROINTESTINAL ASSESSMENT

Abdominal Assessment
Correct order of assessment of the abdomen should start with inspection, followed by auscultation, percussion, and then palpation. Much information can be gleaned about the patient's injuries as well as other underlying medical conditions with keen observation.

Inspection: Inspect the abdomen to assess for distention and ecchymoses, such as seat belt sign. The presence of any scars or umbilical, ventral, or inguinal hernias provides knowledge to the surgeons if they need to provide emergent intra-abdominal surgery. Observe for the presence of any pulsations, which may indicate an aortic aneurysm or dissection. The presence of an aortic pulsation is a normal finding in thin people and can be observed in the epigastric area. Inspection can also provide insight into other medical problems. For example, the presence of a protuberant abdomen with caput medusae and fluid wave in a stable patient may indicate the presence of cirrhosis or other liver disease. Underlying liver disease in a traumatically injured patient has serious implications. Liver dysfunction can cause underlying thrombocytopenia and coagulopathy, inhibiting appropriate clotting. Additionally, a patient with liver disease or a patient who is frail and thin with a flat abdomen may be malnourished at baseline, and thus wound healing will be impeded.

Auscultation: Auscultation of bowel sounds has limited usefulness in the trauma bay. Presence of abdominal sounds, if they can be heard in the noisy trauma bay, does not preclude injury. Nor does the absence of bowel sounds indicate absence of bowel function. Bowel function is assessed by the presence of passing flatus or stool.

Percussion: Percussion can elicit peritoneal signs indicating bowel injury and may be useful to identify fluid in the abdomen, such as blood or ascites. The focused assessment with sonography for trauma (FAST) is a useful tool for assessing fluid in the abdomen. The FAST cannot distinguish between blood and ascites. An unstable patient with a positive FAST exam that is not responsive to fluid will likely go directly to the operating room (OR) for an exploratory laparotomy.

Palpation: Palpation is the last assessment method for the abdomen. Initially palpate with light touch. Gently palpate all four quadrants with one hand. Watch the patient's face for grimacing. Pay particular attention to any abdominal tenderness and guarding. Advance to deeper palpation with two hands. Use the palmar surfaces of the fingers to deeply palpate abdominal structures such as the liver, spleen, kidneys, and any abdominal masses. In severely injured patients, assessment of the gastrointestinal (GI) tract may require a digital rectal exam (DRE) and placement of a nasogastric tube (NGT).

Rectal Exam

Assessment of the rectum is part of the complete GI tract assessment. In awake patients, asking them to squeeze their buttocks together will demonstrate intact musculature. Inspect for blood at the anus. In severely critically injured patients who can't follow commands, a DRE may be needed. A DRE is especially important to assess for rectal tone when spinal cord injuries are suspected.

Nasogastric Tube Assessment

Placement of an NGT may be required if the patient is vomiting, to prevent aspiration. Assess NGT effluent for blood. Remember that patients with oral or facial injuries may swallow blood, thus causing bloody drainage from the NGT. Ongoing active bleeding from the NGT or rectum requires additional diagnostic testing. Specific patients are at risk for gastric bleeding while hospitalized. Specifically, patients with traumatic brain injuries or spinal cord injuries and those who require mechanical ventilation for longer than 48 hours are at greatest risk for GI bleeding. This subset of trauma patients should receive stress ulcer prophylaxis.

Diagnostic Testing

A few diagnostic tests are commonly performed at the bedside by providers at the time of presentation. The extended FAST (eFAST) is an ultrasound performed to assess for intra-abdominal bleeding, cardiac tamponade, and pneumothorax. The five areas assessed by this point-of-care ultrasound are the right upper quadrant of the abdomen (perihepatic view); left upper quadrant of the abdomen (perisplenic view); and pelvic, cardiac, and bilateral lung views. A positive eFAST and signs of shock are indications for immediate operative exploration.

A diagnostic peritoneal lavage (DPL) can also be performed to detect hemoperitoneum. A DPL involves a catheter inserted into the peritoneal cavity; IV fluid is infused into the peritoneum, and the effluent is assessed for blood. This diagnostic tool has fallen out of favor with the availability the eFAST and CT scans.

A CT scan with IV contrast is the best diagnostic test to view specific intra-abdominal injuries and assess for bleeding. Oral or rectal contrast may be needed to assess for specific injuries. A CT scan is not necessary if the patient is in hemorrhagic shock. Unstable patients, especially those who are refractory to transfusion, are likely to be taken directly to the OR for exploratory laparotomy.

Serial Abdominal Exams

Subsequent exams should be performed to monitor for increasing size; worsening distention; and development of rebound tenderness, guarding, and/or rigidity. Rebound tenderness is indicated by tenderness noted in an area when the examiner is pressing down and suddenly releases their hand. Guarding is the voluntary contraction of the abdominal wall, usually accompanied by pain expressed in the face. Rigidity is the involuntary contraction of the abdominal wall that is consistent throughout the abdominal exam.

FAST FACTS

The nurse must report worsening pain, abdominal distention, nausea, and/or vomiting to providers to evaluate for missed intra-abdominal injuries.

GASTROINTESTINAL INJURIES

Solid Organ Injuries

Solid organs include the spleen, liver, and kidney. Kidney injuries are reviewed in Chapter 12. Injury to solid organs in patients who are hemodynamically stable can be managed nonoperatively but require hospitalization for ongoing observation and bleeding. Surgeons must be consulted and available in case the patient requires operative intervention.

Spleen

The spleen is located in the left upper quadrant/flank area. Thus, patients who present with pain in the left upper quadrant should be suspected of having a splenic injury. Splenic injury pain can radiate to the ipsilateral shoulder, referred to as the Kehr sign. The most common mechanism causing splenic injuries is blunt force trauma to the left upper quadrant from motor vehicle crashes, sports injuries, and so forth. Splenic injuries may also occur with penetrating injuries, either due to direct impact from a projectile or from high-velocity bullets causing a "shock wave" that creates a temporary cavitation and injures surrounding tissues. Splenic injuries are graded from 1 to 5 with grade 1 being the least injured and grade 5 being shattered. Nonoperative management is preferred to preserve splenic tissue, which is a vital component of the immune system. Higher grade injuries may require intravascular embolization to control bleeding. The most severe cases, patients who remain hemodynamically unstable despite resuscitation, require surgical splenectomy.

Frequent reassessment and monitoring are required, with conservative management, because the rebleeding risk is highest within the first 48 hours following injury and delayed rupture can occur. Delayed rupture can occur even up to 2 weeks after injury or with repeated trauma, such as falls or sports impacts. Nurses should continuously monitor for patient reports of progressive pain in the left shoulder that worsens with inspiration (Kehr sign). Increasing abdominal tenderness and distention, pallor, tachycardia, and orthostatic hypotension are all signs of ongoing bleeding and should be reported to the team immediately.

Overwhelming Postsplenectomy Infection

Patients who require splenectomy are at an increased risk of severe infections for the duration of their lives. Overwhelming postsplenectomy infection (OPSI), also known as postsplenectomy sepsis, is the most severe form of infection, occurring most commonly within the first 3 years after splenectomy. Common signs and symptoms include fever, chills, malaise, headache, vomiting, and abdominal pain. Patients can rapidly progress to sepsis, with fulminant septic shock occurring within 24 to 48 hours. Mortality rates for OPSI are upward of 50%. Common pathogens include pneumococcus, *Neisseria meningitidis,* and *Haemophilus influenzae.* Less common organisms include gram-negative bacteria such as *Pseudomonas aeruginosa.*

Vaccines

Prevention of OPSI includes administration of vaccines 2 weeks after the splenectomy. Vaccines vary by age. Most hospitals administer the vaccines before discharge to ensure the patient receives them in the event they are lost to follow-up. Postsplenectomy vaccines for adults include the following on the day of discharge or day 14, whichever comes first:

- Pneumococcal 13-valent conjugate (PCV13: Prevnar 13)
- Haemophilus influenza type B vaccine (Hib: ActHIB)
- Meningococcal vaccine (Menactra)
- Meningococcal serogroup B (Bexsero)

Subsequent vaccines include:

- Pneumococcal polysaccharide (PPSV23: Pneumovax 23)—2 months after initial vaccines
- Meningococcal vaccine (Menactra)—2 months after initial vaccines
- Meningococcal serogroup B (Bexsero)—2 months after initial vaccines
- Seasonal flu vaccine—annually
- Pneumococcal polysaccharide—every 5 years.
- Meningococcal vaccine—every 5 years

FAST FACTS

Nurses must ensure the patient who has had a splenectomy receives their vaccines on the day of discharge or hospital day 14, whichever comes first.

Liver

The liver is the most commonly injured solid organ because of its size and location in the abdomen. Liver injuries are commonly caused by both blunt and penetrating injuries. Liver injuries are graded on a scale of 1 to 5, with 1 being least injured and 5 being the worst. Grade 1 and 2 liver injuries comprise more than 80% of all liver injuries. However, severe liver injuries carry a 10% to 15% mortality risk. Patients with liver injuries who are hemodynamically unstable require immediate surgical intervention. Those who are hemodynamically stable can be managed nonoperatively as long as an OR and surgeon are immediately available. Patients with higher grade injuries are at greater risk for failure of nonoperative management. Intravascular intervention with hepatic artery embolization may be an effective means to stop bleeding. Intraoperatively, hemostatic agents may be applied to the liver, or the liver may be packed to apply direct pressure to bleeding tissue. If the liver is packed, the abdomen will be left open, with negative-pressure wound therapy and a plan to return to the OR in 24 to 48 hours.

Complications of liver injury include bile leak, and hepatic necrosis and/or abscess may occur after hepatic artery embolization. Clinical signs of these complications include fever and/or leukocytosis. Bile draining from surgical drains indicates a bile leak. A CT scan is needed to identify these complications. Treatment may include percutaneous drainage of the bile, and endoscopic retrograde cholangiopancreatography and stent placement may stop the leak. Percutaneous drainage and antibiotics treat the abscess.

Nursing Care of Solid Organ Injuries
Nurses should perform serial abdominal examinations, assessing for worsening distention, increasing pain, and ecchymoses. Monitor vital signs frequently for tachycardia, narrowing pulse pressure, tachypnea, pallor, and anxiety, indicating that the patient is progressing into shock. Serial hemoglobin and hematocrit are essential to trend values to observe for stability versus ongoing bleeding. Keep these patients nil per os (NPO) in the event they require an intravascular embolization or surgical intervention. Ensure the patient has an active type and cross with blood readily available in the blood bank.

For patients who have had arterial embolization, assess for complications including hematoma, arteriovenous fistula, and arterial occlusion with limb ischemia. The nurse should assess the arterial access site for ecchymosis, hematoma, pulsations, and thrills. Assess distal pedal pulses and compare them to the contralateral extremity, and check capillary refill. Assess the patient for ongoing abdominal pain and distention. Ensure repeat blood counts are ordered to ensure bleeding has ceased and to assess appropriate response to transfusions.

Patient teaching is a critical component of the nurse's role. Educate patients about delayed rupture, which can occur days or weeks later. Inform patients and families of signs and symptoms of recurrent bleeding, including pain, abdominal distention, light-headedness, dizziness, and so forth. Teach parents and youth to avoid contact sports for at least 8 weeks to avoid reinjuring and rebleeding.

HOLLOW ORGAN INJURIES

Hollow organs include the esophagus, stomach, small bowel, and colon. Hollow organ injuries are less common, occurring in about 5% of patients who have concomitant solid organ injuries. Duodenal injuries may be seen in unrestrained drivers who are involved in frontal impact motor vehicle crashes or handlebar injuries from bicycles. These deceleration injuries to the small bowel are referred to as "bucket handle" injuries. Bowel injuries may be associated with distraction lumbar fractures, called Chance fractures (see Chapter 13). Hollow organ injuries may be difficult to diagnose because they may not be accompanied by hemorrhage and may take hours to a day to develop symptoms from ischemic bowel or spillage of intestinal contents into the peritoneum.

Esophageal Injuries
Esophageal injuries, although part of the GI tract and hollow, are associated with neck and thoracic trauma. Penetrating injury to the neck is the most common mechanism of esophageal injury. Blunt esophageal injury may occur from a direct blow to the upper abdomen and can cause pressure to

force stomach contents to reflux into the esophagus and cause an esophageal rupture or tear in the lower esophagus. Leakage of oral or gastric contents may cause mediastinitis. Esophageal injuries may be occult and not manifest until mediastinitis occurs. Clues to esophageal rupture include mediastinal air on CT scan or a new unilateral pleural effusion. Confirmation of the diagnosis may require esophagoscopy or contrast studies such as a barium swallow. Suspect esophageal injuries in patients with odynophagia (painful swallowing), fevers, chills, chest pain, shortness of breath, and signs of sepsis.

Treatment of esophageal perforation includes strict NPO status to minimize spillage of oral intake into the mediastinum. Microperforations can be managed conservatively, allowing spontaneous healing. Esophageal rupture can be endoscopically stented or may require minimally invasive or open surgical repair. If open surgery is required, expect the patient to have a pleural chest tube and/or mediastinal drainage tubes. See Chapter 10 for pleural tube management.

Bowel Injuries

Bowel injuries include contusions, edema, mesenteric injury, bowel lacerations, acute rupture, and delayed rupture. Signs of bowel injury differ from those of liver and spleen injuries. Bowel injuries commonly have a delayed presentation. Clinical signs include fever, leukocytosis, and increased pain. The development of peritonitis represents a bowel perforation. Signs of peritonitis include rebound tenderness, guarding, and rigidity. Sudden jarring, such as a bump to the stretcher or side rail adjustment, may produce severe pain. Suspected peritonitis should be confirmed by the surgical team. An upright chest x-ray may show free air under the diaphragm. A repeat CT scan is not always needed to make this diagnosis. Anticipate that the patient will need emergent surgical intervention.

FAST FACTS

Hollow organ injuries are not always easily diagnosed. Patients who develop peritonitis in the first 24 to 48 hours should be suspected of having a missed bowel injury.

Rectal Injuries

Approximately 90% of rectal injuries occur from penetrating trauma, including gunshot wounds and stabbings, along with sex-related and foreign body injuries. The remainder of rectal trauma is due to blunt trauma, with a portion directly related to anterior/posterior pelvic fractures compressing the pelvis. Pelvic fractures that penetrate the rectum are considered open fractures and require immediate antibiotics. Nursing should ensure prompt administration of antibiotics to avoid the development of osteomyelitis.

OTHER INTRA-ABDOMINAL ORGAN INJURIES

Pancreatic Injuries

Pancreatic injuries can occur due to blunt force trauma to the epigastric region, when the pancreas is compressed against the spine. Such injuries are more common in young, healthy, thin persons. Pancreatic injuries result from handlebar impact from bicycles or motorcycle crashes to the epigastric area. Pancreatic injuries may not initially be evident, and diagnosis may be delayed. The patient's amylase or lipase may not be elevated initially. Patients will have persistent epigastric pain and may have nausea and vomiting along with other signs of pancreatitis, such as tachycardia and third spacing of fluids. Additional imaging with MRI may be needed, or surgical exploration may be warranted.

Diaphragm Injuries

Diaphragm injuries can range from subtle findings on a chest x-ray to obvious herniation of abdominal contents into the chest cavity. Blunt force injury to the upper abdomen can cause a tear in the diaphragm, with the left hemidiaphragm being injured most often. Penetrating injury to the lower chest or upper abdomen should lead the team to suspect a diaphragm injury. Diaphragm injuries require surgical exploration to correct the deficit.

Adrenal Injuries

Injuries to the adrenal gland are rare because of its positioning in the retroperitoneal space and protection by the ribs, muscles, and soft tissues. Adrenal injuries typically occur on one side and are caused by direct blunt force trauma to the abdomen, flank, or back. Most adrenal trauma involves other injuries as well. Increasingly, adrenal glands are managed conservatively. The adrenal gland is vascular, which may result in significant bleeding.

FAST FACTS

Patients with persistent epigastric pain with associated nausea or vomiting may have a pancreatic injury or hollow viscus injury. The nurse should report these symptoms to providers for further evaluation.

SURGICAL INTERVENTION

Not all trauma patients require surgery, but when they do, it is commonly emergent. Patients who are hypovolemic or in shock are frequently thirsty. The nurse should ensure the patient remains NPO in case surgery is necessary.

Indications for Surgery

Indications for emergent laparotomy include blunt abdominal trauma in a patient with:
1. Hypotension and positive FAST or positive DPL.
2. Hypotension in a patient with a penetrating injury that invades the fascial layer.
3. Gunshot wounds that traverse the peritoneal cavity.
4. Any evisceration of abdominal contents.
5. Bleeding from the NGT, rectum, or genitourinary tract.
6. Intra-abdominal free air.
7. Rupture of the diaphragm.
8. Peritonitis or CT scan that reveals gastrointestinal perforation, bladder injury, olr severe visceral injury.

Damage Control Surgery

Critically injured and unstable trauma patients may require emergent surgery. These patients are unstable and typically require mass transfusions. Damage control surgery is used to avoid the "triad of death," which includes hypothermia, acidosis, and coagulopathy and can ensue quickly in patients are exposed to prolonged surgery. Thus, the principle of damage control surgery is to obtain immediate control of the hemorrhage and minimize intraperitoneal contamination as quickly as possible. The concept of "get in and get out quickly" applies in this situation. The patient is transferred to the ICU to stabilize the patient, correct metabolic acidosis, provide ongoing resuscitation, correct coagulopathies, and rewarm the patient. Definitive surgery occurs once the patient has stabilized in 24 to 48 hours. During damage control surgery, the abdominal fascia is left open, and negative-pressure wound therapy is applied. This is referred to as an "open abdomen," and patients are at risk for evisceration if too much intra-abdominal pressure (IAP) is exerted, such as with coughing or getting out of bed.

FAST FACTS

The nurse should always inquire as to whether the fascia is open or closed. Do not rely on the color of the foam to indicate if the fascia is closed.

Nursing Care of the Patient With an Open Abdomen
Nursing care of the patient with an open abdomen includes ensuring the dressing remains sealed and to negative pressure. Monitor output in the canister. Expected drainage should be serosanguinous. A change to sanguineous indicates ongoing bleeding. A change to green or bile output indicates a missed injury to the stomach, small bowel, or gallbladder structures, or an enterocutaneous fistula. A change to brown or feculent material indicates a colonic perforation. Record the volume of output. Initial output may be substantial but should taper off after a few hours to a day. Patients can be

extubated when medically it is appropriate, before definitive surgery; however, other injuries may preclude extubation. Patients with open abdomen should not be gotten out of bed or ambulated due to the risk of evisceration. Patients with an open abdomen are a relative contraindication to the prone position if they develop acute respiratory distress syndrome (ARDS) or transfusion-related acute lung injury (TRALI). After definitive surgery, routine care should be resumed.

Nursing Care of Patients with Abdominal Trauma
Patients with blunt abdominal trauma may experience an ileus. Patients may be nauseous, vomit, and not tolerate oral or tube feedings. Keep these patients NPO and await return of bowel function, including passing flatus or stool. Early mobility, including ambulation, can assist the ileus to resolve more quickly. Minimize narcotics to prevent narcotic-induced constipation. An expected ileus should resolve in 3 to 4 days. Prolonged or new ileus after an oral diet is tolerated can indicate an intra-abdominal abscess. Monitor for signs of infection, including tachycardia, tachypnea, leukocytosis, and oliguria.

NGT Management
Patients who have had an exploratory laparotomy must be kept NPO. Keep the NGT or orogastric tube (OGT) functioning properly. The NGT/OGT should be to low intermittent suction. Keep the vent/air port patent to ensure the tube can function appropriately. The nurse should be able to hear atmospheric air being suctioned from the vent into the stomach and out the suction port. Clearance of gastric contents may be required, because food particles from recent meals can clog the NGT/OGT. Flush the NGT with 30 mL of saline to clear the gastric lumen. Flushes may need to be repeated. Do not flush any fluids through the vent. Do not obstruct the vent by leaving the catheter tip syringe attached or tie it in a knot, because this renders the tube ineffective. If the vent cannot be cleared, the NGT/OGT may need to be replaced.

FAST FACTS

Maintaining patency of the NGT/OGT is a very high priority. Do not obstruct the vent, and if it has fluid in it, clear the air port with saline.

COMPLICATIONS OF ABDOMINAL TRAUMA

Abdominal Compartment Syndrome
Abdominal compartment syndrome (ACS) can occur in patients with severe trauma, including bowel injuries, burns, massive fluid resuscitation, and so forth (Table 11.1). The inflammatory process allows for

TABLE 11.1

Risk Factors for IAH

Category	Etiology/Contributing Factors
Capillary leak processes	- Sepsis - Major trauma - Bowel injury - Pancreatitis - Burns
Increased abdominal contents	- Distended abdomen - Hemoperitoneum, pneumoperitoneum - Ascites - Intra-abdominal tumors - Laparoscopy with excessive insufflation - Peritoneal dialysis - Misplaced femoral venous catheter - Ruptured abdominal aneurysm
Increases intraluminal contents	- Gastric dilatation - Gastroparesis - Ileus - Volvulus - Bowel obstruction
Decreased abdominal wall compliance	- Prone positioning - Recent abdominal surgery - Rectus sheath hematoma
Patient factors	- Obesity - Shock, hypotension - Age - Acidemia - Coagulopathy - Hypothermia
Pulmonary etiology	- PEEP >10 cm H2O

IAH, intra-abdominal hypertension; PEEP, positive end-expiratory pressure.

capillary permeability and third spacing of fluids into the abdominal tissues. This intra-abdominal edema leads to intra-abdominal hypertension (IAH). The added pressure of the abdomen impedes venous return to the heart. Thus, decreased preload worsens cardiac output and hypotension. Hypotension causes additional ischemia to the bowels; thus, more edema ensues. This vicious cycle continues until the patient dies from multisystem organ failure (Table 11.2). Treatment of ACS involves opening the abdomen tissues and fascia. This can be done in the OR or at bedside in the ICU.

Measurement of Intra-Abdominal Pressure

IAH can be measured by placing the patient in the supine position with their arms by their side. Ensure the patient is sedated and not coughing or

TABLE 11.2

Clinical Signs of IAH by System and Etiology

System	Clinical Signs	Etiology
Gastrointestinal	▪ Decreased abdominal wall compliance ▪ Elevated LFTs ▪ Decreased lactic acid clearance	▪ Increased intestinal permeability ▪ Decreased perfusion to bowels ▪ Decreased portal blood flow
Respiratory	▪ Increased peak and plateau pressures ▪ Compressive atelectasis at lung bases ▪ Elevated diaphragm ▪ Decreased chest wall compliance	▪ V/Q mismatching, resulting in hypoxia
Neurologic	▪ Altered mental status ▪ Encephalopathy ▪ Increased intracranial pressure ▪ Decreased cerebral perfusion pressure	▪ Increased thoracic pressure prevents jugular drainage to SVC
Cardiovascular	▪ Decreased venous return ▪ Decreased cardiac output ▪ Increased CVP, PAOP, SVR, PVR	▪ Inferior vena cava compression
Renal system	▪ Progressive oliguria ▪ Acute kidney injury	▪ Decreased renal blood flow ▪ Decreased renal perfusion

CVP, central venous pressure; IAH, intra-abdominal hypertension; LFTs, liver function tests; PAOP, pulmonary artery occlusion pressure; PVR, pulmonary vascular resistance; SVC, superior vena cava; SVR, systemic vascular resistance.

straining. Next, clamp the Foley and instill 50 mL sterile saline into the bladder. Ensure no air is in the catheter and continuous fluid is present from the clamp to the patient. Connect a transducer to the monitor and the other into the Foley. Level the transducer with the mons pubis and record the number. Normal IAP is 0 to 12 mmHg. IAH is an IAP >12 mmHg. ACS is defined as sustained IAP >20 mmHg with new organ dysfunction or abdominal perfusion pressure (APP) <50 mmHg. The APP is measured by subtracting the IAP from the mean arterial pressure (MAP) as follows:

$$APP = MAP - IAP$$

All high-risk patients should be screened for IAH. Obtain an IAP if two or more risk factors are present. Serial measurements every 4 hours should be obtained to monitor trends in the IAH. APP should be maintained 50 to 60 mmHg to ensure adequate perfusion to the organs.

FAST FACTS

Patients who present with a distended and firm abdomen, oliguria, high peak airway pressures, tachycardia, and hypotension should be suspected for ACS. The nurse should notify providers of these symptoms.

Treatment of Abdominal Compartment Syndrome
Treatment goals of ACS include reducing IAP and contents, such as ensuring the NGT is working properly, evacuating any excess blood or fluid by paracentesis, and evacuating stool from the colon and rectum. Additionally, abdominal muscle resistance should be reduced with analgesics and sedatives. Paralytic agents may be required. Surgical decompression may be warranted. Surgeons should be apprised of the IAP trends. Alternatively, patients who are at high risk and have had abdominal surgery may be preemptively left open. Tertiary compartment syndrome can occur when the laparotomy incision is insufficient to allow the bowels to expand.

Respiratory Complications

Early respiratory complications of abdominal trauma include ARDS, TRALI and transfusion-associated circulatory overload, and acute hypoxic respiratory failure. Later complications include atelectasis, hospital-acquired or ventilator-associated pneumonia, and failure to wean from the ventilator.

Other

Other complications of abdominal trauma include acute kidney injury, malnutrition, skin breakdown, enterocutaneous fistula, and venous thromboembolism, including deep vein thrombosis and pulmonary embolism.

SUMMARY

In summary, abdominal trauma requires nurses to perform frequent reassessment to monitor for ongoing clinical signs of bleeding and complications. Maintaining patency and functioning of NGTs is imperative to prevent vomiting and aspiration. Postoperatively, nurses must monitor surgical drain color and quantify the volume of output to recognize complications early. Any changes should immediately be reported to the team.

REVIEW QUESTIONS

1. Which of the following is a sign that bowel function has returned after surgery?
   a. Bowel sounds present
   b. Absence of nausea
   c. Passing flatus
   d. Absence of bowel movements

2. Patients who have had a splenectomy are at high risk for:
   a. Renal failure
   b. ST-elevation myocardial infarction
   c. Bowel obstruction
   d. Overwhelming postsplenectomy infection
3. A trauma patient has blood at the urethral meatus. The provider writes an order to place a Foley catheter. What is the nurse's best course of action?
   a. Place the Foley
   b. Challenge the order
   c. Call urology to place the Foley
   d. Place a coude catheter
4. A patient involved in a head-on collision hit his head on the windshield. Sixteen hours later, he reports right lower quadrant pain and nausea. Exam reveals a distended abdomen, tender to palpation, with guarding. What is the most likely diagnosis?
   a. Bowel injury
   b. Liver injury
   c. Splenic injury
   d. Pancreatic injury
5. A patient involved in a bicycle crash with the handlebars impacting his epigastric area is diagnosed with pancreatic and splenic injuries. He has had his splenic artery embolized. He required 4 units of packed red blood cells, 4 units fresh frozen plasma, and 1 unit of platelets, as well as 6 L of fluid resuscitation. His abdomen is distended and firm. He has progressively become more oliguric, tachycardic, and tachypneic on the ventilator. The ventilator keeps alarming high-peak airway pressures. The most likely diagnosis is:
   a. ARDS
   b. Bowel injury
   c. Acute kidney injury
   d. Abdominal compartment syndrome

References

Al-Thani, H., El-Matbouly, M., El-Menyar, A., Al-Hassani, A., Jogol, H., El-Faramawy, A., Siddiqui, T., & Abdelrahman, H. (2021). Adrenal gland trauma: An observational descriptive analysis from a level 1-trauma center. *Journal of Emergencies, Trauma, and Shock*, *14*(2), 92–97. https://doi.org/10.4103/JETS.JETS_63_20

American College of Surgeons: The Committee on Trauma. (2018). *ATLS: Advanced Trauma Life support student course manual* (10th ed.). American College of Surgeons.

Engelsgjerd, J. S., & LaGrange, C. A. (2023, January). *Ureteral injury*. [Updated July 5, 2022]. StatPearls Publishing. https://www.ncbi.nlm.nih.gov/books/NBK507817/

Habrat, D. (2023). *How to do diagnostic peritoneal lavage (DPL)*. Merck Manual. https://www.merckmanuals.com/professional/

critical-care-medicine/how-to-do-other-emergency-medicine-procedures/how-to-do-diagnostic-peritoneal-lavage-dpl

Hsu, J. M., & Pham, T. N. (2011, January). Damage control in the injured patient. *International Journal of Critical Illness and Injury Science, 1*(1), 66–72. https://doi.org/10.4103/2229-5151.79285

Kang, L., & Geube, A. (2023, January). *Bladder trauma*. [Updated May 22, 2023]. StatPearls Publishing. https://www.ncbi.nlm.nih.gov/books/NBK557875/

Kirkpatrick, A. W., Roberts, D. J., De Waele, J., Jaeschke, R., Malbrain, M. L., De Keulenaer, B., Duchesne, J., Bjorck, M., Leppaniemi, A., Ejike, J. C., Sugrue, M., Cheatham, M., Ivatury, R., Ball, C. G., Reintam Blaser, A., Regli, A., Balogh, Z. J., D'Amours, S., Debergh, D., Kaplan K., Kimball E, Olvera C; Pediatric Guidelines Sub-Committee for the World Society of the Abdominal Compartment Syndrome. (2013). Intra-abdominal hypertension and the abdominal compartment syndrome: Updated consensus definitions and clinical practice guidelines from the World Society of the Abdominal Compartment Syndrome. *Intensive Care Medicine, 39*, 1190–1206.

Mahan, M. E., & Toy, F. K. (2023, January). *Rectal trauma*. [Updated July 4, 2022]. StatPearls Publishing. https://www.ncbi.nlm.nih.gov/books/NBK551636/

McQuillan, K. A., & Flynn-Makic, M. B. (2020). *Trauma nursing: From resuscitation through rehabilitation* (5th ed.). Elsevier.

Singh, S., & Sookraj, K. (2023, January). *Kidney trauma*. [Updated July 18, 2022]. StatPearls Publishing. https://www.ncbi.nlm.nih.gov/books/NBK532896/

Taghavi, S., & Askari, R. (2023, January). *Liver trauma*. [Updated April 27, 2023]. StatPearls Publishing. https://www.ncbi.nlm.nih.gov/books/NBK513236/

Tahir, F., Ahmed, J., & Malik, F. (2020, February 6). Post-splenectomy sepsis: A review of the literature. *Cureus, 12*(2), e6898. https://doi.org/10.7759/cureus.6898

Genitourinary and Gynecologic Injuries and Care
Dawn Carpenter

Genitourinary and gynecologic injuries are rare but may be serious. The mechanism of injury and injury pattern can increase suspicion and prompt further assessment for such injuries. Most are the result of blunt mechanism of injury from direct impact to the back, flank, or abdomen.

In this chapter, you will learn:
1. Key components of genitourinary (GU) assessment.
2. How to identify common causes of GU trauma.
3. How to identify etiology of gynecologic (GYN) injuries.
4. How to articulate the care of patients with GU injuries.

INTRODUCTION

GU trauma occurs in about 10% of all trauma patients, with most affecting the kidney. The GU tract is divided into the upper and lower tracts. The upper GU tract comprises the kidney and ureters, whereas the lower tract comprises the bladder, urethra, penis, scrotum, and testes. GYN injuries include injuries to the vagina, uterus, and ovaries. Additionally, the patient interview may include sensitive topics such as sexual assault as well as sensitive assessments, including GYN exams.

GENITOURINARY ASSESSMENT

Inspection
Inspect for abrasions, ecchymosis, and hematoma on the posterior chest, flanks, and upper abdomen to identify renal injuries. Inspect for ecchymosis, edema, laceration, or wounds to the testes, mons pubis, labia, vagina, perineum, buttocks, and rectum. Be sure to inspect between skin folds and under buttocks for bleeding, abrasions, and open wounds. Pelvic fractures and penetrating projectiles can invade the vagina or rectum and are considered open fractures with contaminated wounds. Observe for blood at the

meatus. A Foley catheter should not be placed by nursing if blood is noted at the meatus. Inspect the color and quality of urine, if produced.

> **FAST FACTS**
>
> Nurses should not place a Foley catheter in a trauma patient who has blood at the urethral meatus.

Palpation

Palpate the abdomen and flanks, including the costovertebral angle for bulges. A digital rectal exam is part of the gastrointestinal exam but includes palpation of the prostate. A high-riding prostate might indicate a urethral injury in men. Assess for costovertebral angle tenderness.

Adjuncts to Assessment

In severely injured patients, assessment of the GU/GYN tract may require placement of a Foley catheter. Bleeding noted from the urethra, penis, or vagina requires additional diagnostic testing and may require surgical intervention. Gross hematuria in the setting of a blunt trauma causing pelvic fractures is an absolute indication for further diagnostic tests of the lower GU tract. A urinalysis will show microscopic hematuria and can clue the team in to subtle injuries.

Diagnostic Testing

A pelvic x-ray done during the secondary survey can identify life-threatening pelvic fractures that can cause injury to the GU system. All trauma patients with child-bearing organs should have a urine human chorionic gonadotropin (HCG) level. If positive, a serum HCG test should be performed to confirm the pregnancy and identify the gestation of the pregnancy.

CT scans of the abdomen and pelvis are required in severely injured trauma patients. Additional studies, including a CT cystogram, may be needed to evaluate the bladder for contrast extravasation. If present, this is highly suggestive of bladder rupture. Consultation with a urologist is commonly required to evaluate for possible urethral injury or transection.

GYNECOLOGIC ASSESSMENT

A detailed history surrounding the injury is important to provide thorough care. Careful questioning in a one-on-one format can be useful to elicit whether a sexual assault occurred. Pay careful attention to the relationship and interactions with visitors. Visitors or family refusing to leave the patient's side can provide clues to potential sexual assault and sex trafficking of individuals. Ask visitors to step out of the room during interview and examinations. Critically appraise whether injury patterns correlate with the given history of the injury.

Inspection

For patients with a history and mechanism of injury that includes straddle injuries and sexual assault, a GYN assessment should be performed. A GYN assessment includes inspection of the mons pubis, labia majora, labia minora, clitoris, vagina, cervix and ovaries, as well as rectum if not already done during the gastrointestinal assessment.

Trauma to the female genitalia may have psychological implications if the mechanism of injury is the result of sexual abuse or assault. Any patient with genital injury should be screened for sexual abuse. The nurse should offer appropriate police reporting and engage social services to support the patient. Assessment includes a detailed history and thorough physical exam. If available, nursing should engage a specially trained sexual assault nurse examiner (SANE) to assist with performing a "rape kit" and evidence collection.

The GYN exam starts by inspecting the external genitalia, looking for ecchymosis, edema, contusions, hematomas, or lacerations. An internal speculum exam should then be completed by the trauma team or gynecology to assess for lacerations or injuries from pelvic bone fractures. Consultation with obstetrics and/or gynecology (OB/GYN) may be indicated. These exams may be done in the operating room following other more urgent procedures.

GENITOURINARY INJURIES

GU injuries include injuries to the kidney, ureter, bladder, and urethra. Classic signs of renal trauma include ecchymosis, contusions, and hematomas on the back or flank areas. Frank hematuria and microscopic hematuria both warrant further investigation for GU injuries.

Kidney

Renal trauma is rare, with only 1% to 5% of trauma patients experiencing it, and over 80% of cases are the result of blunt force trauma. The kidneys are protected by the rib cage and are seated deep in the retroperitoneal space. Renal injuries are graded on a scale of 1 to 5, with 1 being least injured and 5 being the worst. The most severe form of renal injury is caused by sudden deceleration, which can cause an avulsion of the renal pedicle, resulting in devascularization of the kidney. Penetrating injuries may cause other vascular injuries to the kidney, including pseudoaneurysm or arteriovenous fistula. Over 85% of patients with renal injuries have other concomitant injuries that are associated with mortality. Clinical signs of renal injury include tenderness, pain, or ecchymosis in the flank, abdomen, or back.

The patient's posterior chest, abdomen, and flank should be thoroughly assessed. The presence of hematoma, abrasions, and ecchymosis elevates the suspicion for renal trauma. Hematuria is suspicious for renal injury but is not definitive, as other parts of the GU tract may be injured. A CT scan of the abdomen with IV contrast will demonstrate the injury and the extent.

Nonoperative management with observation is most common with grade 1 to 3 injuries. Selective arterial embolization is preferred to preserve kidney function and prevent surgical nephrectomy. Complications of renal injury include ongoing bleeding. Additionally, delayed bleeding, although rare, may be noted 2 to 3 weeks after injury and is likely related to an arteriovenous malformation or pseudoaneurysm.

Ureter

Ureteral injuries are rare, but when they occur, they are caused primarily by penetrating trauma. Clinical signs of ureteral trauma are quite subtle, with few outward signs. Ureteral injuries are graded from 1 to 5, with grade 1 being the least injured, with a hematoma, and grade 5 being completely avulsed and devascularized. Ureteral injuries are often very difficult to notice but can be identified during an exploratory laparotomy. Delayed diagnosis is common when patients report persistent flank or abdominal pain, prolonged ileus, or urinary tract infection. Laboratory values may demonstrate elevated blood urea nitrogen and creatinine. Hydronephrosis may be seen on CT scan or renal ultrasound. If a surgical drain is present, the fluid can be sent for creatinine and compared with serum creatinine. Creatinine in the fluid will usually be much higher than serum creatinine, ranging widely from 25 to 450 mg/dL. If the fluid is serous, it will be similar to the serum creatinine. Complications of missed ureteral injuries include intra-abdominal urinoma, abscess, ureteral stricture, and potential loss of the affected kidney.

Bladder

Injury to the bladder is rare, occuring in about 1.6% of trauma patients. Bladder injuries are divided into intraperitoneal and extraperitoneal injuries. Intraperitoneal injuries are caused by impact to a full bladder, rupturing at the dome of the bladder, requiring surgical intervention to close the defect. Extraperitoneal injuries are typically the result of pelvic fractures and can be managed by an indwelling Foley catheter for 10 to 14 days. Bladder injuries should have consultation with a urologist and follow-up with a urologist in the clinic before the Foley catheter is removed. Extraperitoneal injuries comprise 60% of all bladder injuries. Retrograde CT cystography is indicated for stable patients who have blood at the meatus; gross hematuria; pelvic fracture with microscopic hematuria; or penetrating injury to the pelvis, buttock, or lower abdomen to assess the bladder for extravasation.

Urethra

Urethral injuries are rare. Urethral injuries include bruising, laceration, transection, and crush injuries. They commonly present with blood at the urethral meatus, urinary retention, or suprapubic fullness. Perineal ecchymosis or hematoma can represent a straddle injury. Urethral injuries are graded on a scale of 1 to 5, with 1 being least severe to 5 being most severe. Urethral injuries include contusions, stretch injuries, partial or complete disruption, and complete transection. Grade 1 injuries do not typically require treatment. Grades 2 and 3 are typically treated nonoperatively with Foley catheterization for 10 to 14 days. Grades 4 and 5 commonly require surgical repair. Consultation with urology is required for surgical repair of urethral injuries. Suprapubic diversion of urine is commonly required to allow for healing.

FAST FACTS

Patients who have urethral injuries should not be on the nurse-driven protocol for Foley catheter removal, because the catheter may need to stay for 10 to 14 days.

Nursing Care of Patients with Kidney, Ureter, Bladder, and Urethral Injuries

For patients with kidney injuries, the nurse should monitor for signs of ongoing bleeding, including increased abdominal, flank, and back pain. Serial hemoglobin and hematocrit levels may be warranted for higher grade injuries. Monitor for other concomitant injuries, such as bowel injuries that may not readily be apparent on initial presentation. Signs of peritonitis include abdominal pain, nausea, vomiting, distention, rebound tenderness, and guarding.

Hematuria is expected with injury to the GU system. However, frank hematuria and clots should be reported to the providers. Nurses are responsible for maintaining patency of the Foley catheter. Irrigation may be required to keep the catheter patent. In patients with traumatic injuries to the bladder and urethra, especially those with surgical repairs, be sure to discuss with the providers the appropriateness of any irrigation, to avoid further injury or disruption of the surgical repair. The most severe cases of hematuria may require a continuous bladder irrigation via a three-way catheter. Irrigation flow should be sufficient to keep the catheter free from clots.

Penile Injury

Penile injuries are rare but are mostly associated with motorcycle and bicycle crashes. Penile injuries are graded on a scale of 1 to 5, with 1 being least severe and 5 being most severe. Penile injuries include lacerations, avulsions, partial or total penectomy, and penile fractures.

Penile fracture is mostly associated with sexual intercourse and is described as an acute bending of the penis, followed by a pop, acute pain, and immediate detumescence. These patients may have a delayed presentation due to embarrassment. Edema of the penis is common, with the penis having an "eggplant deformity." The penis typically deviates to the contralateral side of the injury. Ultrasound of the penis may be indicated if the history of the injury is not consistent with penile fracture and can help identify the location of the tear.

Traumatic amputation of the penis is extremely rare. The severed penis should be rinsed with sterile saline, wrapped in a saline-moistened gauze, placed in a plastic bag, and immersed in a second bag containing icy cold water. Avoid placing directly on ice. Reimplantation is possible within 16 hours of cold ischemic time or 6 hours of warm ischemic time.

FAST FACTS

Never place a severed limb or organ directly on ice. Rather, rinse with sterile normal saline, wrap in a moist saline gauze, and place in a plastic bag. Immerse in a second bag containing icy cold water.

Scrotal Injury

The scrotum contains the testes, vas deferens, and epididymis. Scrotal injuries include contusion, lacerations, and avulsions and are graded on a scale of 1 to 5, with 1 being least severe and 5 being most severe. Scrotal injuries commonly require exploration and evacuation of hematomas.

Testicular Injury

Testicular injuries are rare because of their location and mobility, occurring mostly with sporting injuries or motorcycle crashes in which the testes are impacted by the pelvic bones into the gas tank. Eighty percent of testicular injuries are associated with other injuries in the region. Most often, testicular injury occurs unilaterally and rarely bilaterally. Testicular injuries are graded on a scale of 1 to 5, with 1 being least severe and 5 being most severe. Types of injuries include contusions, hematomas, lacerations, and testicular avulsion. Blunt scrotal trauma may result in a ruptured testis. The most common symptom is extreme pain, rapid swelling, and nausea. Ecchymosis is variable. The degree of injury does not correlate with the size of the hematoma. Pain and blood in the tunica vaginalis compartment commonly limit the physical exam. Testicular ultrasound is the study of choice to assess for injury. The priority of the ultrasound is to determine testicular integrity and blood flow.

Nursing Care of Patients with Penile, Scrotal, and Testicular Injuries

Nursing care of the patient with penile, scrotal, or testicular injuries includes elevation. Use towel rolls under the scrotum to support it. Alternatively, a pillowcase or towel can be used as a sling. Apply ice packs for pain control, but do not apply ice directly to the tissues. Maintain the Foley catheter as directed by the team. These patients may require prolonged catheterization and should not be on a nurse-driven protocol for removal, because reinsertion may be exceptionally difficult. Consultation with urology is common, and the urology team will guide the decision for catheter removal.

GYNECOLOGICAL INJURIES

GYN injuries are less common because the organs are protected by the pelvis. Vaginal and vulvar injuries are the most common. Injury to the uterus and ovaries is rare in nonpregnant individuals. Pregnancy-related injuries are covered in Chapter 18. The term *vulva* refers to all external female structures, including the mons pubis, labia majora, labia minora, clitoris, and vestibule. Lacerations to the labia minora and posterior fourchette commonly occur during both consensual and nonconsensual sexual intercourse. Whereas straddle injuries most commonly result in vulvar hematomas.

Vaginal and Vulvar Injuries

Trauma to the vagina and vulva may occur due to assault or accidentally. Vaginal and vulvar trauma is rare, occurring in less than .2% of all trauma victims. Over two thirds of these injuries occur to the vagina, with less than one third injuring the vulva. Anterior pelvic ring fractures may cause vaginal lacerations. These are considered open fractures and require antibiotics within the first hour after injury. Vaginal trauma is susceptible to hemorrhage due to the internal pudendal arterial blood supply. The primary causes of non–obstetric-related vaginal and vulvar trauma include sporting-related injuries, with bicycle-related injuries being the most common, followed by straddle/saddle injuries, crush injuries, penetrating injuries, and burns. Causes of nonaccidental trauma include sexual assault, rape, and/or abuse.

> **FAST FACTS**
>
> Anterior pelvic ring fractures may cause vaginal lacerations and are considered open fractures that require antibiotics within the first hour after injury.

Nursing Care of Patients with Genitourinary Injuries

Nursing care of patients with GYN injuries, includes asking patients the date of their last menstrual period and possibility of pregnancy. The nurse should obtain a urine HCG test for all patients with child-bearing organs. If the result is positive, a serum HCG test should be performed to identify the gestation of the pregnancy. HCG levels can remain elevated in the postpartum period, returning to normal in 4 to 6 weeks. A fetus is deemed viable if it is over 24 weeks.

> **FAST FACTS**
>
> The nurse should obtain a urine HCG test for all persons with child-bearing organs.

SUMMARY

In summary, GU trauma is less common than injuries to other body systems. GU trauma commonly has other concomitant injuries. Renal and vaginal trauma may cause significant blood loss. Pelvic fractures that lacerate the vagina are considered open fractures and require antibiotics immediately. Nursing care of patients with GYN trauma requires attention to body language and relationships. Nurses are on the front line to recognize sex trafficking and assaults.

REVIEW QUESTIONS

1. Nurses who are caring for an adult who has been sexually assaulted should:
   a. Consult psychiatry
   b. Refer to social work
   c. Report it to the police
   d. Plan for discharge home
2. A trauma patient presents after a bicycle crash, and the secondary exam reveals blood at the meatus. The nurse should:
   a. Consult urology
   b. Place a Foley catheter
   c. Place a three-way catheter
   d. Notify the trauma team leader
3. The nurse is caring for a patient who was struck by a vehicle and sustained a pelvic fracture and associated urethral injury. The Foley catheter was placed by urology in the operating room after surgical repair. On hospital day 2, the nurse should:
   a. Initiate continuous bladder irrigation
   b. Remove the Foley catheter per the nurse driven-protocol
   c. Assess the urine output for color, quantity, and presence of clots
   d. Place the Foley catheter to gentle traction to tamponade any bleeding

References

American College of Surgeons: The Committee on Trauma. (2018). *ATLS: Advanced Trauma Life Support student course manual* (10th ed.). American College of Surgeons.

Coccolini, F., Moore, E. E., Kluger, Y., Biffl, W., Leppaniemi, A., Matsumura, Y., Kim, F., Peitzman, A. B., Fraga, G. P., Sartelli, M., Ansaloni, L., Augustin, G., Kirkpatrick, A., Abu-Zidan, F., Wani, I., Weber, D., Pikoulis, E., Larrea, M., Arvieux, C., & Catena, F. (2019). Kidney and uro-trauma: WSES-AAST guidelines. *World Journal of Emergency Surgery, 14*(1), 1–25.

Coppola, M. J., & Moskovitz, J. (2019). Emergency diagnosis and management of genitourinary trauma. *Emergency Medicine Clinics, 37*(4), 611–635.

Engelsgjerd, J. S., & LaGrange, C. A. (2023, January). *Ureteral injury*. [Updated July 5, 2022]. StatPearls Publishing. https://www.ncbi.nlm.nih.gov/books/NBK507817/

Gambhir, S., Grigorian, A., Schubl, S., Barrios, C., Bernal, N., Joe, V., Gabriel, V., & Nahmias, J. (2019). Analysis of non-obstetric vaginal and vulvar trauma: Risk factors for operative intervention. *Updates in Surgery, 71*, 735–740. https://doi.org/10.1007/s13304-019-00679-4

Kang, L., & Geube, A. (2023, January). *Bladder trauma*. [Updated May 22, 2023]. StatPearls Publishing. https://www.ncbi.nlm.nih.gov/books/NBK557875/

Singh, S., & Sookraj, K. (2023, January). *Kidney trauma*. [Updated July 18, 2022]. StatPearls Publishing. https://www.ncbi.nlm.nih.gov/books/NBK532896/

Tullington, J. E., & Blecker, N. (2022). *Lower genitourinary trauma*. StatPearls Publishing.

West, A., & Gan, C. (2022). Genitourinary trauma. *Surgery (Oxford), 40*(8), 540–549.

Musculoskeletal Injuries and Care
Alexander Menard

> The musculoskeletal (MSK) system encompasses the skeletal system (bones and joints) and the skeletal muscles, ligaments, and tendons. The bones and joints provide protection and support. In addition, the bones are reservoirs for mineral salts and fats, and produce red blood cells (hematopoiesis). MSK injuries may be life- or limb-threating. Nurses have a large role in assessment and management.

In this chapter, you will learn to:
1. Identify key elements of a musculoskeletal (MSK) exam.
2. Discuss nursing care of the patient with a pelvic fracture.
3. Identify complications associated with MSK injuries.

INTRODUCTION

Trauma frequently involves fractures to bones and injury to tendons and ligaments. Nurses commonly assess and care for patients with such injuries. Life-threatening injuries take precedence during initial evaluation and treatment, sometimes placing MSK injury identification and treatment after hemodynamic stabilization. MSK injuries can have long-lasting effects and reduce mobility and independence, thus affecting quality of life.

MUSCULOSKELETAL ASSESSMENT

The first exam of any trauma patient is the primary survey. Bleeding from an extremity is addressed in the circulation phase and may require direct pressure or a tourniquet to control the bleeding. Do not get distracted by extremity deformities if the patient is not hemorrhaging from the extremity. There is an increased focus on the MSK assessment during the secondary survey. During this time, baseline neurovascular and motor functions are assessed and documented. It is crucial to assess and document baseline function to determine whether a patient is improving, worsening, or staying the same. A systematic approach to the MSK exam ensures consistency and reduces the potential for an injury to be missed.

Inspection

Systematic inspection assesses for obvious signs of MSK injury, such as extremity deformity or bone protruding from skin. Other signs indicating potential injury include ecchymosis, edema, and visible muscle spasm, all of which may indicate an underlying MSK injury that needs to be evaluated further. Ecchymosis occurs because of vascular disruption that allows blood to disperse into the soft tissue. Muscle spasms may indicate an underlying MSK injury because they can be the body's response to attempt to splint and realign the underlying injury. Swelling is a result of soft tissue injury that prevents the usual flow of the venous and lymphatic systems, causing a backup of fluids, that is, swelling. Soft tissue injury or damage to cells of the body will trigger an inflammatory response. The inflammatory response triggers the release of inflammatory mediators that act to break down the damaged tissue and increase blood flow to the affected area. This response is directly related to the physical exam findings of redness and warmth in the affected area. There is also a recovery phase of the inflammatory response in which damaged cells are removed by a process called phagocytosis, and eventually cytokines and growth factor are released to begin repair of the damaged tissue.

Alterations in extremity color can be an indication of underlying MSK pathology. A pale-appearing extremity may indicate inadequate arterial blood flow, whereas a dusky/blueish appearance can indicate venous congestion. Importantly, patients with different skin tones/colors require comparison to the unaffected extremity. If the patient can communicate, it is reasonable to ask them to clarify the normal appearance of their extremities and skin.

Palpation

Each extremity must be fully palpated to assess for deformity, pain, crepitus, sensation, pulses, movement, and muscle spasm. Findings must be documented because each evaluation can indicate underlying pathology (Table 13.1).

Circulation, Sensation, and Movement Assessment

Circulation: Circulation is assessed in several different ways. First, a visual inspection: Does the extremity looked well perfused? A poorly perfused extremity will look pale, ashen, or even blue. It may feel cool or cold to the touch. Additional assessment will include the use of a Doppler machine, a device that detects sound waves that correlate to blood flow through a vessel. To detect a pulse, the nurse will place a small amount of petroleum jelly on the tip of the probe, turn on the Doppler, and place the probe on the skin to first detect a pulse and listen to the Doppler sounds, assessing for the quality and presence of the pulse.

Sensation: Sensation can be evaluated by asking the patient what they feel/sense. Does the extremity have paresthesias (tingling), which is a result of pressure on or damage to nerves? Further investigation into sensation

TABLE 13.1

Findings with Palpation of the MSK System

Assess for	Finding	Can Indicate
Deformity	▪ Misshapen, misaligned bone or joint	▪ Fractured bone, joint dislocation ▪ Arthritis, previous injury
Pain	▪ Palpation over site of suspected injury	▪ Fractured bone, damaged tissue, and joint damage
Crepitus	▪ A crunching or grating sound or sensation	▪ Fractured bone, joint damage
Sensation	▪ Inability to differentiate between sharp and dull, or loss of proprioception	▪ Neuronal compression or injury
Pulses and capillary refill	▪ Decreased pulses or capillary filling time <2 seconds	▪ Vascular compromise ▪ Compartment syndrome
Movement	▪ Decreased range of motion from baseline*	▪ Fractured bone, bone/joint dislocation, and neurovascular injury
Muscle spasm	▪ Presence of spasm ▪ Absence of spasm over injury	▪ May represent underlying fracture ▪ May indicate neuronal injury

MSK, musculoskeletal.

*Bones/joints with obvious injury should not be assessed for range of motion due to potential for further neurovascular injury.

---

would include sensing warmth or cold. This can be done by asking the patient to close their eyes, placing a warm or cool cloth onto their skin at various points on the body, and having them determine whether the cloth is warm or cool. Sensation assessment can continue with sharp and dull sensation, which can be done using a wooden cotton swab. Using the cotton side as soft and the bare wood side as sharp, the nurse gently rubs either side of the swab along the patient's skin and asks them to report whether the feeling is sharp (wooden tip) or dull (cotton tip).

Motion assessment: Motor strength must also be assessed and documented. It is important to note that motor function and strength can be limited due to pain. Appropriate pain management should be implemented to achieve an accurate exam. Strength can be assessed and scored by the motor strength grading scale (Table 13.2).

FAST FACTS

A systematic approach to assessing the MSK system ensures consistency in the nurse's assessment and reduces the chance of missing an injury.

TABLE 13.2

Strength Grading Scale

Grade	Description
0	No muscle movement detected in visual inspection or palpation
1	Visible or palpable muscle contractions only
2	Active movement when gravity is eliminated
3	Movement against gravity but without any resistance
4	Active movement against gravity and moderate resistance from the nurse
5	Active movement against gravity and full resistance from the nurse
NT	Unable to assess strength due to severe pain, immobilization, contracture, and so forth

MUSCULOSKELETAL INJURIES

Approximately 66 million MSK injuries occur each year in the United States. The major causes of traumatic MSK injuries are motor vehicle crashes, falls, industrial/home/farming accidents, and interpersonal violence. When a patient presents with an MSK injury, the nurse must also suspect other injuries to the body. MSK injuries encompass strains/sprains, contusions, dislocations, crush injuries, open wounds, and amputations.

Fractures

Fractures are the most common MSK injury and are considered either closed or open. Several other descriptors for types of fractures are used to describe the fracture pattern (Figure 13.1).

FAST FACTS

Common signs of an MSK injury include edema, ecchymosis, hematoma, pain, difficulty moving the affected body part, pain with movement, and altered sensation.

Upper Extremity Injury

Humerus fracture: A humerus fracture is usually a result of a direct or indirect trauma. The patient with a humerus fracture will commonly have erythema to the affected limb and pain with movement and will often support the elbow of the affected limb for support. The treatment for most humerus fractures is nonoperative and includes a sling and progressive rehabilitation.

Chapter 13 Musculoskeletal Injuries and Care 179

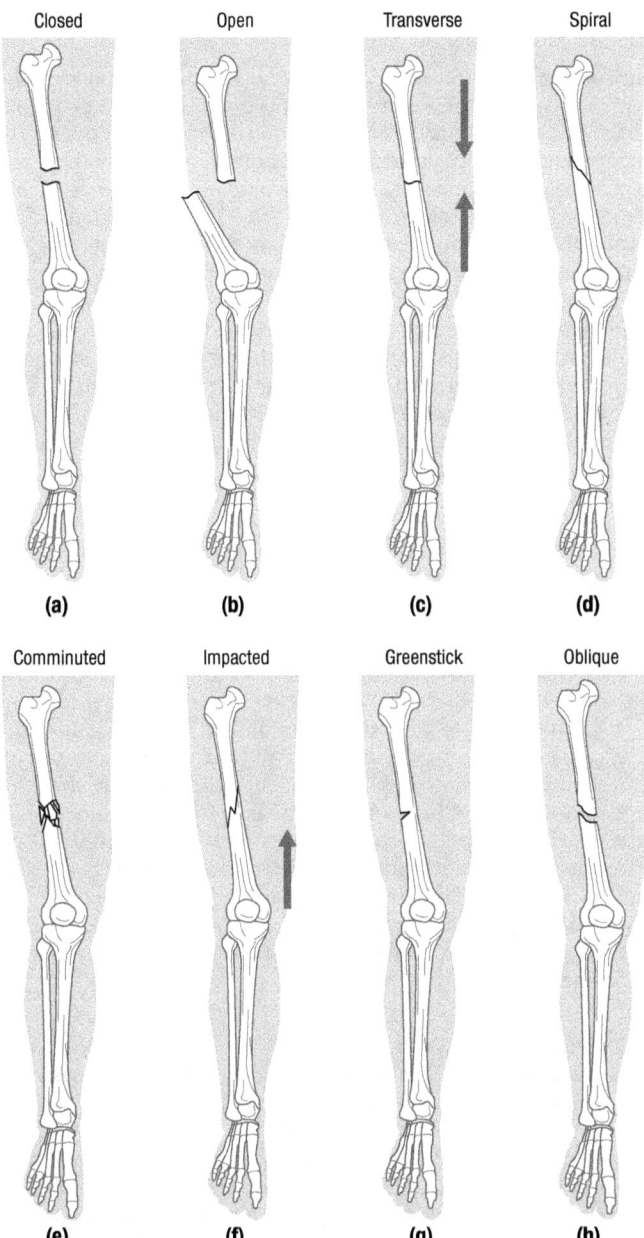

Figure 13.1 Types of fractures.
Source: https://upload.wikimedia.org/wikipedia/commons/3/35/612_Types_of_Fractures.jpg.

More complicated and multilevel fractures may require operative fixation as determined by the orthopedic specialist.

Radius and ulnar fractures: Distal radius fractures are among the most common fractures treated. Radius and ulnar fractures present with pain and sometimes visible deformity. Depending on the fracture, proper alignment and casting may be the treatment; however, more frequently these fractures require surgical correction with plates and screws to return structure and integrity to the bone. A Colles fracture is a break in the distal radius with dorsal comminution, dorsal angulation, dorsal displacement, and radial shortening and may be associated with an ulnar styloid fracture. This is often a result of a fall landing on an outstretched hand with the wrist in dorsiflexion.

Scapula fracture: Scapular fractures are uncommon and indicate high-energy trauma and are accompanied by other multisystem injuries. These fractures often cause pain with shoulder movement. Diagnosis is made with an x-ray and/or CT scan. Most often the treatment for scapula fractures is short-term immobilization with a sling, followed by shoulder exercises to prevent a "frozen shoulder," also known as adhesive capsulitis.

Clavicle fracture: Clavicular fractures are most commonly the result of a direct blow to the clavicle. Most often, the middle third of the clavicle is fractured. Typically, there is an obvious deformity of the affected clavicle, and patients report edema, tenderness, and ecchymosis; at times, crepitus is noted.

Nursing Care of Upper Extremity Injuries

Nursing care for the patient with an upper extremity fracture includes resting the extremity and providing immobility, support, and movement restriction with a sling, brace, or cast. When any device is placed on a patient, it is imperative to complete frequent neurovascular checks, which include testing sensation, movement, capillary refill, and pulse distal to the sling, brace, or cast. Any abnormal finding, such as decreased pulse, capillary refill, and sensation or unintended restriction to movement, should be reported. As swelling occurs, the sling, brace, or cast may become too tight and may need to be loosened or modified by the orthopedic team. Use RICE (rest, ice, compression, and elevation), if not contraindicated, to limit bleeding and edema.

Lower Extremity Injury

Pelvic fracture: The pelvis is a large structure that encompasses several structures (Figure 13.2). *Pelvic fracture* is a broad term referring to fractures of the bones of the pelvis, including the pelvic ring, iliac crest/wing, pubic bone, acetabulum, ischium, sacrum, or coccyx. Pelvic fractures most often occur in the setting of high-impact/energy injuries or in patients with osteoporosis or osteopenia. Pelvic fractures are commonly associated with other injuries. The most severe pelvic fractures often result from motor vehicle collisions, falling from a height, or a pedestrian or cyclist being struck by a vehicle.

Pelvic girdle

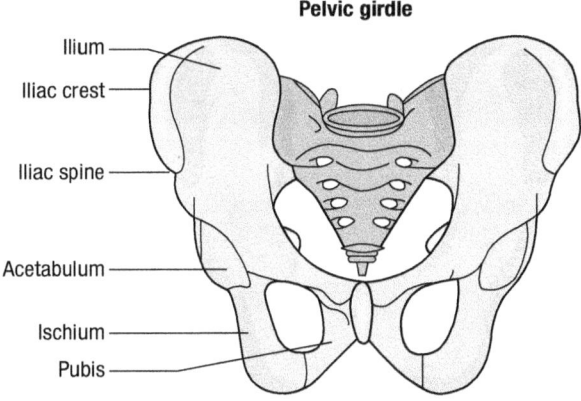

Figure 13.2 The structures of the pelvis.
Source: https://commons.wikimedia.org/wiki/File:Pelvic_girdle_illustration.svg.

The pelvic ring forms from the sacrum, ilium, ischium, and pubis (Figure 13.2). The strong structure of the pelvic ring comes from these bones and the strong ligamentous attachments that maintain the ring's structure. For ring displacement to occur, there must be disruptions in at least two sites. Damage to the pelvic ring is most concerning and leads to unstable fractures. The pelvic bones are highly vascular, and injury to them may lead to significant bleeding and hemorrhagic shock.

A pelvic binder can be placed over the greater trochanter to stabilize the pelvic ring and to help control/tamponade internal bleeding. In cases of vertical shear pelvic injuries, skeletal traction may be used for stabilization. Additionally, patients can be taken to the operating room for external fixation of the pelvis to provide pelvic stability and help staunch the bleeding in those who are hemodynamically unstable.

Hip fracture: A hip fracture is a result of a fracture to one of four areas of the upper femur (Figure 13.3). In the figure, the femoral head is noted as #1, the femoral neck as #2, the intertrochanteric area as #3, and the subtrochanteric area as #4.

Hip fractures, or fractures of the proximal femur, are common in the geriatric population, but high-impact/energy trauma may also cause an acute hip fracture in the younger adult population. Intertrochanteric and femoral neck fractures are the most frequently seen hip fractures. Femoral head fractures are rare and should prompt the nurse to suspect a high-velocity trauma.

Determining the underlying cause of a hip fracture is as important as managing the fracture. For example, for a "fall" causing a hip fracture, it must be determined whether it was a result of a syncopal episode or mechanical fall. A pathologic hip fracture may also be caused by malignancy or

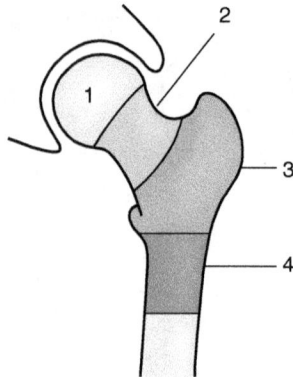

Figure 13.3 Hip fracture types.

Sources: https://upload.wikimedia.org/wikipedia/commons/8/8e/Hip_fracture_types.jpg; Doctodoc, CC BY-SA 4.0 <https://creativecommons.org/licenses/by-sa/4.0>, via Wikimedia Commons.

TABLE 13.3
Blood Loss Cause by Fractures

Humerus	500 to 1,500 mL
Radius/ulnar	250 to 500 mL
Pelvis	750 to 6,000 mL
Femur	500 to 3,000 mL
Tibia/fibula	250 to 2,500 mL
Ankle	250 to 1,000 mL

osteoporosis. Most hip fractures are diagnosed with x-rays, including anteroposterior and lateral views. Less than 10% of hip fractures are not seen on x-ray and are diagnosed by CT or MRI of the hip. The gold standard for diagnosing a suspected hip fracture not seen on x-ray is MRI.

Bleeding is a primary focus of care. Blood loss may be in excess of 1 L of blood from a proximal femur (hip fracture). See Table 13.3 for blood loss volumes by fracture. Thus, nurses must monitor for signs of hemorrhagic shock. Anticoagulants are common in older adults; thus, reversal agents require timely administration. Transfusions are commonly required; thus, it is important to ensure that the patient has an active type and screen in the blood bank. The goal of treatment of hip fractures is to restore the patient's mobility and control pain. Operative repair is the mainstay of treatment.

FAST FACTS

Hip fractures may result in massive blood loss due to the highly vascularized region.

Femur fracture: One of the most common fractures treated by orthopedic surgeons, femur fractures often result from high-energy mechanisms of injury. The components of the femur include the femoral head, neck, intertrochanteric, subtrochanteric, shaft, supracondylar, and condylar regions. Younger patients generally experience high-energy mechanisms of injury such as motor vehicle collisions, whereas older patients sustain osteoporotic femur fractures from ground-level falls. Femur fractures are immobilized temporarily with traction splints. Femur fractures, aside from hip fractures, can induce large amounts of blood loss, in the range of 500 to 3,000 mL.

The gold standard for treatment is intramural nailing. The goal of this treatment is early healing and functional recovery. Given the highly innervated and vascularized area the femur resides in, it is important for nurses to complete neurovascular checks initially, before and after traction is applied, and after surgical stabilization. Any changes must be reported to the primary team.

Knee: For the patient with a knee injury, a knee immobilizer or posterior long-leg plaster splint is effective in maintaining stability and comfort. The knee should not be immobilized in a position less than 10 degrees of flexion to reduce strain on neurovascular structures. Nurses should remove the splint to perform skin assessment, monitoring for pressure injuries and signs of deep vein thrombosis (DVT).

Tibia/fibula: Tibial fractures occur in a bimodal pattern including low- and high-energy mechanisms of injury. Low-energy injury is a result of a torsional force resulting in a spiral fracture with or without an associated fibular fracture at a different level with minimal surrounding soft tissue injury. Conversely, high-energy mechanism injury typically results from direct trauma causing wedge or short oblique fractures. Fractures with significant comminution are associated with increased soft tissue injury, which may lead to compartment syndrome.

Foot and ankle fractures: Foot fractures are among the most commonly missed injuries during the primary survey of the trauma patient. Complex trauma of the foot involves a range of injuries including fractures, fracture dislocations, extensive bone and cartilage comminution, and soft tissue damage. The most common injured site of the hindfoot is the calcaneus, often associated with a fall or jump from height landing on the feet. The foot and ankle are a complex set of bones, ligaments, and joints that require early assessment and intervention with a specialist to maximize recovery.

Nursing Care of Lower Extremities

In the case of pelvic fractures, limiting pelvic motion is essential because the pelvis is highly vascularized. This is also true for all lower extremity fractures because a large amount of blood can pool in the lower extremities, resulting in hemorrhagic shock. It is prudent to measure the lower extremity girth (in a consistent location) if there are concerns for bleeding because an expanding extremity might indicate accumulation of blood, and that, coupled with unstable vital signs, will require prompt notification of the care team.

Neurovascular and pulse assessments are critical for the patient with lower extremity fractures because vasculature and nerve roots/pathways track along with bones, and fractures can cause vesicular or nerve disruption. Standard care of fractures includes RICE, if not contraindicated, to limit bleeding and edema.

Spinal Fractures

Injuries to the spine must always be suspected, regardless of whether patients present disability. Minimize manipulation of the spine until definitive assessment and diagnostics can be done. The spinal column has 7 cervical, 12 thoracic, and 5 lumbar vertebrae as well as the sacrum and coccyx (Figure 13.4).

Spinal fractures can be classified as stable or unstable. A stable fracture is not a threat to the spinal cord, whereas an unstable fracture is at risk of causing paralysis. There are several types of vertebral injuries (Table 13.4). When these injuries are reported, they are denoted by injury type and location within the vertebral column. Vertebral anatomy is depicted in Figure 13.5 and will be helpful in interpreting Table 13.4.

Nursing Care of Spinal Fractures

Strict log roll precautions must be maintained until the spine is cleared and/or specific precautions are clearly ordered (e.g., Thoracic and lumbar spine cleared. Okay to elevate head of bed [HOB] 45 degrees. Must always maintain C-spine precautions and hard cervical collar). Thorough neurologic exams must be completed on the patient with a spinal column injury, particularly before and after any interventions. Patients who require a hard cervical collar must have the pads changed and cleaned, and the skin must be inspected to ensure injuries are not missed and pressure injuries from the collar are avoided or detected early. The HOB should be elevated as soon as possible to avoid aspiration. If the HOB cannot be elevated, it is reasonable to place the patient with cervical, thoracic, and/or lumbar spine precautions in reverse Trendelenberg while awaiting official spine clearance or stabilization to maintain spinal precautions and assist with breathing mechanics. Cervical spinal cord injuries are commonly associated with head injuries, which require the HOB to be at a minimum of 30 degrees.

Complications of Musculoskeletal Injuries

Complications related to MSK injuries vary widely, from venous thromboembolism (VTE), to tetanus, to nerve injury. Prevention is key to avoiding MSK complications. Early detection is the next best course of action to reduce the negative impacts of the following potential complications.

Chapter 13 Musculoskeletal Injuries and Care 185

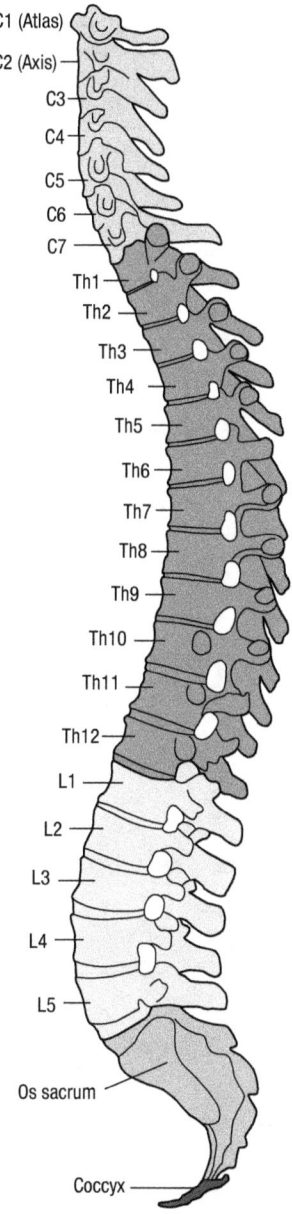

Figure 13.4 The spine.

Sources: Jmarchn, CC BY-SA 3.0 <https://creativecommons.org/licenses/by-sa/3.0>, via Wikimedia Commons; https://upload.wikimedia.org/wikipedia/commons/5/54/Gray_111_-_Vertebral_column-coloured.png.

TABLE 13.4
Vertebral Injuries

Vertebral Injury	Description
Simple fracture	■ Solitary fracture/break most commonly to the spinous or transverse process, pedicles, or facets of the vertebral arch
Wedge fracture	■ Anterior portion of the vertebral body is compressed (axial loading)
Burst fracture	■ Shattered vertebral body as a result of axial loading; may be associated with vertebral disk rupture and can be associated with spinal cord compromise
Teardrop fracture	■ A small triangular portion of bone from the anterior edge of the vertebra breaks off
Chance ("seat belt") fracture	■ A flexion distraction injury; occurs in the setting of rapid deceleration with lumbar restriction and results in a horizontal vertebral fracture due to compressive forces on the vertebral body that are transmitted through the spinous process

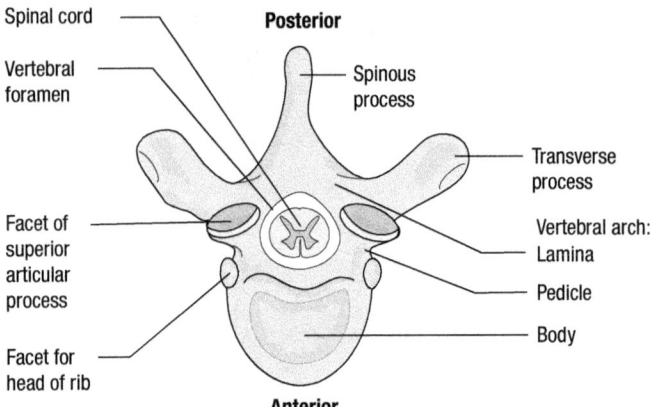

Figure 13.5 Vertebral anatomy.

Source: https://commons.wikimedia.org/wiki/File:Vertebra_Superior_View-en.svg.

Venous Thromboembolism

Venous thromboembolism is a term encompassing both DVT and pulmonary embolism (PE), both of which are preventable complications after trauma. Approximately two thirds of VTE events present as DVT and one third as

PE with or without DVT. Trauma patients are at an increased risk of VTE, which is thought to be related to decreased venous blood flow, diminished fibrinolysis, immobilization, surgery, release of and/or exposure to tissue factor, and depletion of endogenous anticoagulants.

Evidence of DVT includes unilateral localized swelling, erythema, and pain, often noted in the lower extremities. Low-grade fever may also accompany DVT or PE. PE can present with hypoxia and/or tachycardia and in severe cases cause respiratory and cardiovascular collapse. DVT can be diagnosed with venous duplex ultrasound, whereas PE is confirmed by a chest CT angiogram, commonly referred to as CT PE protocol. The treatment for both DVT and PE is anticoagulation. The option to treat with thrombolytic agents (such as tissue plasminogen activator) may be limited in the trauma population, depending on the severity and location of injuries. Massive PEs may cause obstructive shock, for which patients may undergo a thrombectomy or surgical intervention. When patients cannot be anticoagulated, an inferior vena cava filter should be placed.

Nurses should always maintain a high index of suspicion for VTE in the trauma population. All patients should have mechanical DVT prophylaxis. The best method to prevent VTE is a combination of mechanical and chemical prophylaxis. Bilateral sequential compression devices should be routine for all trauma patients. If bilateral lower extremity use is contraindicated, application to an arm has been shown to be effective. Foot pumps are also an option. Timely administration of mechanical and chemical VTE prophylaxis is critical to prevent VTE.

Fat embolism: *Fat embolism* is defined as the presence of fat globules in the peripheral or pulmonary circulation. *Fat emboli syndrome* is the term for the constellation of clinical symptoms that may result and includes respiratory distress, neurologic symptoms, and petechial rash. This most frequently occurs after trauma and during orthopedic procedures to long bones. Fat embolism and fat emboli syndrome are rare but may be life-threatening. The diagnosis can be challenging; relying on clinical symptoms, lab results, and imaging findings is not specific, with fat embolism being largely a clinical diagnosis after excluding other etiologies. Treatment is supportive care focusing on oxygenation and ventilation, optimizing hemodynamics, and resuscitation with fluid and blood products as indicated.

Tetanus: Tetanus is an infection caused by *Clostridium tetani*, a toxin-producing bacterium that is predominantly found in soil, dust, and animal feces. The organisms enter the body through punctures, wounds, lacerations, skin breaks, or infected syringes. The incubation period ranges from 3 to 21 days, with an average of 10 days. The toxins cause painful muscle contractions, particularly of the neck and jaw, which is why it is commonly referred to as lockjaw or trismus. All trauma patients should be asked about their tetanus immunization status upon arrival. The decision to give tetanus prophylaxis is determined by the provider and is influenced by the patient's previous immunization status and risk of wound infection and whether the patient is immunocompromised. If more than 5 years have passed since the last vaccination, a tetanus vaccine should be administered.

Nerve injury: Nerve injuries are often a result of compression or crush injuries, fractures (open or closed), soft tissue injury, and/or dislocations. Symptoms of nerve injury include pain, paresthesia (tingling or pins and needles) and numbness, decreased sensation, and decreased or absent movement. Patients commonly describe the pain as a shooting, stabbing, or burning sensation. Early recognition of neurologic compromise is imperative because timeliness can save function of the extremity, meaning prolonged deficit from neurologic compromise is more likely to remain even if an intervention can be done. Thus, nurses should immediately report symptoms of nerve pain to providers.

Brachial plexus: The brachial plexus provides motor and sensory control to the arm, elbow, forearm, wrist, and hand. Injury to the brachial plexus may be a result of blunt or penetrating trauma. Common mechanisms of injury include trauma in which the arm is pulled or stretched forcefully. The most common cause is motorcycle crashes, motor vehicle collisions, falls, and knife and gunshot wounds. Associated traumatic injuries include traumatic head injuries, subclavian and axillary vein and artery injuries, and shoulder dislocations. Mild brachial plexus injuries do not require treatment, whereas more severe injuries may require surgical intervention to regain function of the hand or arm.

Compartment syndrome: *Compartments* are defined as closed spaces containing nerves, muscles, and vascular structures that are surrounded by fascia. When the pressure increases inside a compartment, a patient may develop compartment syndrome. Pressure can increase for a variety of reasons, including tissue edema, blood accumulation, or fluid infiltration. Inflammation and ischemia of the tissues lead to edema formation, which can increase the pressure in the compartment. Increased pressure then worsens ischemia, causing a vicious cycle of ischemia and edema. *Compartment syndrome* is defined as increased pressure in and around muscles within a compartment that causes pain, decreased blood flow, and tissue or limb loss if left untreated.

Compartment syndrome can affect any compartment within the body but most often affects the compartments of the lower extremities. It is defined by increased pressure within a closed osteofascial compartment that results in decreased circulation. With increasing pressure, the patient can express any of several symptoms, referred to as the six "P's" (Box 13.1).

Box 13.1 The "Six P's"

- Pain
- Paresthesias
- Poikilothermia
- Pallor
- Paralysis
- Pulselessness

Pain is often the first symptom, especially with dorsiflexion of the great toe, and pulselessness is a very late finding. Patients typically report pain that is uncontrolled by escalating doses of pain medications. Providers can measure compartment pressures directly with an intercompartmental pressure monitor device. A normal pressure is 0 to 8 mmHg, and a pressure greater than 30 mmHg is used to aid in the diagnosis of acute compartment syndrome. If a patient has any of the six P's, the team should be notified immediately because this could represent a surgical emergency.

Treatment for acute compartment syndrome requires surgical decompression of the compartment by way of fasciotomy, a surgical incision to the fascia to relieve pressure in the compartment. If left untreated, the patient can lose function and have permanent nerve damage and the limb may die, requiring an amputation.

Over time, the swelling will decrease, and the fasciotomy can be primarily closed or may require secondary closure with skin grafting.

FAST FACTS

Acute compartment syndrome is a surgical emergency. Acute pain, paresthesias, pain with movement, and decreased sensation should be immediately reported.

Rhabdomyolysis: Rhabdomyolysis occurs when muscle tissue is damaged and the muscles release proteins and electrolytes into the circulation. The result is an influx of circulating proteins and electrolytes, which may result in acute kidney injury, electrolyte disturbances, and disseminated intravascular coagulation. The hallmark of rhabdomyolysis is elevated serum creatine phosphokinase (CPK) levels; patients may also exhibit reddish brown urine from myoglobinuria. These signs can be seen in a patient with damage to muscle tissues, making trauma patients at increased risk for rhabdomyolysis, often seen in patients with crush injuries or acute compartment syndrome and in those who had a prolonged downtime related to their trauma. The normal CPK level ranges from 20 to 200 IU/L; an elevation five times that of normal is considered rhabdomyolysis. The mainstay of treatment is volume resuscitation to flush the circulating proteins out of the body through intravenous fluids and increased urine production. Trending CPK levels is a good measure of how well the resuscitation is going; higher levels indicate more volume or alternative intervention is needed, and lower levels indicate clearing/resolution. If volume resuscitation is not effective at lowering the CPK and the patient has persistent decline in kidney function, dialysis may be required. Indications for dialysis include **A**cidosis, **E**lectrolyte abnormalities, toxic **I**ngestions, volume **O**verload, and **U**remia.

FAST FACTS

A E I O U—know your vowels. These are indications for dialysis.

SUMMARY

Although MSK injuries may not be the first injuries assessed in the trauma bay, they do warrant careful assessment and timely interventions to reduce morbidity and mortality. Often the primary focus of an MSK injury will be immobilization to reduce further injury until definitive stabilization or correction can be completed. The nurse plays a key role in early identification of MSK injuries. Nurses spend the greatest amount of time with patients and can pick up on a subtle or dramatic change in status, whether it be an improvement or decline in the patient's clinical exam.

REVIEW QUESTIONS

1. A 45-year-old male was working under a car when the supports failed, and the car fell on the patient crushing his right lower extremity. The patient presents with a taught right lower extremity with pain, pallor, and paresthesia. What might the patient be experiencing?
   a. Spinal cord injury
   b. Acute compartment syndrome
   c. Nerve root injury
   d. Deep vein thrombosis
2. What lab value is most important when monitoring for rhabdomyolysis?
   a. Hemoglobin
   b. Sodium
   c. Creatine phosphokinase
   d. Alanine aminotransferase
3. Physical exam findings concerning for a deep vein thrombosis include:
   a. Redness and ecchymosis
   b. Muscle spasms
   c. Pulselessness and paresthesia
   d. Erythema, edema, and pain
4. This can be applied to stabilize the pelvic ring and tamponade bleeding:
   a. Tourniquet
   b. Pelvic binder
   c. Pressure bandage
   d. Knee immobilizer

References

American College of Surgeons: The Committee on Trauma. (2018). *ATLS: Advanced Trauma Life Support student course manual* (10th ed.). American College of Surgeons.

Bae, C., & Bourget, D. (2023, January). *Tetanus*. [Updated May 31, 2023]. StatPearls Publishing. https://www.ncbi.nlm.nih.gov/books/NBK459217/

Libby, C., Frane, N., & Bentley, T. P. (2023, January). *Scapula fracture*. [Updated Jul 17, 2023]. StatPearls Publishing. https://www.ncbi.nlm.nih.gov/books/NBK537312/

McQuillan, K. A., & Flynn-Makic, M. B. (2020). *Trauma nursing: From resuscitation through rehabilitation* (5th ed.). Elsevier.

Rothberg, D. L., & Makarewich, C. A. (2019, April 15). Fat embolism and fat embolism syndrome. *Journal of the American Academy of Orthopaedic Surgeons, 27*(8), e346–e355. https://doi.org/10.5435/JAAOS-D-17-00571

Torlincasi, A. M., Lopez, R. A., & Waseem, M. (2023, January 16). *Acute compartment syndrome*. StatPearls Publishing.

Yorkgitis, B., Berndtson, A., Cross, A., Kennedy, R., Kochuba, M., Tignanelli, C., Tominaga, G., Jacobs, D., Marx, W., Ashley, D., Ley, E., Napolitano, L., & Costantini, T. (2022). American Association for the Surgery of Trauma/American College of Surgeons-Committee on trauma clinical protocol for inpatient venous thromboembolism prophylaxis after trauma. *Journal of Trauma and Acute Care Surgery, 92*(3), 597–604. https://doi.org/10.1097/TA.0000000000003475

Integumentary Injuries and Care

Alexander Menard

The integumentary system is the body's largest organ and is often injured during trauma. Burn injuries can be a severe source of major trauma, requiring specialized and intensive nursing care, which is covered in this chapter. Other musculoskeletal and integumentary injuries may be life- or limb-threatening, and nurses have a large role in their assessment and management.

In this chapter, you will learn to:
1. Identify key elements of an integumentary assessment.
2. Articulate nursing interventions to manage burn injuries.
3. Identify complications associated with integumentary injuries.

INTRODUCTION

Skin is the protective later between the internal body systems and the environment. It protects the body from injuries, microorganisms, caustic substances, and environmental heat and cold. Skin also helps with temperature and water regulation. The integumentary system is also involved in the functions of the nervous system, aiding in the detection of pressure, pain, heat, and cold. Valuable information can be obtained during the assessment of the integumentary system of a trauma patient.

INTEGUMENTARY ASSESSMENT

Inspection

A thorough and systematic visual inspection of the trauma patient's skin is required. This includes evaluation for discolored skin or open areas. Patients have different skin tones; thus, it is important to compare against expected skin tones and document these differences. Record all lesions; skin breakdown; or unusual findings, such as rashes, petechiae, unusual moles, or burns. Uploading photos into the electronic medical record is recommended for future comparison.

Nurses must be able to differentiate between chronic wounds that were present before the trauma and acute wounds that are related to the current event. Examples of chronic wounds include venous stasis ulcers, pressure ulcers, diabetic foot ulcers, and arterial insufficiency ulcers.

Venous stasis ulcers are typically found on the lower half of the leg between the knee and ankle. The medial and lateral malleoli are the most common locations for venous ulcers. These wounds have concomitant edema that improves with elevation. They are generally shallow and irregular in shape with a wound bed that is lined with granulation tissue (described as beefy red). The surrounding skin often appears with scaling, weeping, and/or crusting.

Pressure ulcers are more prevalent in hospitalized patients and patients residing in long-term care facilities. However, there are other risk factors for the development of pressure injuries, including decreased mobility and malnutrition. These wounds usually develop over bony prominences (sacrum, ischial tuberosities, and calcaneum). Pressure injuries may be a result of medical devices such as nasal gastric tubes, oxygen tubing, or endotracheal tubes. Any medical device that rests or places pressure on the skin is a risk for pressure injury development. Proper precautions should be taken to avoid such injuries by frequent position changes, application of skin protectant, and padding when appropriate. Pressure injuries may be present on admission and should be documented as such. Pressure injuries should be graded on admission and regularly thereafter, noting the stage. Pressure injuries range from nonblanchable erythema to unstageable wounds. Pressure injuries are often a result of the patient being immobile for a prolonged period.

Diabetic foot ulcers are chronic wounds that result from neuropathy secondary to the side effects of diabetes. These ulcers are typically found on the plantar metatarsal heads and dorsal interphalangeal joints. Arterial insufficiency ulcers often present on the distal part of the toes. These ulcers typically have sharply demarcated margins and minimal exudate. Because these wounds are caused by a lack of blood flow (arterial insufficiency), the wound beds are often pale, gray, or yellow and lack granulation tissue.

Palpation

Palpation of the skin must include assessment of temperature, moisture, capillary refill, and presence of any edema. If erythema or rashes are present, firmly touch the skin to determine whether the skin is blanchable or lightens in color with pressure. Skin that is blanchable is at risk for tissue damage, whereas nonblanchable skin indicates the presence of tissue injury. Temperature can be assessed simply by touching the patient's skin. Patients who have an infection or burn injury may feel hot to the touch, whereas patients presenting in shock states may feel cool due to poor perfusion. Moisture should also be assessed; diaphoresis may represent shock. Capillary refill is a good indication of perfusion or the amount of blood flow to tissues local to the area. This assessment is done typically on or near nail beds by firmly depressing the skin or nail to allowing blanching and then timing how long it takes for color to return. The expected finding is less than 2 seconds; longer than 2 to 3 seconds indicates impaired perfusion. Edema can be assessed during inspection and palpation. Edema may be found in the area of an underlying injury and is secondary to swelling of the surrounding tissues.

FAST FACTS

Patients have differing skin tones; thus, it is important to compare against expected skin tones and document these differences. Record all lesions; skin breakdown; or unusual findings, such as rashes, petechiae, unusual moles, or burns.

INTEGUMENTARY INJURIES

Trauma may result in many different types of wounds and soft tissue injuries. The integumentary system comprises the skin, hair, nails, sweat glands, and sebaceous glands. The skin has several layers, and to evaluate injuries to the integumentary systems, these layers must be understood. The outermost layer of skin is called the *epidermis*. The second layer is termed the *dermis*, with the subcutaneous tissues below the dermis (Figure 14.1).

Traumatic Wounds and Soft Tissue Injuries

Traumatic wounds to the soft tissues include contusions, hematomas, abrasions, avulsions, lacerations, and punctures (Table 14.1).

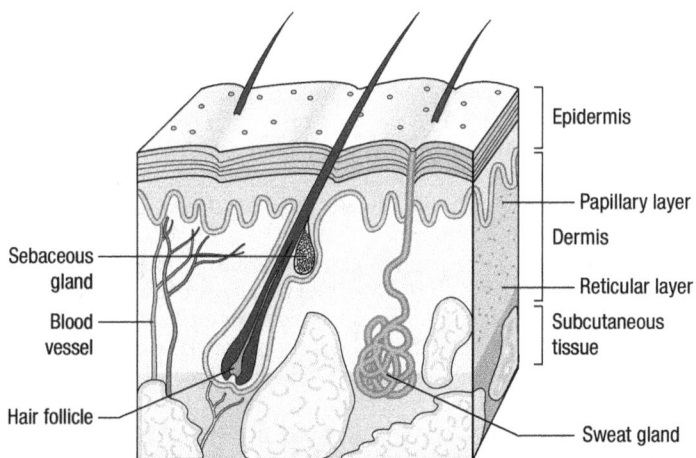

Figure 14.1 Layers of skin.

Source: https://commons.wikimedia.org/wiki/File:Labeled_layers_of_the_skin.jpg.

TABLE 14.1

Types of Traumatic Wounds and Soft Tissue Injuries

Traumatic Wound or Soft Tissue Injury	Description
Contusion	Results from rupture of subcutaneous blood vessels; skin remains intact
Hematoma	Results from rupture of deep or large blood vessels (arterial or venous), causing accumulation of blood into the adjacent tissues
Abrasion	Results from friction and varies in depth (superficial, partial-thickness, or full-thickness abrasion)
Avulsion	Results from stretching or tearing of soft tissues, resulting in a full-thickness loss
Laceration	Results from trauma from a sharp object, resulting in a linear separation of skin, or a blunt impact that causes a more jagged-appearing wound and wound edges
Puncture	Results from a sharp or pointed object that pierces the skin and penetrates beyond deeper layers

Contusions are caused by blunt force trauma and result in a localized region of injury that is defined by ecchymosis, swelling, and pain. X-rays should be performed to assess for underlying fractures. Nurses should assess the patient's circulation, sensation, and motor function at the site and distal to the contusion.

Abrasions result from friction that scrapes and removes the outer layers of skin. An abrasion will never be deeper than the dermis (Figure 14.1). Abrasions should be thoroughly cleansed and foreign material removed. Abrasions are often seen in bicycle or motorcycle crashes and are related to a patient sliding or being dragged across a road or other surface. Abrasions that cover significant portions of the body can significantly increase fluid loss. Patients with large friction injuries may require clinical management similar to a thermal burn injury.

Avulsions result from tearing or ripping, resulting in wound edges that cannot be approximated. A degloving injury is a type of avulsion injury that occurs when a piece of skin and the layer of soft tissue below are partially or completely separated from the body. Degloving injuries commonly occur to the hands and feet. Avulsion injuries vary in severity and may result in the need for both temporary and/or permanent skin grafting.

Lacerations are open wounds that result from tearing or cutting. Lacerations can be classified as superficial (including only the dermis and epidermis) or deep (including the soft tissue or other underlying structures). Lacerations need to be cleaned and evaluated for foreign or retained material. Lacerations that are grossly contaminated or include the bone may require antibiotics. Circulatory, sensory, and motor (CSM) functions must be assessed at and distal to the laceration. Lack of appropriate movement may indicate tendons or ligaments are involved, in which case, surgical repair is often required.

Puncture wounds present with a small opening at the surface but penetrate deep into the underlying tissues. These wounds must be cleansed and evaluated for underlying structural damage.

Nursing Care
All the aforementioned traumatic wounds and soft tissue injuries have a risk for infection, requiring thorough cleansing and foreign material removal. Nurses should continually assess for signs of infection, including fever, wound discoloration, discharge, odor, increased tenderness, warmth, and induration surrounding the wound. In addition, continued monitoring of CSM function is needed to identify complications. Swelling and/or hematoma expansion may persist for days and impair CSM function. Any signs of infection or alterations in the CSM exam must be reported to the trauma team. Bleeding is possible with all these injuries and can be addressed with direct pressure or tourniquet application for arterial hemorrhage. Severe cases may require surgical intervention.

Dressing changes are often completed by nursing with specific instructions/orders provided by the trauma team. Large and/or deep wounds require packing with moist gauze to debride the wound, aiding in the healing process. If a wound requires packing, one continuous piece should be used to reduce the potential for leaving or losing a piece of gauze in the wound.

Burn Injuries

Trauma nurses must be able to identify and treat burn injuries. The first 48 hours of burn care are the most critical and have the greatest influence on morbidity and mortality. Most burn injuries are a result of thermal injury, with fewer than 10% resulting from electrical or chemical sources. Flame and scald burns are considered thermal burns and are the leading cause of burns in adults. Burn injuries differ from other traumas because of the overwhelming inflammatory response that occurs moments after injury.

FAST FACTS

There is a significant difference between burn injuries and all other injuries in that the consequences of burn injuries are directly related to the extent of inflammatory response to injury.

The extent of a burn injuries is expressed as a percentage of total body surface area (TBSA) involved. Adults and children have different considerations to determine the TBSA given that children have different body proportions.

TABLE 14.2
Methods to Estimate TBSA in Adults

Method	Description	
Rule of nines	Head = 9% Each arm = 9% Anterior chest and abdomen = 18%	Posterior chest and back = 18% Each leg = 18% Perineum = 1%
Lund and Browder chart	Each arm = 10% Anterior trunk = 13% Posterior trunk = 13% Head and legs: percentage varies based on patient's age	
Palmar surface	For small burns, the patient's palm surface (excluding the fingers) represents approximately .5% of their body surface area, and the hand surface (including the palm and fingers) represents about 1% of their body surface area.	

TBSA, total body surface area.

Note: Used with permission from Carpenter Menard Adult-Gerontology Acute Care Nurse Practitioner (AGACNP) review book.

See Table 14.2 for methods to determine adult burn TBSA. Determining TBSA in the pediatric population can be done with the rule of nines but has different allocation for percent burn (head, 18%; chest, 18%; back, 18%; right arm, 9%; left arm, 9%; perineum, 1%; right leg, 12.5%; and left leg, 13.5%). It is important to note that determining TBSA in all burn patients is challenging, particularly in the pediatric population. Burn injuries are classified into several categories (Table 14.3).

Nursing Care

It is essential to stop the burning process as soon as possible. It may be difficult to remove clothing because it may have adhered to the underlying tissues, but clothing needs to be removed to fully assess the extent of the burns. When removing the patient's clothing, it is important to remember that burn patients lose tremendous amounts of heat and become hypothermic due to the loss of skin integrity. The room temperature must be increased in an attempt to counter hypothermia and other warming measures implemented once it is safe to do so.

The first 24 to 48 hours are critical for fluid resuscitation of the burn patient. For patients with TBSA greater than 20%, the Parkland formula (Box 14.1) is often used to calculate the amount of volume resuscitation needed. Resuscitation protocols may vary depending on institution and patient-specific clinical needs. It is important to remember when instituting fluid resuscitation that the first 24 hours starts from the time of injury and NOT the time the patient arrives to the facility.

Burn care and management are nursing intensive. Nurses may be required to perform dressing changes on the burn patient or frequently

TABLE 14.3

Classification of Burns

Classification of Burn	Level of Burn Injury	Signs and Symptoms
SB First degree	Epidermis only	- Burns are red - Blanch with light pressure - Painful and tender - No vesicles or bullae
SPTB Second degree	Papillary dermis	- Burns blanch with pressure - Painful, tender - Vesicles and bullae develop within 24 hours - Bases of the vesicles and bullae are pink and develop fibrinous exudate
DPTB Second degree	Reticular dermis Involves hair follicles and sweat glands	- Burns may be white, red, or mottled white and red - No blanching with pressure and are less painful and tender than the more superficial burns - Patient has difficulty discerning pinprick and will describe it as pressure instead of sharp - Vesicles or bullae may develop - Burns are usually dry
FTB Third degree	Below the dermal layers of the skin into adipose	- Burns may be white or pliable, black or charred, brown or leathery, or bright red secondary to fixed hemoglobin in the subdermal region - Pale FTB may appear to be normal skin except that the skin does not blanch to pressure - May lack sensation, or be reduced - Hairs can be pulled easily from follicles - Vesicles and bullae do not usually develop
SDB Fourth degree	Extends through the skin and subcutaneous tissue into the fascia, muscle, or bone	- Burn goes through both layers of skin and involves underlying adipose, muscle, and/or bone - Hypoesthesia exists in the area because the nerve endings are destroyed

DPTB, deep partial-thickness burn; FTB, full-thickness burn; SB, superficial burn; SDB, subdermal burn; SPTB, superficial partial-thickness burn.

Note: Modified with permission from Carpenter Menard AGACNP review book (modified from page 496).

wet dressings that are in place. Burn dressing changes are performed using aseptic technique. Care of the burn wounds will depend on the depth, size, and location of the burns. Detailed instructions are provided by the trauma, burn, plastic surgery, and/or other consulting teams regarding timing and specifics of dressing changes.

> **Box 14.1 PARKLAND FORMULA AND EXAMPLE**
>
> **Parkland Formula**
>
> **Total fluid to be given in the first 24 hours = 4 mL of LR × patient actual weight (kg) × %TBSA**
> (50% of fluid to be given in the first 8 hours, with the remaining 50% to be given over the remaining 16 hours)
>
> **Example:**
> A 75-kg passenger in a motor vehicle crash, in which the car was engulfed in flames, presents with a 35% TBSA burn.
> 4 mL of LR × 75 kg × 35 = 10,500 mL
> 10,500 × .5 = 5,500 mL in the first 8 hours
> 10,500 × .5 = 5,500 mL over the remaining 16 hours
>
> LR, lactated Ringer (solution); TBSA, total body surface area.

Burn care requires interdisciplinary collaboration. It is recommended that any burn over 20% TBSA, circumferential burns, burns involving the face, genitals full thickness burn, or electrical injury be transferred to a certified burn center.

Patients with deep partial-thickness or full-thickness burns require timely surgical intervention to remove eschar (necrotic tissue). An escharotomy is a surgical incision into eschar that is performed on presentation, after the primary and secondary surveys, to temporarily allow expansion of the compartments. Escharotomies may be needed for full-thickness burns that include the chest, abdomen, and extremities, because third spacing of fluid occurs during the immediate resuscitation phase.

Burn injuries are very painful, particularly during dressing changes. Adequate pain control is required. Patient needs can vary from as-needed doses of analgesics to conscious sedation and even general anesthesia for repeated surgical debridement in the operating room.

The primary goal of burn wound care is to obtain full permanent coverage of the burn wounds. Until the wounds are permanently covered, the patient is at high risk for infections. Surgical intervention and wound care are the mainstay of burn care. This process involves multiple debridements of the nonviable tissue while protecting newly formed dermis or epidermis. After the wound is cleaned, antimicrobial topical agents are applied to limit bacterial growth. Silver sulfadiazine (Silvadene) and sulfamylon are common agents used to prevent burn wound infections. Bacitracin or polysporin ointments are commonly used on facial burns on initial presentation or facial burns that do not require surgical intervention. Antimicrobial agents may differ depending on patient factors, such as allergies and burn care center preferences.

Following debridement, skin grafting may be needed to restore skin covering over the burned area. Either allografting or autografting may be performed.

- Allograft—Tissue from a donor used to cover the burn wound (temporary coverage).
- Autograft—Tissue from another part of a patient used to cover the burn wound (permanent coverage).
- Xenograft—Skin graft from an animal, commonly a pig. Xenografts are common due to limited supply and cost of human skin; they are temporary coverage until an autograft is available.

Inhalation Injury

Inhalation injuries may result from smoke or chemical inhalation as well as thermal injury. To definitively confirm an inhalation injury is present, direct visualization must occur. This can be done by visual inspection of the oropharynx as well as bronchoscopy to evaluate the airway and lungs. Nurses should have high suspicion of an inhalation injury with every burn patient. Soot around the mouth and or nose, facial burns, and singed nasal passages or facial hairs are highly suggestive of an inhalation injury. Inhalation injuries can result in significant airway edema that can progressively worsen from the time of the burn to hours after the injury. Nurses must be ready to immediately intubate these patients. Keep difficult airway supplies by the patient's room. Bronchoscopy may be needed to clear the airway of soot and debris.

Nurses must also be concerned about carbon monoxide) or cyanide poisoning. A patient with carbon monoxide and/or cyanide poisoning may report headache, dizziness, weakness, dyspepsia, vomiting, chest pain, and confusion. If left untreated, the patient can progress to a depressed mental status and cardiac arrest.

Nursing Care

If an inhalation injury is present, careful and continuous monitoring of the patient's respiratory status is essential. Airway swelling may occur hours after the initial insult. Signs of airway swelling and/or respiratory compromise include stridor, inability to speak in full sentences, and a rapid respiratory rate. Any of the previous signs of respiratory compromise must be reported to the team. It is expected the nurse will stay with the patient, apply supplemental oxygen, and call for help if any of these signs are present.

Hypothermia

Hypothermia is defined as an involuntary reduction in body temperature to <35°C (95°F). This can have major implications for a trauma patient given that hypothermia is part of the "lethal triad" of hypothermia, acidosis, and coagulopathy. Removal from the cold source and removal of clothing that may be contributing (e.g., wet and cold clothing) are essential Hypothermia must be immediately addressed, but caution must be taken when rewarming a patient. Dramatic changes to body temperature may result in peripheral vasodilation and hypotension, arrhythmias, and/or heart failure.

Nursing Care
The first priority of care for cold trauma patients is addressing the ABCDEs (airway, with restriction of cervicalspine motion; breathing; circulation; disability; and exposure. The patient should be removed from the source of cold. Wet clothes must be removed, and the patient dried. Rewarming can be achieved through active and passive means (Table 14.4).

Cold Injuries

Cold injuries are a result of exposure to low temperatures and are related to the duration of the exposure. Frostbite is a freezing injury that is seen when the ambient temperature or environment is below freezing (32°F or 0°C). In contrast, nonfreezing injuries result from exposure to damp/wet conditions when temperatures are low. Examples of nonfreezing injuries include trench foot and chilblains. Chilblains cause inflamed, swollen areas and blisters on the feet and hands. Frostbite typically results in permanent tissue damage, whereas nonfreezing injuries result in inflammatory lesions on the skin that can heal.

The treatment for nonfreezing injuries is supportive care. This includes keeping the injured area warm, dry, and elevated and continually monitoring for signs of infection. Treatment for frostbite depends on the degree of injury (Table 14.5). Third- and fourth-degree frostbite requires surgical debridement.

Nursing Care
Nursing care for cold injuries always includes removing the patient from the cold source/environment and institution of rewarming procedures. Continuous assessment for infection is critical for both freezing and nonfreezing injuries because of the high risk for infection. Nursing care of

TABLE 14.4

Active and Passive Methods for Rewarming

Active Rewarming Methods	Passive Rewarming Methods
■ Heating devices (pads, blowers) ■ Warm blankets ■ Warm intravenous fluids ■ Gastric, colonic, peritoneal, and mediastinal lavage ■ Warmed inhaled air or oxygen ■ Hemodialysis ■ Continuous arteriovenous rewarming ■ Continuous venovenous rewarming	■ Warm ambient air ■ Dry the patient ■ Shivering (patient compensatory mechanism)

TABLE 14.5
Frostbite Injury Classification

Classification	Description
First degree	Numbness, central pallor with erythema and edema, peeling skin, and dysesthesia (unpleasant feeling, pain)
Second degree	Blisters with erythema and edema
Third degree	Entire thickness loss of skin and hemorrhagic blisters
Fourth degree	Loss of entire thickness of skin, deep structures; affected area will be nonviable

Note: Modified from Tintinalli et al. *Emergency Medicine*, Table 208-3.

Source: Paddock, M. T. (2020). Cold injuries. In: J. E. Tintinalli, O. Ma, D. M. Yealy, G. D. Meckler, J. Stapczynski, D. M. Cline, & S. H. Thomas (Eds.), *Tintinalli's emergency medicine: A comprehensive study guide* (9th ed.). McGraw Hill. https://accessmedicine-mhmedical-com.umassmed.idm.oclc.org/content.aspx?bookid=2353&sectionid=220746407.

nonfreezing injuries involves keeping the wounds dry, clean, and elevated. Restrictive dressings should be avoided. Nursing care of freezing injuries depends on the degree of the injury (Table 14.5). These injuries may be painful, and administration of analgesics is essential. Topical aloe vera cream may be applied to the affected area. After the rewarming phase of a frostbite injury, intravenous or intra-arterial thrombolytic therapies may be used to revascularize vessels. These agents are administered based on institutional protocols.

Wound Healing

Many factors affectt wound healing, including age, smoking status, nutritional status, and preexisting health conditions. Burn injuries can induce a hypermetabolic state that is proportional to the extent of the burn. This hypermetabolic state may persist for months after the injury. The target for burn patients' caloric requirements is calculated using this formula:

20 to 30 kcal/kg body weight/day

Daily protein intake is set at a goal of 1.5 to 2 g of protein per kilogram of body weight. The nurse plays a critical role in ensuring burn patients meet optimal nutritional intake. The preferred method is enteral feeding. In awake patients, this includes oral intake and high-protein supplements and may even require nocturnal tube feedings via small-bore feeding tubes.

Integumentary Injury Complications

Complications related to integumentary injuries include venous thromboembolism (VTE), tetanus, nerve injury, infection, contractures, stress ulcers, disfigurement, compartment syndrome, and rhabdomyolysis. Prevention is key to avoiding integumentary injury complications. Early detection is the next best course of action to reduce the negative effects of the following potential complications.

Venous thromboembolism: *Venous thromboembolism* is a term that encompasses deep vein thrombosis (DVT) and pulmonary embolism (PE). Both are complications after trauma that can be prevented by mechanical and chemical DVT prophylaxis combined with early mobility. For patients who cannot receive anticoagulation, an inferior vena cava filter should be considered to prevent DVTs from becoming PEs.

Approximately two thirds of VTE events present as DVT and one third as PE with or without DVT. Trauma patients are at an increased risk of VTE, which is thought to be related to decreased venous blood flow, diminished fibrinolysis, immobilization, surgery, release of and/or exposure to tissue factor, and depletion of endogenous anticoagulants.

Evidence of DVT includes unilateral localized swelling, erythema, and pain, often noted in the lower extremities. Low-grade fever may also accompany DVT or PE. PE can present with hypoxia and/or tachycardia and in severe cases cause respiratory and cardiovascular collapse. DVT can be diagnosed with venous duplex ultrasound, whereas PE is confirmed by a chest CT angiogram, commonly referred to as CT PE protocol. The treatment for both DVT and PE is anticoagulation. The option to treat with thrombolytic agents (such as tissue plasminogen activator) may be limited in the trauma population because of the risk of bleeding. Massive PEs can cause obstructive shock, for which patients may undergo intravascular or surgical thrombectomy.

Nurses should always maintain a high index of suspicion for VTE in the trauma population. All patients should have mechanical DVT prophylaxis. The best method for preventing VTE is the combination of mechanical and chemical prophylaxis combined with early mobility. Bilateral sequential compression devices should be routine for all trauma patients, although application to an arm has been shown to be effective. Foot pumps are also an option. Timely administration of DVT prophylaxis is critical to prevent VTE. Nurses should hold VTE prophylaxis before operative interventions and question any order, if orders are written to hold doses. In rare situations, DVT prophylaxis may be held because the risk outweighs the benefit. In these circumstances, the primary team must provide adequate documentation to support holding the chemical DVT prophylaxis.

Tetanus: Tetanus is an infection caused by *Clostridium tetani*, a toxin-producing bacterium that is predominantly found in soil, dust, and animal feces. The organisms enter the body through puncture wounds, lacerations, skin breaks, or infected syringes. The incubation period ranges from 3 to 21 days, with an average of 10 days. The toxins cause painful muscle contractions, particularly of the neck and jaw, which is why it is commonly referred to as lockjaw or trismus.

All trauma patients should be asked about their tetanus immunization status upon arrival. The decision to give tetanus prophylaxis is determined by the provider and is influenced by the patient's previous immunization status and risk of wound infection, and whether the patient is immunocompromised. If more than 5 years have passed since the patient's last vaccination, a tetanus vaccine should be administered.

Contractures: Contractures are a common complication of burn injuries and result from normal skin being replaced with scar tissue. This scar tissue results in loss of motion and tissue alignment and may result in misalignment of a joint or other anatomic structure. Interventions to reduce and manage scar tissue start in the hospital and continue through rehabilitation. Physical and occupational therapy must be involved with the care of the burn patient early on. Patients will often require a splinting schedule to help prevent joint contractures. Patients with burns to the hands require aggressive hand therapy by specialized occupational therapists.

Disfigurement: Integumentary injuries may result in permanent disfigurement. The nurse spends the greatest amount of time with the patient and will be the front-line support for the patient with disfigurements. These patients commonly require additional supportive services, including but not limited to social workers, psychologists or psychiatrists, and clergy/faith workers.

Stress ulcers: Burn patients are at high risk for stress ulcers and gastrointestinal bleeding. These ulcers are referred to as Curling ulcers. Additionally, a severely burned patient commonly requires ventilatory support, and the ventilator can further increase the risk for stress ulcers. These ulcers are best prevented with early initiation of a histamine-2 antagonist (H2 blocker) or a proton pump inhibitor combined with early enteral feedings.

Nerve injury: Nerve injuries are often observed with compression or crush injuries, fractures (open or closed), soft tissue injuries, and/or dislocations. Symptoms of nerve injury include pain, paresthesia (tingling or pins and needles), numbness, decreased sensation, and decreased or absent movement. Patients commonly describe the pain as a shooting, stabbing, or burning sensation. Early recognition of neurologic compromise is imperative, because time can preserve function of the extremity and digits, meaning the longer the neurologic compromise lasts, the more likely the deficit will remain, even if an intervention is done. Thus, nurses should immediately report symptoms of nerve pain to providers. Nerve pain is commonly managed with gabapentin (Neurontin) or pregabalin (Lyrica). Nurses can suggest these agents to the team when nerve injury is suspected or confirmed.

Compartment syndrome: *Compartments* are defined as closed spaces containing nerves, muscles, and vascular structures that are surrounded by fascia. When the pressure increases inside a compartment, a patient can develop compartment syndrome. Pressure can increase for several reasons, including tissue edema, blood accumulation, and fluid infiltration. Inflammation and ischemia of the tissues lead to edema formation, which can increase the pressure in the compartment. Increased pressure then worsens ischemia, causing a vicious cycle of ischemia and edema. *Compartment syndrome* is defined as increased pressure in and around muscles within a compartment that causes pain; decreased blood flow; and, if left untreated, tissue or limb loss.

Compartment syndrome can affect any compartment within the body but most often affects the compartments of the lower extremities. It is defined by increased pressure within a closed osteofascial compartment that results in decreased circulation. With increasing pressure, the patient can express any of several symptoms, referred to as the "six P's" of compartment syndrome: pain, pallor, poikilothermia, paresthesia, pulselessness, and paralysis.

Pain is often the first symptom, especially with dorsiflexion of the great toe. Patients typically report pain that is uncontrolled by escalating doses of pain medications. Providers can measure compartment pressures directly with an intercompartmental pressure monitor device. A normal pressure is 0 to 8 mmHg, and a pressure greater than 30 mmHg is used to aid in the diagnosis of acute compartment syndrome. If a patient has any of the six P's, the team should be notified immediately because this could represent a surgical emergency. Pulselessness is a very late finding, and the limb is likely to be unsalvageable and may require amputation. Thus, recognition of compartment syndrome must occur before loss of or diminished pulses. Nurses should perform hourly CSM assessment with severe limb burns or injuries.

Treatment for acute compartment syndrome requires surgical decompression of the compartment with fasciotomy, a surgical incision through the skin and soft tissues to the fascia covering the muscles to relieve pressure in the compartment. If left untreated, the patient can lose function and have permanent nerve damage and the limb may die, requiring an amputation.

Over time, the swelling will decrease. Closure of the fasciotomy can be performed by primarily closing the wounds. If the swelling does not completely resolve, secondary closure may be required with skin grafting.

FAST FACTS

Acute compartment syndrome is a surgical emergency. Acute pain, paresthesia, pain with movement, and decreased sensation should be immediately reported to the trauma team.

Rhabdomyolysis: Rhabdomyolysis occurs when muscle tissue is damaged and the muscle releases proteins and electrolytes into the circulation. The result is an influx of circulating proteins and electrolytes into the bloodstream. This process may cause acute kidney injury and electrolyte disturbances; specifically concerning is the threat of hyperkalemia. Hyperkalemia may present with peaked T waves on EKG. Patients at risk for rhabdomyolysis should be monitored with telemetry. The hallmark of rhabdomyolysis is an elevated serum creatine phosphokinase (CPK) level. Patients may also exhibit reddish brown urine from myoglobinuria. This can be seen in a patient with damage to muscle tissues and is often seen in patients with crush injuries or compartment syndrome and/or those who had prolonged downtime. The normal CPK level ranges from 20 to 200 IU/L; an elevation five times that of normal is considered rhabdomyolysis. The mainstay of treatment is volume resuscitation to flush out the circulating proteins. Trending serial CPK levels are a good measure of how well the resuscitation is going. Rising CPK levels indicate more volume is needed, whereas decreasing levels indicate clearance of the proteins. If volume resuscitation is not effective to lower the CPK levels and the patient has progressive decline in kidney function, then continuous renal replacement therapy or hemodialysis is required.

FAST FACTS

Rising CPK levels indicate more volume is needed, whereas decreasing levels indicate clearance of the proteins.

SUMMARY

Traumatic injuries to the integumentary system are common among trauma patients. Burn injuries are less common but carry the most significant mortality and morbidity and require specialized care. Cold injuries are related to the degree of cold exposure, and management will vary depending on the classification of the injury. Care of integumentary injuries requires significant nursing care time to prevent scars and infections.

REVIEW QUESTIONS

1. This formula can aid in the fluid resuscitation of a burn patient with >20% TBSA:
   a. Wells criteria
   b. Parkland formula
   c. Harris formula
   d. Heat formula
2. Stridor in a patient with an inhalation injury is an indication of:
   a. Respiratory compromise
   b. Carbon monoxide poisoning
   c. Cyanide poisoning
   d. Inadequate resuscitation
3. A degloving injury falls under which type of skin and soft tissue injury?
   a. Puncture
   b. Abrasion
   c. Laceration
   d. Avulsion
4. Severe burn patients require this amount of protein:
   a. 1 to 1.5 g of protein per kilogram of body weight
   b. 3 to 4 g of protein per kilogram of body weight
   c. 1.5 to 2 g of protein per kilogram of body weight
   d. 2.5 to 3 g of protein per kilogram of body weight

References

American College of Surgeons: The Committee on Trauma. (2018). *ATLS: Advanced Trauma Life Support student course manual* (10th ed.). American College of Surgeons.

Bae, C., & Bourget, D. (2023, January). *Tetanus.* [Updated May 31, 2023]. StatPearls Publishing. https://www.ncbi.nlm.nih.gov/books/NBK459217/

Bush, J. S., Lofgran, T., & Watson, S. (2023, January). *Trench foot.* [Updated August 8, 2023]. StatPearls Publishing. https://www.ncbi.nlm.nih.gov/books/NBK482364/

Duong, H., & Patel, G. (2023, January). *Hypothermia.* [Updated January 24, 2022]. StatPearls Publishing. https://www.ncbi.nlm.nih.gov/books/NBK545239/

Latenser, B. A. (2014). Critical care of the burn patient. In J. B. Hall, G. A. Schmidt, & J. P. Kress (Eds.), *Principles of critical care* (4th ed.). McGraw Hill. https://accessmedicine-mhmedical-com.umassmed.idm.oclc.org/content.aspx?bookid=1340&sectionid=80027724

McQuillan, K. A., & Flynn-Makic, M. B. (2020). *Trauma nursing: From resuscitation through rehabilitation* (5th ed.). Elsevier.

Paddock, M. T. (2020). Cold injuries. In J. E. Tintinalli, O. Ma, D. M. Yealy, G. D. Meckler, J. Stapczynski, D. M. Cline, & S. H. Thomas (Eds.), *Tintinalli's emergency medicine: A comprehensive study guide* (9th ed.). McGraw Hill. https://accessmedicine-mhmedical-com.umassmed.idm.oclc.org/content.aspx?bookid=2353&sectionid=220746407

Shubert, J., & Sharma, S. (2023, January). *Inhalation injury.* [Updated June 12, 2023]. StatPearls Publishing.

Torlincasi, A. M., Lopez, R. A., & Waseem, M. (2023, January). *Acute compartment syndrome.* [Updated January 16, 2023]. StatPearls Publishing.

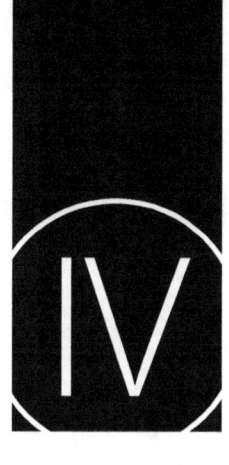

POSTRESUSCITATIVE PHASE OF CARE

Triage, Admission, and Transfer Criteria

Dawn Carpenter

> *Trauma patients must be treated at hospitals that can accommodate their specialized needs. Thus, early identification of who can stay and who must be transferred starts with the prehospital report. All hospitals are obligated to assess, resuscitate, and stabilize patients before transfer to higher levels of care or admission. Failure to assess and stabilize is a violation of the Emergency Medical Treatment and Labor Act. Rapid transfer to a definitive care facility is the next highest priority. Once at a definitive care facility, trauma patients require frequent reassessment to determine the appropriate level of care at time of admission. Therefore, nurses must understand institutional admission, internal transfer, and discharge criteria to ensure appropriate resource utilization to positively impact optimal patient outcomes. Discharge disposition can vary depending on patient needs. This chapter also reviews discharge disposition and trauma patient admission criteria.*

In this chapter, you will learn:
1. Criteria for transfer to a higher level of care.
2. Criteria for admission to intensive care, intermediate care, and ward.
3. Considerations for triaging patients.
4. Options and criteria for posthospital discharge facilities.

INTRODUCTION

Triage is the process of initial assessment and determination of patient acuity and need for a higher level of care. This includes specialty care, nursing care, facility capabilities, and need for surgical intervention. Triage is a collaborative process involving nurses, emergency medical professionals, and physicians. Triage is completed at multiple phases of care, including prehospital, emergency department, in hospital, and decision to discharge and/or transfer.

TRIAGE

Emergency medical service (EMS) personnel ideally need to transport trauma patients to the nearest trauma center for assessment, resuscitation, and stabilization. If a trauma center is not readily available, EMS may need to stop at a critical access hospital or community hospital. The decision to transfer care should be made as early as possible and can be made at any time during the assessment or resuscitative phase but should be decided within 15 minutes of the patient's arrival. Decision to transfer is based on the local facility's capabilities, hemodynamic status of the patient, severity of injuries, mechanism of injury, number of patients, and weather.

Although the team leader ultimately makes the decision to transfer, nurses can suggest or inquire about transfer. A handoff report from the sending to receiving team should occur. Provide patient name and age (if known), mechanism of injury, hemodynamic variables, resuscitative interventions completed, any procedures that were performed, medications administered, and mode of transport. Ensure the medical record is copied or faxed and copies of all radiographs and CT scans are sent on a disc or uploaded to an image-sharing program for the receiving facility to view. Determine what level of personnel needs to travel with the patient (advanced cardiovascular life support vs. basic). If transfer is delayed due to lack of transportation, staff, or weather, a contingency plan should be developed. Seek guidance from the receiving team on additional care that should be provided to help optimize patient outcomes.

The mode of transport, via ground versus air, is also determined by these factors. Time spent at nontrauma centers as well as level III and IV trauma centers should be kept to a minimum. Diagnostic testing should be limited to items needed to treat life-threatening injuries, where the patient may die en route to the higher level of care. Avoid unnecessary testing if the patient will be transferred. The transfer process can start before the patient's arrival.

FAST FACTS

The decision to transfer care should be made as early as possible and within 15 minutes of the patient's arrival. Limit diagnostic testing to items needed to treat life-threatening injuries.

ADMISSION AND TRANSFER CRITERIA

Acute and critical care nurses must know the hospital's specific admission and transfer criteria as well as the triage policies to match patient-specific needs to available institutional resources. Institutional resource limitations and therapeutic capabilities must be considered. Specifically, ICU admission decisions should be made based on the need for the highest level of patient care/monitoring and/or interventions that can be done only in the ICU setting. Teams must prioritize according to the patient's condition, diagnoses, bed availability, vital signs, laboratory values, need for life-supporting therapies, and prognosis. Available clinical expertise and the potential for the patient to benefit from these interventions must also be considered. Triage decisions should be performed in conjunction with the trauma and ICU providers. When resources are limited, a huddle with involved providers, ICU charge nurse, and hospital administrators collaboratively can strategize how best to accommodate patients. In the absence of sufficient resources, the decision to transfer outside the institution can be made.

Decision of where to admit a patient is guided by hospital criteria. Typical levels of care for hospitals are reviewed in Table 15.1; Table 15.2 presents a ranking system for triaging to different levels of care. The triaging process may vary based on institutional policies and protocols.

TABLE 15.1

Types of Inpatients by Level of Care

Level and Nursing Ratio	Type of Patients	Interventions
Intensive care 1:1 to 1:2	Critically ill patients who require care that can be provided only by ICU nurses who may not be available in other areas of the hospital, have clinical instability (e.g., status epilepticus, hypoxemia, and shock), are at high risk for imminent respiratory decline (e.g., impending intubation), or require hourly and/or invasive monitoring	Invasive interventions not provided elsewhere in the hospital, such as CSF drainage or ICP monitoring, invasive mechanical ventilation, vasopressors, ECMO, or CRRT
Intermediate care <1:3	Unstable patients who need nursing interventions, laboratory workup, and/or monitoring every 2 to 4 hours	Noninvasive ventilation, IV infusion, or titration of vasodilators or antiarrhythmic agents
Telemetry <1:4	Stable patients who need close cardiac monitoring for stable arrhythmias or laboratory work every 2 to 4 hours	IV infusions with minimal titration
General care <1:5	Stable patients who need testing and monitoring no more frequently than every 4 hours	IV antibiotics, laboratory and/or radiologic workup

CRRT, continuous renal replacement therapy; CSF, cerebral spinal fluid; ECMO, extracorporeal membrane oxygenation; ICP, intracranial pressure; ICU, intensive care unit; IV, intravenous.
Source: Used with permission from Carpenter. Fast Facts for Adult-Gerontology Acute Care Nurse Practitioners (AGACNPs), p. 22.

TABLE 15.2

Prioritizing ICU Patients

Level of Care	Priority	Type of Patient
ICU	1	Critically ill patients with organ failure who require intensive monitoring and interventions provided only in the ICU environment. Life, limb, and/or organ saving interventions include invasive ventilation, CRRT, invasive hemodynamic monitoring, ECMO, IABP, and other situations requiring critical care (e.g., patients with severe hypoxemia and/or shock)
ICU	2	Priority 1 patients who have lower probability of recovery but will accept intensive care interventions, but not CPR (e.g., patients with metastatic cancer and respiratory failure secondary to pneumonia or in septic shock requiring vasopressors)
IMCU/SDU	3	Patients with organ dysfunction who require close observation and/or interventions, or who could be managed at a level of care less than ICU, such as postop patients who need close monitoring for risk of deterioration, respiratory insufficiency with NIV. If aggressive management is successful, the patient will not need the ICU
IMCU/SDU	4	Patients, as above, but with low probability of recovery/survival (i.e., patients with metastatic disease) and want to be DNR/DNI. If the hospital does not have an IMCU, these patients could be considered for ICU
Palliative	5	Terminal or moribund patients with no possibility of recovery; such patients, in general, are not appropriate for ICU (unless they are potential organ donors). For persons who have clearly declined ICU therapies or have irreversible processes, palliative care should be offered

CPR, cardiopulmonary resuscitation; CRRT, continuous renal replacement therapy; DNI, do not intubate; DNR, do not resuscitate; ECMO, extracorporeal membrane oxygenation; IABP, intra-aortic balloon pump; IMCU, intermediate care unit; NIV, noninvasive ventilation; SDU, step-down unit.

Source: Used with permission from Carpenter. Fast Facts for the AGACNP, p. 23.

Tips for Triaging ICU Level of Care

- Trauma patients should be admitted or discharged to the ICU based on their potential to benefit from advanced care.
- Triage decisions should never be based on age, race, ethnicity, social status, gender, sexual identity, preference, and/or finances.
- Over-triage of trauma patients is preferable to under-triaging patients and risking rapid response activations and escalation of care.
- Critically ill trauma patients should be admitted to the ICU in <6 hours.

- Patients with risk factors for decompensation should be monitored more closely in a higher level of care than the ward.
- Decisions to admit older adult patients to the ICU are based on the patient's comorbidities, severity of illness, functional status, preference regarding life-sustaining treatment, and likelihood to benefit from interventions.
- Routinely reassess the benefit of ICU interventions and discuss continuation or de-escalation of life-sustaining interventions with the patient and legal decision-maker.

Transfer out of ICU

Transfer of trauma patients from the ICU to a lower acuity area should occur once the patient's physiologic status has been stabilized and the need for advanced monitoring and treatment has been resolved. Transfer parameters should be based on ICU criteria, criteria of the lower levels of care, availability of these resources, patient prognosis, hemodynamic stability, and requirement of ongoing interventions. Avoid transfer of patients from the ICU "after hours" ("night shift" or after 7 p.m.). Transfer of patients who are at high risk for death and/or readmission should be carefully considered and coordinated with the multidisciplinary team. Hospitals should have standardized processes, for both provider and nursing, when transferring patients from the ICU to reduce risk of readmission.

SUMMARY

In summary, nurses must know the institutional capacity and capabilities as a whole and of each department. This includes the skills, knowledge and experience of nurses and other staff, number of beds, and the criteria for admission and transfer to and from these units. Early transfer to a higher level of care should not be delayed for extensive diagnostic testing.

REVIEW QUESTION

1. All hospitals are obligated to _____ before transfer to higher level of care.
   a. Collect insurance information
   b. Obtain complete trauma workup imaging
   c. Assess, resuscitate, and stabilize the trauma patient
   d. Provide pain medications

References

Agency for Healthcare Research and Quality. (2020, February). *Re-engineered discharge (RED) toolkit*. https://www.ahrq.gov/patient-safety/settings/hospital/red/toolkit/index.html

American College of Surgeons, Committee on Trauma. (2015). *Rural trauma team development course* (4th ed.). American College of Surgeons.

Nates, J. L., Nunnally, M., Kleinpell, R., Blosser, S., Goldner, J., Birriel, B., Fowler, C. S., Byrum, D., Miles, W. S., Bailey, H., & Sprung, C. L. (2016). ICU admission, discharge, and triage guidelines: A framework to enhance clinical operations, development of institutional policies, and further research. *Critical Care Medicine, 44*(8), 1553–1602. https://doi.org/10.1097/ccm.0000000000001856

Stefanacci, R. (2015). Admission criteria for facility-based post-acute services. *Annals of Long-Term Care Clinical Care Aging, 23*, 18–20.

Best Practices in the Care of Trauma Patients
Dawn Carpenter

Best practices refer to care common to all trauma patients and should be addressed every shift and every day. Adherence to these best practices reduces complications and shortens length of stay. In the ICU, these practices are referred to as the ABCDEF bundle. In this chapter, they are modified to the trauma population and are the A to J bundle. Discharge planning begins at admission; as such, every day and every shift, nurses must ask what needs to happen to get this patient prepared for discharge. Weaning medications, maintaining nutrition and strength, mobilizing the patient, and preventing complications are the mainstay of nursing care.

In this chapter, you will learn:
1. Acute pain management strategies.
2. Criteria for spontaneous breathing trials (SBTs) and extubation.
3. Delirium prevention.
4. Indications for stress ulcer prophylaxis (SUP).
5. How nurses can engage family in the care of the trauma patient.

INTRODUCTION

Trauma patients have injuries to multiple tissues, including muscle, bone, nerves, and organs. Each of these have specific types of pain symptoms. The trauma nurse should be familiar with the types of pain and treatments to ease the patient's pain. Analgesia is the *A* in the A to J bundle of care for trauma patients. See Box 16.1 for the A to J bundle elements.

A: ANALGESIA

Types of Pain
Trauma patients will have pain, which may be superimposed on chronic pain. Nurses must be able to differentiate between types of pain (Table 16.1).

Box 16.1 A TO J BUNDLE ELEMENTS

A: Analgesia, sedation
B: Breathing trial, pulmonary hygiene
C: Circulation—bleeding, H&H, anticoagulation, and DVT prophylaxis
D: Delirium prevention
E: Early mobility
F: Fluids, Foley, and family
G: Gastric/stress ulcer suppression, GI: Nutrition, and goals of care
H: Hospital stay—how to shorten—consult therapies (PT/OT/ST/WOCN)
I: Infections and IPV, elder mistreatment, and child abuse/neglect
J: Just remember other medical problems and associated medications

DVT, deep vein thrombosis; GI, gastrointestinal; H&H, hemoglobin and hematocrit; IPV, intimate partner violence; OT, occupational therapy; PPx, prophylaxis; PT, physical therapy; ST, speech therapy; WOCN, wound ostomy continence nurses.

TABLE 16.1

Types of Pain

Pain Category	Description/Sensation	Localization
Neuropathic: ■ Central ■ Peripheral nerves	■ Burning ■ Hyperesthesia ■ Stabbing ■ Shooting ■ Intense	■ Stocking/glove pattern ■ Radiates down nerve
Somatic: ■ Skin ■ Subcutaneous tissue ■ Joints ■ Connective tissue ■ Muscle ■ Fascia	■ Aching ■ Cramping ■ Throbbing ■ Constant ■ Dull ■ Gnawing ■ Aching	■ Localized ■ Sometimes radiates to surrounding areas
Visceral: ■ Organs ■ Organ capsule ■ Connecting structures	■ Cramping ■ Heaviness ■ Stabbing ■ Squeezing ■ Intense	■ Diffuse ■ Radiates to adjacent or supporting structures

Source: Modified and used with permission. Carpenter. Fast Facts for Adult-Gerontology Acute Care Nurse Practitioners (AGACNPs), p. 84.

Some medications are better at targeting and treating the different types of pain. Thus, multimodal pain regimens are widely used.

Pain is also described as acute, chronic, or acute on chronic. The duration of pain is the primary factor between acute and chronic pain, as defined below.

- **Acute pain**—Is the abrupt onset of pain with a known cause, such as trauma. Acute pain improves as the body heals. Acute pain lasts <3 months.
- **Chronic pain**—Is pain that lasts >3 months. Chronic pain can be caused by inflammation, chronic disease, a previous injury, or medical treatment.
- **Acute on chronic pain**—Occurs when an acute pain occurs simultaneously with a chronic pain. Acute on chronic pain requires additional interventions to address both the acute and chronic pain.

Treatment Strategies

A multimodal approach to analgesia is recommended for all trauma patients. A multimodal pain regimen includes both nonpharmacologic interventions and multiple pharmacologic agents from different classifications of medications. Multimodal pain regimens use several medications to target multiple pain types and pain pathways. Multimodal strategies can also potentiate other interventions and reduce the use of narcotics (Table 16.2). The goal of multimodal pain regimens is to reduce opioid use and prevent physical dependence and substance use disorders.

TABLE 16.2

Multimodal Pain Regimen Strategies

Nonpharmacologic Strategies	Pharmacologic Strategies

- Elevation
- Cold or warm packs
- Compression (Ace wrap)
- Bracing (TLSO)
- Stretching
- Guided imagery or distraction
- Massage
- Relaxation techniques
- Breathing techniques
- Music therapy
- Spiritual practices
- Control of the environment
   - Reduce hospital noise and lighting
   - Reduce stimulation from family/visitors
- Reiki
- Acupuncture
	- Acetaminophen (Tylenol) or Ofirmev IV
	- Muscle relaxants
	   - Methocarbamol (Robaxin)
	   - Cyclobenzaprine (Flexeril)
	   - Tizanidine
	   - Diazepam (Valium)
	- Local anesthetics
	   - Lidocaine patches
	   - Lidocaine infusion
	- NSAIDs (works well for MSK)
	   - Ibuprofen (Motrin)
	   - Ketorolac (Toradol)
	   - Diclofenac cream
	- Antiepileptics (work well for nerve pain)
	   - Gabapentin (Neurontin)
	   - Pregabalin (Lyrica)

(continued)

TABLE 16.2 (continued)
Multimodal Pain Regimen Strategies

Nonpharmacological Strategies	Pharmacological Strategies
	■ Serotonin/norepinephrine reuptake Inhibitors 　■ Duloxetine (Cymbalta) 　■ Venlafaxine (Effexor) ■ Regional blocks ■ Epidural catheter infusions ■ NMDA antagonists 　■ Ketamine bolus (for procedural sedation) 　■ Ketamine infusion ■ Alpha2-receptor agonists 　■ Clonidine (Catapres) 　■ Dexmedetomidine (Precedex) infusion ■ Opioids 　■ Fentanyl 　■ Morphine 　■ Hydromorphone 　■ Oxycodone 　■ Hydrocodone 　■ Tramadol 　■ Oxycontin

MSK, musculoskeletal; NMDA, N-methyl D-aspartate; NSAIDs, nonsteroidal anti-inflammatory drugs; TLSO, thoracic lumbar sacral orthotic.

Opioids are commonly used to manage acute pain in the trauma population. Opioids are highly addictive; thus, the goal is to minimize opioid use. Fentanyl, hydromorphone, and morphine are the most common IV opioids used for trauma patients. Morphine should be avoided in patients with renal dysfunction because metabolites can accumulate, which can cause oversedation.

Upon presentation, a trauma patient requires IV formulations of analgesics for pain control. Surgical stabilization of fractures aids in reducing pain. Once admitted, oral agents are preferred when a patient has a functioning gastrointestinal tract. This allows for longer duration of analgesic effects. IV pro re nata (PRN) doses should be second-line agents, reserved for turning patients, mobilization, and breakthrough pain.

Patients with a substance use disorder, including use or misuse of prescribed narcotics, heroin, or methadone, may have a tolerance to opioids. These patients likely require higher than usual doses to treat their pain. The trauma team should consider consultation with an acute pain service. Nurses can obtain history from the patient, family, and visitors and suggest consultation (if available).

Older adults have physiologic changes (see Chapter 17), causing them to be less sensitive to painful stimuli. Combine these changes with chronic conditions, polypharmacy, and alterations in pharmacokinetics, and older patients can become very sensitive to medications. Thus, extreme caution must be used when administering analgesics to older adults. Reduced doses are required to prevent oversedation and delirium. Nurses must follow the motto "Start low and go slow!!!" Administer small doses and repeat if needed, rather than risking oversedation from larger doses. Patients with obstructive sleep apnea who have had recent general anesthesia are also at risk for oversedation. Oversedation can cause hypercarbia, respiratory acidosis, and obtundation, which could trigger a rapid response activation.

FAST FACTS

"Start low and go slow" when administering analgesics for to older patients.

Sedation

Sedation is commonly required in the ICU. Keep sedation at the lowest possible level to allow the patient to engage in their care. Titrate doses to target Richmond Agitation Sedation Scale goal of 0 to −1 or Riker Sedation-Agitation Scale goal of 4, which is described as calm, cooperative, and following commands. Every patient should have a complete sedation awakening trial (SAT), in which 100% of the analgesics and sedatives are stopped, except if they are on a paralytic agent, have active cardiac ischemia, have an unstable spine pending fixation, are receiving multiple vasopressors, or have other contraindications. SATs allow the kidney and liver time to clear the medications and prevent drug accumulation in the tissues. SATs help prevent delirium and post–intensive care syndrome (PICS).

FAST FACTS

A sedation awakening trial is essential to minimize the accumulation of medication in the body.

Post–Intensive Care Syndrome

PICS is defined as new or worsening cognitive, psychiatric, or physical function after critical illness and/or injury. Physical impairments include decreased physical strength and neuromuscular and pulmonary function. Cognitive changes include decline in memory, attention, executive function, and mental processing speed, and mimics Alzheimer dementia. Mental health changes include the development of anxiety, depression, and posttraumatic stress disorder. Family is also affected by PICS by the development of anxiety, depression, posttraumatic stress disorder, and complicated grief. These symptoms may be present for more than a year after discharge. Reduction of sedation and analgesics reduces these symptoms.

B: BREATHING TRIAL AND PULMONARY HYGIENE

Initially, trauma patients who are in shock require oxygen to enhance oxygen delivery to the tissues to preserve organ function. Once patients are stabilized, weaning of oxygen is important to minimize atelectasis and oxygen toxicity. Patients should be weaned from ventilatory support and extubated promptly to avoid ventilator-associated events, which can occur in 48 hours. Patients who are intubated should have their oxygen weaned to 50% before weaning positive end-expiratory pressure (PEEP). PEEP should be increased to facilitate weaning oxygen. Once the ventilator is weaned to ≤50% and ≤8% of PEEP, then a SAT and SBT can commence. The SAT and SBT are coordinated between nursing and respiratory therapy, stopping sedation and analgesia 30 to 60 minutes before starting the SBT. Patients must meet specific criteria to be eligible for an SBT, including:

- Ventilator settings of ≤50% and ≤8% of PEEP
- The shock state has resolved or is resolving
- Bleeding has ceased or is controlled
- Vasopressors are being weaned
- Vital signs are in acceptable range

Extubation criteria include:
- Resolution of the reason for intubation
- Minimal pulmonary secretions or strength sufficient to cough and expectorate secretions
- Sufficient mental capacity to follow commands (neurologically injured patients require a Glasgow Coma Scale score of 9 or higher, or neuro critical care expertise to determine extubation)
- Sufficient muscle strength (the patient can lift their head off the bed)
- A successful SBT of at least 30 minutes
- A rapid shallow breathing index <105, which is predictive of successful extubation

For patients with facial and neck trauma, a cuff leak check may be requested and is completed by the respiratory therapist. A cuff leak is noted as positive when the exercise tolerance test cuff is deflated and air is heard moving around the cuff. If air is not heard moving around the cuff, further investigation is warranted. Some providers desire a negative inspiratory force where the end of the endotracheal tube is occluded to assess the patient's muscle strength during inhalation. The minimum considered acceptable for extubations is −20 cm H2O. Patients with obesity or weaker muscles may be extubated to bilevel positive airway pressure as a transition to prevent atelectasis.

Pulmonary Hygiene

All patients, including those recently extubated, require aggressive pulmonary hygiene. These techniques include hourly incentive spirometry, positive expiratory pressure (PEP) therapy, and coughing and deep breathing exercises. All patients should be mobilized to be out of bed unless absolutely contraindicated. Advancement to ambulation should occur as soon as possible. Nurses do not need to wait for physical therapy (PT) to begin mobilization. Even patients who are still ventilated must be out of bed and in a chair and can ambulate to maintain mobility and functional status as injuries allow. Additional therapies, if needed, include an insufflator-exsufflator to augment inspiration and aid in mobilizing secretions. The percussive vest is helpful for patients who have secretions to mobilize. Quad coughing can be performed for patients with spinal cord injuries or diaphragm paralysis. These therapies should continue throughout the hospital stay. Nursing should record the incentive spirometry readings and report decreases to the team. Nurses play a key role in educating and empowering family members to prompt the patient to perform incentive spirometry and PEP therapies.

FAST FACTS

Nurses need to encourage patients to perform incentive spirometry and PEP therapy and engage the family to coach the patient.

C: CIRCULATION—BLEEDING, MONITORING, DEEP VEIN THROMBOSIS PROPHYLAXIS, AND ANTICOAGULATION

Initial Resuscitation

Assessment of bleeding is a high priority for trauma patients. Reversal of anticoagulation should be done immediately in the trauma bay, operating room, or ICU. Bleeding can be obvious or more subtle. Patients presenting in hemorrhagic shock require transfusion despite the results of the complete blood count. Whole blood is preferred. Alternatively, transfusions should occur at a ratio of 1 unit of packed red blood cells (PRBCs) to 1 unit of fresh frozen plasma and 1 unit of platelets. Trauma patients may also receive a tranexamic acid bolus followed by an infusion.

Thromboelastography or rotational thromboelastometry is used to evaluate the effectiveness of resuscitation and indicate what other products may be required. Cryoprecipitate may be required to replace clotting factors.

IV calcium gluconate or calcium chloride is needed with massive transfusion because the citrate in the PRBCs will bind with the patient's calcium, causing hypocalcemia. Typically, 1 g of calcium gluconate is given with every fourth unit of PRBCs. If calcium is not administered in the trauma bay or operating room, the ICU nurse should suggest this intervention.

Postresuscitation

Once the initial resuscitation is complete, trend serial hemoglobin levels and monitor drain output to assess for ongoing bleeding. The hemoglobin level should increase by 1 g for every unit of PRBCs administered. If this is not occurring, the patient may either still require resuscitation or be still actively bleeding. Notify the trauma team, and they should repeat the primary and secondary surveys, inspecting for other injuries. Some bleeding is in the form of oozing, such as from bone, as happens with hip fractures. Bones are highly vascular and can ooze for a day or so. Nurses should monitor for new ecchymosis and hematoma formation in the soft tissues, which can indicate other injuries. Compression of soft tissues with Ace wraps can be helpful to tamponade bleeding.

FAST FACTS

Hemoglobin should increase 1 g for each unit of PRBCs. A hemoglobin level that fails to respond indicates ongoing bleeding.

Deep vein thrombosis (DVT) prophylaxis: Trauma patients are at high risk for venous thromboembolism (VTE). All trauma patients should have mechanical DVT prophylaxis. Once all bleeding is stopped and hemoglobin is stable, chemical DVT prophylaxis should be initiated. If the nurse suspects ongoing bleeding, they should discuss their concern with the trauma team to determine whether to hold the chemical prophylaxis. Patients with head injuries should be started on chemical DVT prophylaxis within 24 hours of having a stable head CT scan. Spinal cord injuries should have chemical DVT prophylaxis started within 24 hours of surgical stabilization. The nurse should consult the team on rounds if DVT prophylaxis is not started within these time frames.

Anticoagulation: Many trauma patients are on anticoagulation for atrial fibrillation, VTE, or mechanical valves. A discussion with the patient, trauma team, and specialists should ensue as to if and when to resume the anticoagulation. For older patients who fall frequently, a frank discussion should occur with the trauma surgeon, primary care provider, patient, and family about the potential risk of additional falls, injury with life-threatening bleeding, or head injury before anticoagulants are resumed. For patients who already have a head injury, discussion with neurosurgery should include guidance on resumption of anticoagulation. When anticoagulation is initiated, nurses should monitor for recurrent bleeding. Subtle neurologic changes can indicate recurrent bleeding.

D: DELIRIUM PREVENTION

Trauma patients, especially older adults, are at risk for delirium while hospitalized. Multiple factors can trigger delirium, including history of dementia, a new environment, head injury, general anesthesia, analgesics, sedation, and lack of sleep. Delirium can be either hyperactive or hypoactive, with the former being more common. Family frequently finds delirium disturbing. Nurses can ease family's anxiety with education about delirium and encourage family presence and interaction with the patient. Keeping the patient awake and active during the day helps to promote sleep at night. Nurses should facilitate an environment conducive to sleep, including a quiet environment: Dim the lights, turn off the TV at night, offer eye masks and earplugs, and block patient care interventions to allow for uninterrupted periods of rest. Quiet-time protocols have been proven helpful in preventing delirium, which can reduce ICU and hospital length of stay and mortality.

E: EARLY MOBILITY

Critically ill and injured patients who are on bed rest lose around 16% of their muscle mass in a week. A prolonged ICU stay is associated with neuromuscular dysfunction in about 45% of patients. Early mobility of patients maintains their strength, improves functional capacity, prevents atelectasis, increases number of ventilator-free days, reduces delirium, and decreases the need for rehabilitation. Several forms of early mobility exist, including dangling at the bedside, progressing to standing, sitting in the chair, and ambulation. For patients who are bedbound, stationary bed-level pedaling is effective to maintain leg strength. Use of small hand weights, elastic bands, and squeeze balls maintains strength of upper extremities. Nurses must not rely solely on PT to mobilize patients. Ventilated as well as nonventilated patients can and should be mobilized regularly. Hospitals should have a mobility program, and daily goals for mobilization should be established on rounds. Nurses should document mobilization progress and report to providers any barriers to mobilization, including patient refusal, so the team can reinforce the importance of mobility. Tracking progress with a standardized mobility scale is helpful for teams to measure progress.

F: FLUIDS, FOLEY, AND FAMILY

Fluids

The patient's fluid status should be assessed and addressed every day. Does the patient need more or less fluid? After the initial resuscitation, the patient commonly needs less. When calculating total fluid intake, infusions, antibiotics, and enteral flushes should be calculated into the hourly intake. Maintenance fluids should be decreased to accommodate these infusions. Nurses play a keen role in questioning whether fluids can be decreased. Conservative fluid management strategies lead to decreased ventilator days and ICU length of stay.

Foley

Prolonged use of Foley catheters leads to increased risk of catheter-associated urinary tract infections (CAUTI). Prevention of CAUTIs has been demonstrated with the use of nurse-driven catheter removal protocols. If the nurse-driven protocol is not in place, nurses should discuss the Foley catheter during rounds. Evaluate the need on a daily and even shift-by-shift basis. Indications for keeping the catheter in place should be clearly documented in the record.

Family

The family's presence during trauma resuscitation can facilitate their understanding of the severity of injuries and appreciate all that was done to salvage their loved one's life. If the patient doesn't survive, this may be the family's last opportunity to see them. Have one person assigned to attend the family during resuscitation, which doesn't need to be a nurse who may be engaged in care of the patient. A nursing supervisor, clergy member, or social worker may fulfill this role. Family presence during resuscitation may also be useful to provide patient medical history and medications, which can guide interventions.

Family presence during the patient's admission is beneficial to the patient's recovery. Nurses should routinely engage family in the care of the patient, provide education, and encourage family to motivate the patient during therapies. Families can encourage incentive spirometry, perform range of motion, and encourage strength training. Nurses play a pivotal role by notifying the trauma team of the family at bedside to allow the team to provide a medical update and facilitate formal family meetings to discuss injuries, goals of care, and disposition.

As stated in Chapter 2, trauma patients can be victims of their social situations; as such, "trauma drama" may occur. Nurses must ensure they and the patient are always safe. Open communication among nurses, security, nursing leadership, and the trauma team is essential. Additionally, nurses should refrain from engaging in family disputes or disagreements and remain neutral in the family dynamics that spill over to the hospital.

G: GASTRIC/STRESS ULCER SUPPRESSION, NUTRITION, AND GOALS OF CARE

Gastric/Stress Ulcer Prophylaxis

A select population of patients should be on SUP while hospitalized. Patients who are on a ventilator more than 48 hours, have a head or spinal cord injury, have coagulopathy, or are on steroids require SUP. Either histamine-2 receptor antagonists (H2 blockers) or proton pump inhibitors (PPIs) can be used for SUP. Providers should continue H2 blockers or PPIs if patients were on them at home to treat gastroesophageal reflux disease. Nurses can encourage discontinuation of these agents to prevent side effects of unnecessary use. Side effects of PPIs in the hospital setting include risk of pneumonia, *Clostridium difficile* infection, and hypomagnesemia.

Nutrition

Many trauma patients present in a malnourished state. Older adults, persons with alcohol or other substance use disorders, unhoused persons, persons with lower socioeconomic status, and medically complex patients routinely do not have a nutritionally sound diet. Traumatically injured patients also require higher protein levels to heal wounds. Nurses should consult a dietitian to evaluate the nutritional state of all trauma patients. Nutritional supplements are encouraged to meet caloric needs. Burn patients and those with significant tissue destruction have especially high caloric needs.

Nutrition should be started within the first 24 to 48 hours of admission. Enteral nutrition is preferred over parenteral nutrition. Patients must have an intact and functional gastrointestinal tract for either oral or tube feedings. Trauma patients who have had abdominal surgery are at risk for ileus due to the trauma or presence of blood in the abdominal cavity, including those who have had intra-abdominal injuries embolized.

> **FAST FACTS**
>
> Enteral nutrition should be initiated within 24 to 48 hours of admission.

Nurses can ensure accurate calorie counts, which can be useful to determine whether patients are meeting their intake goals. Nurses should ensure tube feedings are not stopped for prolonged periods of care. Volume-based feeding protocols can help ensure the patient receives their caloric needs. Volume-based tube feeding calculates the total daily dose of feedings and adjusts the tube feeding rate to catch up for periods when the feedings were held. Nurses can collaborate with dietitians to create unit or hospital protocols as quality improvement projects or for clinical ladder projects.

Goals of Care

Every patient who is admitted should have an initial discussion regarding goals of care, including the status of do not resuscitate. Additional conversations may be needed to address the possible need for intubation and ventilator support or other life-sustaining treatments. Further in-depth conversations regarding goals of care include but are not limited to:

- Whether a patient with severe traumatic brain injuries or failure to wean from the ventilator would desire a tracheostomy and percutaneous gastrostomy tube placement
- Necessity for intubation and ventilation in a patient who develops progressive respiratory failure
- Initiation of dialysis in a patient with acute kidney injury
- Requirement for long-term acute care hospitalization and rehabilitation and possible long-term care post discharge
- Functional status before injury and during recovery, and what the patient's new baseline may be after recovery
- Any change in patient status, such as upgrade to a step-down unit or ICU.

H: HOSPITAL STAY—HOW TO SHORTEN—CONSULT THERAPIES (PHYSICAL THERAPY/OCCUPATIONAL THERAPY/SPEECH THERAPY/COGNITIVE THERAPY/WOUND OSTOMY CONTINENCE NURSE)

Discharge planning begins at the time of admission. A thorough history of a patient's home environment is helpful to envision whether the patient can return home. Considerations include location of the bathroom, bedrooms, use of patient's extremities, and presence of head injuries, and combined with frailty score or functional scores at time of admission can provide a general sense.

Trauma patients should receive evaluation by PT and occupational therapy (OT) to assess their strength and ability to care for themselves at home or if rehabilitation services are required. Nurses should premedicate the patient with pain medication before PT and OT evaluation and mobilization. Nurses should not wait for PT to get a patient out of bed and mobilized; early mobilization is desired. Nurses, PT, and OT should engage family to assist with mobilizing patients. Commonly, patients decline rehabilitation, relying on their family to provide care. Family needs to be taught how to safely mobilize patients. Families who desire to support the wishes of patients to avoid rehabilitation must be able to safely demonstrate they can get the patient in and out of bed and chair and to and from the bathroom. Nurses may also need to teach patients and families how to do dressing changes or care for external fixation pins.

For patients who have had a loss of consciousness, a cognitive evaluation is required. Patients may have a concussion and need supervision at home until symptoms resolve, or they may require inpatient or outpatient traumatic brain injury rehabilitation. Patients with a severe brain injury can benefit from coma stimulation programs to enhance recovery. Both cognitive evaluations and coma stimulation programs can be provided by either a speech language pathologist or OT depending on the institution.

All patients who are extubated should receive a bedside swallow by the nurse before a diet is instituted. Patients who have a cervical spine injury and are required to wear a cervical spine collar may have difficulty with swallowing, especially the older population. These patients and any patients who have difficulty swallowing should receive a swallow evaluation by a speech language pathologist. Older patients may have had difficulty before admission from previous injuries or strokes and can benefit from swallow therapies and techniques.

Many trauma patients have reasons for consultation with a wound ostomy continence nurse (WOCN). All burn patients, patients with spinal cord injuries that require firm mattresses until surgical repair can occur, those requiring high vasopressors, those with complex wounds, whose who required an ostomy, and those who developed an enterocutaneous fistula all should have a consult placed with a WOCN. Nurses routinely perform skin assessments on all tubes, lines, and drains for pressure points. In the trauma population, cervical collars, nasogastric tubes, and tracheostomies can all cause pressure ulcers.

The patient's mental health should be considered while the patient is hospitalized. The trauma team should conduct mental health screenings on all admitted trauma patients. If the nurse notes a patient is struggling to cope with the illness and injuries, has flashbacks, or develops anxiety or depression while admitted, the team should obtain a psychiatric consult.

I: INFECTIONS, INTIMATE PARTNER VIOLENCE, ELDER MISTREATMENT, AND CHILD ABUSE

Infections

Trauma patients are at risk for infections because many of their wounds are contaminated with debris from the ground, clothing, foreign objects, glass, or other penetrating objects. Additionally, as with all hospitalized patients, trauma patients are at risk for nosocomial infections, including hospital- and/or ventilator-associated pneumonia, urinary tract infections, central line–associated bloodstream infections, and *C. difficile* infections. Nurses play a key role in preventing these infections and thereby reducing morbidity, mortality, length of stay, and cost. Pulmonary hygiene, daily SATs and SBTs, nurse-driven catheter removal protocols, thorough central line care, and maintenance of dressings reduce these complications.

Intimate Partner Violence, Elder Mistreatment, and Child Abuse or Neglect

Nurses spend the most amount of time with a patient and are skilled communicators. Trauma patients need thoughtful communication to elicit additional details from patients about their injuries. Nurses should observe interactions with visitors and create the opportunity to spend time alone with each patient. Inquire whether they were harmed and if they feel safe. Nurses must have a high index of suspicion that traumatic injuries may not have been caused by the stated mechanism. Consider whether injury patterns are consistent with the stated events. Assess for ecchymosis in various stages of healing. Radiology reports may also report other now-healed fractures.

Intimate Partner Violence

IPV is behavior in an intimate relationship that causes physical, sexual, or psychological harm. It may include controlling behaviors, physical aggression, psychological abuse, and sexual coercion. Both women and men, straight and same-sex partners who are dating, living together, or married can be victims of IPV. Overall, IPV affects women more than men, with male partners being the perpetrators.

Depending on the state, persons aged 18 to 50 years may not be considered a protected group. Those younger than 18 or older than 50 years are considered children and elders, respectively, and thus have special protections with mandatory reporting. IPV in persons aged 18 to 50 years can be reported, but services may not be available. Social work should be engaged with all patients to provide information on community resources and shelters. They can help the patient form a plan to get out of the situation.

Elder Mistreatment
Elder mistreatment is the intentional act or failure to act that causes harm to an older adult (see Chapter 17).

Child Maltreatment
Children are frequently injured. Nurses should confirm and document how a child was injured (see Chapter 19).

J: JUST REMEMBER: OTHER MEDICAL PROBLEMS AND ASSOCIATED MEDICATIONS

Many trauma patients present emergently and are registered as an unknown patient to facilitate more efficient emergency care. Patients are often sent to trauma centers out of the healthcare system where they routinely receive care. Thus, their medical history may not be immediately known. Once the patient is admitted and stabilized, obtaining a detailed medical history and medication record is essential. Nurses can ask families to bring in all medications, including prescription and over-the-counter drugs as well as vitamins and herbal supplements, that the patient is currently taking. This brown bag approach to medication reconciliation can provide accurate data. Additionally, the nurse can ask the family which pharmacy the patient uses and gather a medication list from them. The nurse can also acquire this information by consulting with the pharmacist. Medication reconciliation is a key component to providing thorough and holistic care for the patient.

The trauma team needs to ensure that all the patient's preexisting medical conditions are managed throughout the hospital stay. Commonly, patients who are in shock upon admission are not started on some of their home medications. This may lead to patients having complications such as rapid atrial fibrillation from withholding antiarrhythmic agents or pulmonary edema from withholding diuretics, among others. The nurse plays a key role on rounds by inquiring if any home medications can be restarted or voicing family concerns if medications have not yet been resumed.

FAST FACTS

Nurses play a key role in performing medication reconciliation at the time of admission. Ask the family to bring a list of medications or a bag of all medications the patient takes.

SUMMARY

Nurses play a vital role in ensuring trauma patients receive the best possible care. The list of A to J should be addressed every day on rounds. The nurse should keep a checklist to ensure the team addresses these items throughout the stay.

REVIEW QUESTIONS

1. A patient with rib fractures becomes hypoxic to 88%. What is the nurse's first intervention?
   a. Obtain a chest x-ray
   b. Apply oxygen
   c. Notify the provider
   d. Have the patient perform incentive spirometry
2. An adult patient with a femur fracture is on call to the operating room for surgical repair of his fracture. He's reporting 10/10 pain. Which of the following PRN orders should the nurse administer?
   a. Tylenol 650 mg PO
   b. Dilaudid .5 mg IV
   c. Oxycodone 2.5 mg PO
   d. Fentanyl 25 mcg patch
3. A patient newly admitted with a severe head injury and elevated intracranial pressure should have:
   a. Heavy sedation
   b. Lovenox for DVT prophylaxis
   c. Pepcid for SUP
   d. Visits from family and friends

References

American College of Surgeons Committee on Trauma. (2020). *ACS trauma quality programs: Best practice guidelines for acute pain management in trauma patients.* American College of Surgeons.

Devlin, J. W., Skrobik, Y., Gélinas, C., Needham, D. M., Slooter, A. J., Pandharipande, P. P., Watson, P. L., Weinhouse, G. L., Nunnally, M. E., Rochwerg, B., Balas, M. C., van den Boogaard, M., Bosma, K. J., Brummel, N. E., Chanques, G., Denehy, L., Drouot, X., Fraser, G. L., Harris, J. E., ... Alhazzani, W. (2018). Clinical practice guidelines for the prevention and management of pain, agitation/sedation, delirium, immobility, and sleep disruption in adult patients in the ICU. *Critical Care Medicine, 46*(9), e825–e873.

Escalon, M. X., Lichtenstein, A. H., Posner, E., Spielman, L., Delgado, A., & Kolakowsky-Hayner, S. A. (2020). The effects of early mobilization on patients requiring extended mechanical ventilation across multiple ICUs. *Critical Care Explorations, 2*(6), e0119.

Ley, E. J., Brown, C. V. R., Moore, E. E., Sava, J. A., Peck, K., Ciesla, D. J., Sperry, J. L., Rizzo, A. G., Rosen, N. G., Brasel, K. J., Kozar, R., Inaba, K., & Martin, M. J. (2020). Updated guidelines to reduce venous thromboembolism in trauma patients: A Western Trauma Association critical decisions algorithm. *The Journal of Trauma and Acute Care Surgery, 89*(5), 971.

McClave, S. A., Saad, M. A., Esterle, M., Anderson, M., Jotautas, A. E., Franklin, G. A., Heyland, D. K., & Hurt, R. T. (2015). Volume-based feeding in the critically ill patient. *Journal of Parenteral and Enteral Nutrition, 39*(6), 707–712.

McLaughlin, K. H., Friedman, M., Hoyer, E. H., Kudchadkar, S., Flanagan, E., Klein, L., Daley, K, Lavezza, A., Schechter, N., & Young, D. (2023). The Johns Hopkins activity and mobility promotion program: A framework to increase activity and mobility among hospitalized patients. *Journal of Nursing Care Quality, 38*(2), 164.

Nehra, A. K., Alexander, J. A., Loftus, C. G., & Nehra, V. (2018, February). Proton pump inhibitors: Review of emerging concerns. *Mayo Clinic Proceedings, 93*(2), 240–246.

Silversides, J. A., Major, E., Ferguson, A. J., Mann, E. E., McAuley, D. F., Marshall, J. C., Blackwood, B., & Fan, E. (2017). Conservative fluid management or deresuscitation for patients with sepsis or acute respiratory distress syndrome following the resuscitation phase of critical illness: A systematic review and meta-analysis. *Intensive Care Medicine, 43*, 155–170.

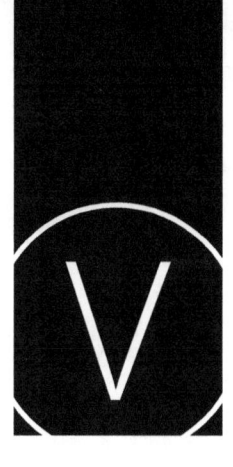

SPECIAL POPULATIONS AND CIRCUMSTANCES

Older Adult Trauma Patients
Dawn Carpenter

> Older adult patients comprise a significant portion of trauma patients. Trauma nurses must recognize physiologic changes that occur with aging, including lack of physiologic reserve. Medical problems and polypharmacy reduce older adult patients' ability to survive injuries.

In this chapter, you will learn:
1. Normal physiologic changes associated with aging.
2. Pharmacokinetics in the aging trauma population.
3. Tips for medication administration in older adult trauma patients.
4. Drugs to avoid with older adult trauma patients.
5. Causes of falls in the older adult.

INTRODUCTION

Older adult trauma patients are at higher risk for complications. Physiologic changes associated with aging and chronic comorbid conditions can be exacerbated secondary to the trauma and associated diagnostic testing. For example, acute kidney injury is common given the physiologic decrease in glomerular filtration rate and inability to compensate for shock states. This can be further complicated by administration of IV contrast used during CT scans to diagnose injuries.

PHYSIOLOGIC CHANGES WITH AGING

Aging decreases physiologic reserve, rendering older adult trauma patients unable to recover from relatively minor injuries. Additionally, multiple comorbid conditions affect their ability to tolerate injuries. Even patients with low injury severity scores are prone to complications that can lead to death in the frail population. To understand assessment of the older adult, nurses must recognize physiologic changes that occur with aging (Table 17.1).

These physiologic changes predispose older adults to more severe injuries and worse outcomes than younger patients. Even minor injuries in a younger person can prove fatal to an elder. Preexisting medical conditions

TABLE 17.1

Physiologic Changes with Aging

Organ System	Changes	Implications
Neurologic	■ Autoregulatory capabilities ■ Brain atrophy ■ Short-term memory loss	■ Susceptibility to injury ■ Atrophy allows increased blood accumulation before neurologic changes are present ■ May not recall how injury occurred ■ Risk of delirium
Pulmonary	■ Vital capacity ■ Forced expiratory volume ■ Smaller alveolar surface area ■ Chest wall compliance	■ Respiratory reserve ■ Rib fractures and pulmonary contusions are not well tolerated; increases mortality
Cardiac	■ Cardiac output ■ Sensitivity to catecholamines	■ Cardiac reserve ■ Normal BP may be hypotensive for older adult ■ May not be tachycardic due to certain medications
Renal	■ GFR ■ Renal mass	■ May have baseline renal impairment ■ Risk of contrast-induced nephropathy ■ Susceptibility to fluid overload ■ Clearance of certain medications
Hepatic	■ Hepatic function	■ Clearance of certain medications
GI	■ Pain sensation ■ Laxity of ABD wall ■ Difficulty swallowing/chewing	■ Need less medication to treat pain ■ Potential for significant intra-abdominal trauma without clinical signs ■ Risk for aspiration and malnutrition
Immune	■ Impaired immune response	■ Risk of infections
Musculoskeletal	■ Loss of muscle mass ■ Osteoporosis ■ Arthritis	■ Risk of falls ■ Risk of fractures ■ Difficulty of intubation
Integumentary	■ Decreased adipose ■ Thinning skin	■ Risk for hypothermia ■ Risk of pressure injuries ■ Risk of skin tears

ABD, abdominal; BP, blood pressure; GFR, glomerular filtration rate; GI, gastrointestinal.
Source: Modified with permission from Carpenter, Fast Facts for the Adult-Gerontology Acute Care Nurse Practitioners (AGACNP).

TABLE 17.2

Pharmacokinetics in Aging

Process	Physiologic Change	Pharmacokinetic Effect
Distribution	▪ Total body mass, increased proportion of body fat ▪ Proportion of body water ▪ Plasma albumin, disease-related increase in alpha-1 acid glycoprotein ▪ Altered tissue perfusion	▪ Volume of distribution of highly lipid-soluble drugs ▪ Volume of distribution of hydrophilic drugs ▪ Changes % of free drug, volume of distribution, and measured levels of bound drugs
Metabolism	▪ Liver mass, liver blood flow, and hepatic metabolic capacity	▪ Accumulation of metabolized drugs
Excretion	▪ Glomerular filtration, renal tubular function, and renal blood flow	▪ Accumulation of metabolized drugs

Source: Modified with permission from Carpenter, Fast Facts for the AGACNP.

can be worsened by the trauma, the diagnostic workup, and/or the treatments required. Medications to treat chronic conditions can mask signs of shock, worsen bleeding, cause electrolyte and volume disturbances, and alter interpretation of vital signs. These changes require astute trauma nurses to take these factors into account in an attempt to preserve organ function and improve functional outcomes.

Physiologic changes associated with aging can affect pharmacokinetics (Table 17.2). A foundational tenet of administering medications in the older adult is to "start low and go slow." Emphasis should be on avoiding potentially inappropriate medications in the older adult. Older adult patients are also at greater risk for delirium, which increases length of stay, complications, and even mortality.

Tips for Administering Medications to Older Adult Trauma Patients

- Analgesic goals are to achieve tolerable pain levels so the patient can be functional.
- Perform a detailed medication reconciliation prior to providers prescribing.
- Hold all anticoagulant and antiplatelet agents until bleeding has ceased and hemoglobin is stable.
- Patients on anticoagulants with intracranial bleeding should immediately receive reversal agents.
- Avoid drugs that have known deleterious effects in older adult patients (see "Beers Criteria").

- Start low, go slow; start with one fourth to one half of a dose; it is easy to add more, but can't be reduced once it's been given.
- Minimize opioids by using nonpharmacologic treatments, including cold, heat, compression, and splints and bracing to provide pain relief.
- Consider whether a change in the patient's condition is an adverse drug reaction; if so, avoid administering additional medications. Less is more in the older adult!
- Monitor the creatinine clearance rather than creatinine in the older adult.
- Avoid benzodiazepines because of the high risk of delirium; also, do not abruptly stop if chronically taken, because the patient may experience withdrawal symptoms.
- Acetaminophen (Tylenol) doses are to a maximum of 3 g/d, 2 g/d in those with liver injuries.
- Delirium—consider whether delirium is related to current medications versus a new acute problem, such as an infection. Avoid requesting additional medications to treat delirium. Nurses should implement a sleep protocol or add a sitter.

FAST FACTS

When administering opioid analgesics to older adult trauma patients, start low, go slow!!! You can always add more but can't get it back once it's been given!

MEDICATION RECONCILIATION

The medication reconciliation on admission is a critical process for all trauma patients but especially for elders who commonly have a multitude of comorbid conditions. Older adults and patients with complex medical histories commonly have several prescribers in multiple health systems, and then a trauma can add new diagnoses and places them at higher risk for medication errors and omissions. The "brown bag" method allows for review of each medication, dosage, and administration timing and adherence. The brown bag method engages the patient and family to bring in all prescribed and over-the-counter medications and supplements. The nurse should review these with the patient and family and update the medication list in the electronic medical record.

BEERS CRITERIA

The Beers criteria are medications or types of medications that are "potentially inappropriate" for older adults. The Beers list outlines three classifications of medications: (1) potentially inappropriate medications in older adults, (2) potentially inappropriate medications in older adults from drug–disease or drug–syndrome interactions, and (3) drugs to avoid in older adults. These agents all have higher risks of side effects in the older adult (see BEERS criteria: https://agsjournals.onlinelibrary.wiley.com/doi/epdf/10.1111/jgs.18372).

FAST FACTS

Avoid benzodiazepines in the older adult as they can precipitate delirium, which could lead to prolonged hospital stay and increased mortality. If benzodiazepines are taken chronically, they should not be abruptly stopped, or the patient may experience benzodiazepine withdrawal.

FALLS VERSUS SYNCOPE

Falls are the most common mechanism of injury in the older adult. Trauma team members must explore whether the patient had a mechanical fall, meaning they recall tripping over an object or losing their balance, or whether they lost consciousness and then fell.

Syncope in the older adult is common and has many causes, such as:
- Orthostatic hypotension from dehydration and/or hypovolemia.
- Infection, which can lead to sepsis.
- Cardiac arrhythmias, including heart block, bradycardia, or tachyarrhythmia.
- Severe aortic stenosis.
- Ischemic or hemorrhagic stroke or hypoperfusion due to atherosclerotic arteries.
- Hypotension due to medications.

The causative factor(s) should be elicited during the hospitalization to prevent further events and risk for additional injuries and adverse events, including rehospitalization and/or death. The events immediately before the patient fell are critical to determine whether they fell and then lost consciousness or lost consciousness and then fell. Family or friends who were present may be able to contribute this information if the patient is amnestic to the event.

On admission, telemetry monitoring is needed during the first 24 hours, at a minimum, to identify arrhythmias. A transthoracic echocardiogram (TTE) should be completed if a recent study is not available or there is suspicion of a new cardiac cause. The TTE will evaluate for critical aortic stenosis and other abnormalities that could precipitate syncope. If witnesses describe any seizure-like activity, an EEG should be obtained.

Physical assessment should include auscultation of the carotid arteries for possible bruits, which can indicate carotid stenosis that might lead to syncope. Nurses should obtain orthostatic or postural vital signs to determine whether a change in position caused the syncope. Assess the patient's weight and compare it to previous readings to assess for weight loss. Weight loss can indicate malnutrition and muscle wasting, which can lead to weakness. Weight loss can also cause patients to not require the same level of antihypertensive medications.

ELDER MISTREATMENT

Elder mistreatment is the intentional act or failure to act that causes harm to an older adult. Elder mistreatment may be in the form of neglect; physical, emotional, financial, or sexual abuse; or abandonment. Injury patterns that are not congruent with the stated mechanism of injury should raise suspicion. Signs of elder mistreatment include unexplained ecchymosis, fractures, abrasions, pressure ulcers, contact burns, and scald injuries, which might indicate physical abuse. Ecchymosis or injuries to the breasts or genitalia can represent sexual abuse. Elders may seem withdrawn from previously enjoyed activities and unusually depressed. Neglect may be noted as poor hygiene, unexplained weight loss, or failure to address medical needs. Psychological abuse can be noted by the abuser belittling, threatening, or having frequent arguments. Notify the trauma team, which should reassess and inspect records and diagnostic reports for other injuries or injuries at various stages of healing. As mandated reporters, nurses must document and report to proper authorities when elder mistreatment is suspected. Trauma providers and social workers can assist with reporting.

SUMMARY

In summary, older adults, and especially frail elders, require considerable attention to medication reconciliation. Pay special attention to pharmacokinetics and pharmacodynamics because of the pathophysiologic changes that occur during the aging process. The medication principle of starting low and going slow is critical to prevent overmedication! Nurses should maintain a high index of suspicion for elder abuse.

REVIEW QUESTIONS

1. An older adult trauma patient becomes delirious. The nurse should:
   a. Call the provider for a dose of Ativan
   b. Institute a sleep protocol
   c. Administer pain medication
   d. Turn on the lights
2. The nurse is assessing a newly admitted trauma patient. The nurse notes she has multiple ecchymoses in varying stages of healing. The patient reports that she falls frequently. The nurse should:
   a. Discuss with social work
   b. Call the provider
   c. Report to elder services
   d. All of the above

References

Alpert, J. S. (2019). Syncope in the elderly. *The American Journal of Medicine, 132*(10), 1115–1116.

American College of Surgeons, Committee on Trauma. (2015). *Rural trauma team development course* (4th ed.). American College of Surgeons.

McKearney, K., & Coleman, J. J. (2020). Prescribing medicines for elderly patients. *Medicine, 48*(7), 463–467.

Milton, J. C., Hill-Smith, I., & Jackson, S. H. (2008). Prescribing for older people. *British Medical Journal, 336*(7644), 606–609.

2019 American Geriatrics Society Beers Criteria® Update Expert Panel, Fick, D. M., Semla, T. P., Steinman, M., Beizer, J., Brandt, N., Dombrowski, R., DuBeau, C. E., Pezzullo, L., Epplin, J. J., Flanagan, N., Morden, E., Hanlon, J., Hollmann, P., Laird, R., Linnebur, S., & Sandhu, S. (2019). American Geriatrics Society 2019 updated AGS Beers criteria® for potentially inappropriate medication use in older adults. *Journal of the American Geriatrics Society, 67*(4), 674–694.

Pregnant Trauma Patients
Dawn Carpenter

> Trauma is the leading cause of death for pregnant women in the United States. The most common mechanism of injury in the trauma patient is motor vehicle collision, accounting for nearly 50% of injuries, followed by falls, assault, gunshot wounds, and burns. Intimate partner violence increases during pregnancy and is frequently underreported. Although the primary and secondary survey process remains unchanged, providers need to recognize that both the physiologic changes that occur during pregnancy and the gestational age can alter response to injuries. Additionally, U.S. maternal mortality rates are due to multifactorial socioeconomic factors and pregnancy-related conditions. Thus, this chapter reviews common obstetric urgencies and emergencies and respective care.

In this chapter, you will learn:
1. Normal physiologic and anatomic changes with pregnancy.
2. Nursing care of the injured pregnant patient.
3. Common obstetric emergencies.

INTRODUCTION

The pregnant trauma patient is unique because the trauma team is caring for two patients: the mother and the fetus. To improve fetal outcomes, trauma management focuses on aggressive resuscitation of the mother. The trauma team should consult with obstetricians as soon as possible, which can occur before the patient's arrival. Anticipate early transfer to a level I trauma center. When a trauma patient is known to be pregnant, staff should bring an infant warmer with infant resuscitation system to the trauma bay/ICU in the event of emergent delivery.

Positioning
Trauma patients commonly present to the ED with a cervical collar applied and the patient strapped to a rigid backboard in the supine position. The weight of a gravid uterus over 20 weeks' gestation in the supine position

compresses the inferior vena cava and reduces the venous return to the heart, with up to a 30% decrease in cardiac output. Thus, upon completion of the primary survey, position the patient with the right side elevated while maintaining spinal precautions. This can be done by placing a pillow under the right side of the spinal backboard 15 to 30 degrees or 4 to 6 inches under the right hand side of the backboard or a blanket roll under the right hip once the spines are cleared. Alternatively, manual displacement of the uterus upward to the left side can temporarily relieve the pressure while ongoing life-saving care is given. Given the challenges to adequate displacement when the uterus is at/above the umbilicus, if CPR is necessary, early Cesarean delivery (within 4 minutes of arrest) may be needed to support maternal survival, even if the fetus is previable.

Anatomic Changes in Pregnancy

The greater the gestational age, the higher the location of the uterine fundus, leading to displacement of intra-abdominal organs from their typical/expected locations. At around 12 weeks of gestation, the uterus is starting to rise out of the pelvis; by 20 weeks, the uterus may be at or near the level of the umbilicus. This in turn pushes the intestines higher, now being partially protected by the thoracic cage. However, the uterus is now less protected as it has risen from the pelvis but remains below the protective rib cage, increasing vulnerability to traumatic injury.

Physiologic Changes in Pregnancy

Trauma nurses must be aware of physiologic changes during pregnancy (Table 18.1). Many changes happen during the first trimester, when pregnancy may not be obvious. Thus, all persons with female anatomy who are of child-bearing years should be tested immediately for pregnancy.

FACT FACTS

Pregnant patients should be positioned onto the left side to enhance venous return to the heart.

An important concept for pregnant trauma patients is that their circulating blood volume increases; thus, they can lose large quantities of blood before clinical signs of hypovolemia are present. Additionally, their heart rate is elevated at baseline, complicating providers' assessment of volume status.

Gestational Age

The team should immediately establish the gestational age. Initial triage determines whether the fetus is of viable gestation if delivery is required and whether the fetus is still currently alive. Gestations under 20 weeks are

TABLE 18.1

Physiologic Changes in Pregnancy

	Changes	Impact
Reproductive system	■ Uterus extends out of the pelvis after the 12th week of gestation ■ At 20 weeks, the uterus is at the umbilicus ■ At 34 to 36 weeks, the uterus is at the costal margins ■ Increased blood flow to uterus (600 mL/min)	■ Uterus displaces bowel superiorly, protecting the bowel; however, as the uterus becomes more exposed, it is more vulnerable to injury ■ Increased likelihood of hemorrhage ■ Susceptible to shearing injury
	■ Placenta is not elastic ■ Placental vasculature is normally dilated ■ Uteroplacental circulation cannot autoregulate	■ Sensitive to hypovolemia and catecholamine stimulation ■ Hypovolemia results in ↑ placental vasoconstriction and fetal hypoxia
	■ ↓ Vaginal pH ■ ↑ Glycogen in vaginal epithelium	↑ Risk of chorioamnionitis
Cardiovascular	↓ Peripheral vascular resistance ↓ SVR and BP in 2nd trimester, returns to prepregnancy levels at term. ↑ Heart rate 10% to 15% over baseline or by 15 to 20 bpm ↓ Arterial pressure Increased cardiac output by 30% to 50% Increased preload, decreased afterload Cardiac flow murmurs ↑ Plasma volume by 50% ↑ Red cell volume by 30%	Masks initial signs of sepsis/hypovolemia, leading to delays in stabilization ↑ Hypoperfusion Uteroplacental circulation cannot autoregulate Can lose 1,200 to 1,500 mL blood before showing signs of hypovolemia

(continued)

TABLE 18.1 (continued)

Physiologic Changes in Pregnancy

	Changes	Impact
Respiratory	↑ Tidal volume ↑ Respiratory rate ↑ Minute-ventilation by 30% to 40% ↑ AP diameter ↑ PaO$_2$ and pH ↓ Functional residual capacity and residual volume ↓ PaCO$_2$ ↑ Oxygen consumption ↑ Diaphragm, up to 4 cm	Limited pulmonary reserve ↓ Ability to respond to acidosis Becomes hypoxic more quickly ↑ Risk of pneumothorax from CVC Chest tubes placed 1 to 2 ribs higher (between 3rd and 4th intercostal space)
Renal	↑ Renal blood flow, GFR ↑ Creatinine clearance ↓ BUN and creatinine Renal pelvis and ureteral dilation and ↓ ureteral pressure due to smooth muscle relaxation Bladder displaced out of pelvis ↑ Intravesical pressure ↑ Vesicoureteral reflux ↑ Renal plasma flow Asymptomatic bacteriuria	Normal BUN/creatinine can signify AKI, which can delay identification of AKI ↑ Risk of pyelonephritis ↑ Risk of bladder injury

(continued)

TABLE 18.1 (continued)

Physiologic Changes in Pregnancy

	Changes	Impact
Gastrointestinal	Displacement of abdominal organs ↓ Tone of lower esophageal sphincter ↓ Muscle tone across the GI tract ↓ Perfusion of gastric mucosa Delayed gastric emptying Changes in bile composition ↑ Production of proinflammatory cytokines by Kupffer cells ↑ Increased abdominal pressure	Altered patterns of pain ↑ Risk of regurgitation and aspiration ↑ Risk of bacterial translocation ↑ Risk of aspiration pneumonia ↑ Risk of cholestasis, hyperbilirubinemia, and jaundice ↑ Increased venous congestion ↑ Risk for IAH and ACS
Hematologic	↑ Leukocyte count Anemia ↓ Platelet count (usually remains WNL) ↑ Factors VII, VIII, IX, X, XII, von Willebrand, and fibrinogen ↓ Protein S ↓ Fibrinolytic activity	Leukocytosis is unreliable indicator of trauma or sepsis Pregnancy is a hypercoagulable state: ↑ risk of thrombotic events Increased risk of DIC

Source: Modified with permission from Carpenter, Fast Facts for Adult-Gerontology Acute Care Nurse Practitioner (AGACNPs).
ACS, abdominal compartment syndrome; AP, anterior posterior; AKI, acute kidney injury; BP, blood pressure; bpm, beats per minute; BUN, blood urea nitrogen; CVC, central venous catheter; DIC, disseminated intravascular coagulation; GFR, glomerular filtration rate; GI, gastrointestinal; IAH, intra-abdominal hypertension; $PaCO_2$, partial pressure of carbon dioxide; SVR, systemic vascular resistance; WNL, within normal limits.

deemed nonviable, 20 to 23 weeks are "periviable," and over 23 weeks are generally considered viable.

Laboratory Testing

Laboratory testing of pregnant trauma patients remains the same as in other, nonpregnant patients but also includes a baseline serum human chorionic gonadotropin and a Kleihauer–Betke (KB) test. The KB test is used to identify the presence of fetal blood in the maternal circulation, indicating possible placental trauma or placental abruption. A negative test does not exclude minor bleeding and mixing of blood. Thus, all pregnant Rh-negative trauma patients who have abdominal trauma or vaginal bleeding should receive Rh immunoglobulin within 72 hours of injury, unless the injuries are minor and far from the fetus.

FACT FACTS

All pregnant Rh-negative trauma patients should receive Rh immunoglobulin within 72 hours of injury unless the injuries are minor and far from the fetus.

TRAUMATIC INJURIES

Ninety percent of traumautic injuries to pregnant women are the result of blunt mechanisms, with the remaining 10% penetrating injuries. Fetal injuries can occur due to direct trauma to the abdominal wall. With motor vehicle crashes (MVCs), unrestrained pregnant persons have a higher fetal mortality and risk of premature delivery. Isolated lap belt use is associated with uterine compression and uterine rupture or abruptio placentae. The shoulder restraint prevents upper body flexion and decreases direct compression of the uterus. Thus, understanding the type of restraint can predict risk of injuries.

MONITORING

Indications for ongoing maternal and fetal assessments/monitoring:
- Trauma-related indications
  - Mechanism of injury (motorcycle crash, pedestrian struck, high-speed MVC, and ejection from vehicle)
  - Injury severity score >9
  - Maternal tachycardia (maternal heart rate >110 bpm)
  - Maternal serum fibrinogen <200 mg/dL
- Pregnancy/fetal-related indications
  - Auscultation of fetal heart rate (FHR) if <23 weeks; external electronic fetal heart monitoring if 23+ weeks
  - Fetal tachycardia or bradycardia (FHR >160 or <110)
  - Abnormal FHR variability or episodic changes (acceleration/decelerations)

- Vaginal bleeding
- Rupture of membranes
- Contractions: more than one every 10 minutes
- Palpation of uterus for tenderness or rigidity
- Ultrasound

ANALGESICS AND SEDATIVES DURING PREGNANCY

Opioids are commonly used in the treatment of acute pain in trauma patients. If delivery is imminent, anticipate that use of opioids, including fentanyl, morphine, and hydromorphone can cause respiratory depression in the infant and prolonged use can cause withdrawal symptoms in the newborn. Notify the pediatrician and neonatologist of any opioids used. Propofol can cause hypotension in the mother; lower appearance, pulse, grimace, activity, and respiration (APGAR) scores; muscle hypotony; and depressed neuromuscular activity. Benzodiazepines, including midazolam and lorazepam, can cause respiratory depression, floppy infant syndrome, and withdrawal syndrome in the newborn.

FACT FACTS

Routinely consult the obstetric team and pharmacist for any medications before use.

INTIMATE PARTNER VIOLENCE

Intimate partner violence (IPV) is a common cause of traumatic injuries in pregnant women. Nearly 20% of all pregnant persons experience IPV. Nurses should pay careful attention to the interaction between patient and family members. Attempt to interview the patient in private. Note whether partners insist on being present for interviews and examinations or dominate the interview. Assess the patient for signs of depression. Note any self-blame for the injuries. Inspect the chart for frequent ED or urgent care visits. Assess for isolated injuries to the abdomen, breasts, or genitalia. Compare the history of injuries with injury patterns for inconsistencies. Document and report any suspicion of IPV.

OBSTETRIC URGENCIES AND EMERGENCIES

Pregnant trauma patients may experience obstetric emergencies while hospitalized for their injuries. Acute and critical care nurses need to be familiar with common obstetric urgencies and emergencies and their associated management, Including preterm labor, placental abruption, premature rupture of membranes, severe preeclampsia, eclampsia, and anaphylactic syndrome of pregnancy (amniotic fluid embolism). Nearly 40% of pregnant trauma patients will experience contractions. Almost 25% of trauma patients with a viable fetus experience preterm labor. After maternal death, placental abruption is the leading cause of fetal demise.

FACT FACTS

Nurses should prepare the patient and family that any fetal distress may require emergent Cesarean delivery.

SUMMARY

In summary, obstetric trauma patients are complex to manage because of normal changes in maternal physiology, specific pregnancy-related conditions, and both maternal and fetal considerations. Care of these patients requires interprofessional collaboration with obstetric and neonatal nurses and providers as well as intensivists and pharmacists.

REVIEW QUESTIONS

1. An obviously pregnant trauma patient presents after an MVC. Vital signs are as follows: heart rate, 120 bpm; blood pressure, 90/60 mmHg; respiration rate, 24 per minute; oxygen saturation, 94% on room air. What is the initial intervention for this patient?
    a. Place on left side
    b. Administer IV bolus of normal saline 1 L STAT
    c. Transfuse 1 unit of whole blood
    d. Tilt right side of the backboard up
2. A severely injured pregnant trauma victim with blood type A negative should receive:
    a. Covid booster
    b. Tetanus booster
    c. O negative blood
    d. Rh immunoglobulin

References

American College of Surgeons, Committee on Trauma. (2015). *Rural trauma team development course* (4th ed.). American College of Surgeons.
American College of Surgeons: The Committee on Trauma. (2018). *ATLS: Advanced Trauma Life Support student course manual* (10th ed.). American College of Surgeons.
Buscher, M., & Edwards, J. H. (2020). Obstetric emergency critical care. *Emergency Department Critical Care*, 30, pp. 503–532. https://doi.org/10.1007/978-3-030-28794-8_30
Kaur, M., Singh, P. M., & Trikha, A. (2017). Management of critically ill obstetric patients: A review. *Journal of Obstetric Anaesthesia and Critical Care*, 7(1), 3.

Kilpatrick, S. J. (2023). Initial evaluation and management of major trauma in pregnancy. In T. W. Post (Ed.), *UpToDate*. Wolters Kluwer.

McQuillan, K. A., & Makic, M. B. F. (2020). *Trauma nursing from resuscitation through rehabilitation* (5th ed.). Elsevier.

Ruth, D., & Mighty, H. E. (2019). Trauma in pregnancy. In N. H. Troiano, P. M. Witcher, & S. M. Baird (Eds.), *High-risk and critical care obstetrics* (4th ed., pp. 331–343). Wolters Kluwer.

Pediatrics

Alexander Menard

Pediatric patients are a unique subset of trauma patients for several reasons, including their size and developmental differences. Traumatic injuries to children over the age of 1 year are the leading cause of death and disability to this population in the United States. The most common cause of death in children between 1 and 19 years of age is a motor vehicle crash. Falls are the leading cause of injury in this same population.

In this chapter, you will learn:
1. Normal physiologic differences in pediatric patients.
2. Assessment considerations in the pediatric population.
3. Resuscitation considerations in the pediatric population.

INTRODUCTION

Most pediatric trauma is preventable (see Chapter 24, Trauma Prevention). Given differences in pediatric anatomy and physiology and that blunt trauma is the most common form of trauma in the pediatric population, injury patterns are predictable. Most traumatic deaths occur due to motor vehicle crashes, and most traumatic injuries are due to falls. Pediatric patients are still developing and should not be considered small adults. They have less muscle, less fat, and less calcified bones, and their organs are in closer proximity compared with adults, causing higher rates of multiorgan injury involvement.

ANATOMIC AND PHYSIOLOGIC

The pediatric population has several differences in their anatomy and physiology compared with the adult trauma population (Table 19.1). Importantly, from a physiologic perspective, cardiac output is most influenced by heart rate as opposed to heart rate and stroke volume as occurs in the adult population. The pediatric population is very responsive to endogenous catecholamines, which allows pediatric patients to alter vascular tone. Given an increased heart rate and robust response to endogenous catecholamines, pediatric patients are better able to compensate for shock states for longer

TABLE 19.1

Anatomic Considerations

Anatomic Location	Difference in Pedi/Infant	Implications
Head	■ Larger head ■ Thinner cranium ■ Open sutures	■ Larger surface area for injury, bleeding ■ Transmission of energy; higher risk of fracture or damage to underlying structures ■ Delayed development of signs/symptoms of increased ICP
Spine	■ Weaker neck muscles, larger cranium, and less calcified vertebral bodies	■ Predisposition to higher cervical spine injuries and ligamentous injuries
Airway	■ Smaller structures and different anatomy: neck and airway	■ Higher risk for airway compromise due to swelling, hematoma, positioning, or other space-occupying pathology
Chest	■ More compliant chest ■ Smaller diameter of respiratory structures	■ Intrathoracic injury without or with minimal chest wall injury (i.e., no rib fractures with significant pulmonary contusion or laceration) ■ Higher chance of respiratory obstruction
Abdomen	■ Less development of abdominal muscles ■ Less intra-abdominal fat content	■ Higher risk for abdominal solid organ injury and hollow viscous injury ■ Higher risk for acceleration/deceleration injuries from seat belts or handlebars ■ Higher risk of chance fracture with seat belt injuries
Musculoskeletal	■ Incomplete calcification of bones	■ Allows for bending/bowing/greenstick injuries
Integumentary	■ Higher body surface area to mass	■ Increased risk for hypotension ■ Higher fluid losses in burn patients ■ Hypothermia occurs quickly, even during assessment in the ED

ICP, intracranial pressure.

periods with relatively stable vital signs. For example, pediatric patients might not start to become hypotensive until 25% to 40% of circulating blood volume is lost. From a respiratory standpoint, pediatric patients have a lower functional residual capacity, thus will become hypoxic after short periods of apnea. The pediatric patient has a higher metabolic demand and thus high caloric needs.

FAST FACTS

Avoid passive flexion of the cervical spine in the pediatric patient. Given the larger cranium compared with midface, there is a higher likelihood of airway obstruction/compromise. Placing a 1-inch pad underneath the infant or toddler's entire torso can help maintain alignment of the cervical spine in a neutral position, which then helps maintain a patent airway.

PEDIATRIC ASSESSMENT

Initial care of the pediatric trauma patient follows advanced trauma life support guidelines with completion of the primary, secondary, and tertiary surveys (see Chapters 4–6). Specific to the pediatric patient is the need to determine the child's weight. This can be done with a length-based resuscitation tape, the most common of which is the Broselow Pediatric Emergency Tape. After determining a child's height, an estimation of weight can be made from the Broselow tape, and the tape can be used to guide fluid resuscitation and dosing of medications, as well as determining the size of other equipment, including an oral airway or endotracheal tube, blood pressure cuff, oral/nasogastric tube, and so forth.

The pediatric population has different ranges for normal vital signs based on patient age and weight (Table 19.2). Nurses need to take these norms, by

TABLE 19.2

Vital Signs by Age/Weight

Normal Vital Sign Ranges

Age Range	Weight (kg)	Heart Rate (bpm)	Blood Pressure, Systolic (mmHg)	Respiratory Rate (breaths per minute)	Urine Output (mL/kg/hr)
0 to 12 months	0 to 10	<160	>60	<60	2
1 to 2 years	10 to 14	<150	>70	<40	1.5
3 to 5 years	14 to 18	<140	>75	<35	1
6 to 12 years	18 to 36	<120	>80	<30	1
>13 years	36 to 70	<100	>90	<30	.5

bpm, beats per minute.

age and weight, into consideration when assessing and treating the pediatric trauma patient.

> **FAST FACTS**
>
> Determining pediatric height is essential for estimated weight and selecting appropriately sized equipment. Be sure to use the Broselow tape to aid in the care of pediatric patients.

PEDIATRIC RESUSCITATION

Fluid replacement is weight based for the pediatric population. The pediatric patient can lose up to 25% of circulating blood volume before signs of hemorrhage are obvious, with tachycardia preceding hypotension. The process of resuscitation is to administer 20 mL/kg of isotonic fluid bolus; if further resuscitation is needed based on the vital signs, give 10 to 20 mL/kg of packed red blood cells and 10 to 20 mL/kg of fresh frozen plasma and platelets. If the patient is not at a facility that can support the transfusion of blood products, isotonic fluid administration alone is acceptable until the patient can be transferred to a higher level of care with such capabilities.

Resuscitation is evaluated based on the patient's response to treatment. Indications of successful resuscitation include trends toward hemodynamic norms and broader assessment findings related to improved mental status, improvement of peripheral pulses, return of normal skin color and capillary refill, increased warmth of extremities, blood pressure returning to normal range for age, and urine production of 1 to 2 mL/kg.

OTHER PEDIATRIC CONSIDERATIONS

Interpreting behavior is challenging in the pediatric patient who was involved in a trauma and is now in an unfamiliar place, surrounded by unfamiliar people, and experiencing pain. Developing a rapport with the child is essential. Involvement of the family or caregiver can be helpful to comfort the patient as well as to provide crucial information about the patient's mental status and what might be normal versus abnormal for that child. Nurses should engage child life services if available or consult with pediatric nurses from other areas within the healthcare system.

CHILD MALTREATMENT

Child maltreatment can be in the form of neglect; medical neglect; or physical, emotional, or sexual abuse. Nonaccidental trauma, or child abuse, is the leading cause of death in children with an injury under the age of 1 year. Signs of child maltreatment include unexplained ecchymoses, fractures, abrasions, pressure ulcers, contact burns, or scald injuries. Pediatric trauma patients who present with an intentional or nonaccidental trauma often have higher injury severity as well as greater likelihood of dying from the injuries when compared with patients with accidental trauma.

Nurses should suspect child maltreatment when the history does not align with the injuries. History gathering may reveal repeated presentations with traumatic injuries. If the mechanism of injury seems impossible given the child's developmental stage, further assessment is warranted. A common saying to help remember this in infants is, "Babies who don't cruise (crawling or walking) shouldn't bruise."

Neglect can manifest as being thin, underweight, or hungry; having soiled clothing; or having soggy diapers with diaper dermatitis or *Candida* infection. Medical neglect can manifest as a long duration between the injury and presentation to a healthcare facility, failure to seek care, or noncompliance with medical recommendations/advice.

Nurses are mandated reporters. If there is suspicion of child maltreatment, it must be reported to the appropriate authorities. It is not the nurse's responsibility to determine whether maltreatment is present, rather the nurse identifies any concerning findings and reports to the appropriate authorities to investigate and make the formal determination.

FAST FACTS

Nurses are mandated reporters when it comes to suspicion of child maltreatment.

SUMMARY

Pediatric trauma patients have unique needs related largely to their size, developmental stage, and anatomic and physiologic differences compared with an adult. Taking these factors into consideration when caring for a pediatric trauma patient is essential.

REVIEW QUESTIONS

1. When a nurse suspects child maltreatment, they are required to:
   a. Investigate the home and family of the patient
   b. Report the suspected maltreatment to the appropriate authorities
   c. Ask the caregiver if abuse is present in the home
   d. Render judgment of the caregiver
2. Pediatric fluid resuscitation is based on
   a. Height
   b. Injury severity
   c. Weight
   d. Age

References

American College of Surgeons: The Committee on Trauma. (2018). *ATLS: Advanced Trauma Life Support student course manual* (10th ed.). American College of Surgeons.

Centers for Disease Control and Prevention. (2021, September 22). *Injuries among children and teens*. Centers for Disease Control and Prevention. https://www.cdc.gov/injury/features/child-injury/index.html

Ernst, G. (2020). Pediatric trauma. In J. E. Tintinalli, O. Ma, D. M. Yealy, G. D. Meckler, J. Stapczynski, D. M. Cline, & S. H. Thomas (Eds.), *Tintinalli's emergency medicine: A comprehensive study guide* (9th ed.). McGraw Hill. https://accessmedicine.mhmedical.com/content.aspx?bookid=2353&sectionid=219644072

Lam, T. (2023, June 16). *The 7 most common childhood injuries*. HealthPartners Blog. https://www.healthpartners.com/blog/most-common-childhood-injuries/#:~:text=Falls%3A%20The%20most%20common%20cause,fall%2Drelated%20injuries%20every%20day

McQuillan, K. A., & Flynn-Makic, M. B. (2020). *Trauma nursing: From resuscitation through rehabilitation* (5th ed.). Elsevier.

Veterans
Dawn Carpenter

> Veterans of the armed forces warrant special attention because their previous experiences shape how they respond to traumatic events, injuries, and treatment. Many people who served in the armed services don't consider themselves veterans, especially those who served in the national guard, served during peaceful eras, or didn't engage in combat. Regardless, they may have distinct physical or psychological conditions from their previous experiences and exposures that the average person doesn't encounter.

In this chapter, you will learn:
1. Select specific history questions pertinent to patients who have served in the armed services.
2. Differentiate illness syndromes that are specific to each war/conflict.
3. Understand care of veterans with posttraumatic stress disorder (PTSD).

INTRODUCTION

Veterans' Health and Trauma
Trauma is unpredictable, and as such, most veterans who are injured are not seen in the Veterans Affairs health system. On average, the Veterans Health Administration (VHA) reports that fewer than 20% of all veterans and less than 40% of veterans with service-connected disability receive care from the VHA. In short, nurses in every hospital care for veterans. Thus, every nurse should be asking patients whether they have ever served in the armed services. This knowledge is critical to providing holistic, patient-centered care. Military service is an occupation fraught with hazards, stressors, toxic exposures, and risks that are not usually encountered in the civilian population, making this population unique to care for in the civilian healthcare systems.

ASSESSMENT

Nurses must be aware of their patients' military histories and potential for service-connected health concerns resulting from their military service. Questions to ask to get to know a veteran include:

Have you or has someone close to you ever served in the military?
- When did you serve in the armed forces? Which branch?
- What did you do while you were in the military?
- Were you assigned to a hostile or combative area?
- Did you experience enemy fire, see combat, or witness casualties?
- Were you wounded, injured, or hospitalized?
- Did you have exposure to noise, blasts, chemicals, gasses, demolition or munitions, pesticides, or other hazardous substances?
- Have you ever obtained healthcare service from the VHA?
- Do you have a primary care provider with the VHA?
- What conditions does the VHA provider treat?
- Do you have a service-connected condition or disability?

FAST FACTS

Each patient should be asked whether they've ever served in the armed forces. This includes the coast guard, along with the army or air national guard. Simply asking whether they are a veteran misses opportunities to include populations who have similar exposures.

ILLNESS SYNDROMES BY WAR

A large population of veterans are homeless and do not get any routine healthcare. Thus, when a veteran presents as a trauma patient, many comorbid health conditions may be present but were undiagnosed at admission. Concerning findings may be incidentally found during diagnostic testing.

Certain health concerns are consistent throughout military service, whereas others are unique to a specific conflict. The most common conditions seen with all conflicts include musculoskeletal injuries with chronic pain (especially lower back pain), PTSD, and hearing loss. Common conditions unique to specific conflicts are as follows:
- **Korea:** Cold injuries, such as frostbite.
- **Vietnam:** Agent Orange exposure illnesses include a long list of blood and solid organ cancers, ischemic heart disease, diabetes, early-onset peripheral neuropathy, Parkinson disease, skin disorders, and amyloidosis.
- **Persian Gulf War I:** Unexplained medical symptoms (Gulf War syndrome). Symptoms may include but are not limited to fatigue, cardiovascular disease, respiratory disorders, muscle and joint pain, headache, neurologic and psychological problems, abnormal weight

loss, skin conditions, sleep disturbances, chronic fatigue syndrome, and irritable bowel syndrome.

- **Operation Enduring Freedom (Afghanistan), Operation Iraqi Freedom (Iraq), Operation New Dawn (Iraq, post "end of combat operations in August 2010"):** Traumatic brain injuries including polytrauma; musculoskeletal injuries; mental health disorders; hearing loss; and respiratory problems, along with conditions related to burn pit exposure.
- **Southwest Asia, including Iraq or Afghanistan:** Infectious diseases that may produce symptoms later, including malaria, brucellosis, *Campylobacter jejuni* infection, West Nile virus, *Coxiella burnetii* (Q fever), *Mycobacterium tuberculosis*, *Shigella*, nontyphoidal *Salmonella*, and visceral leishmaniasis.

POSTTRAUMATIC STRESS DISORDER

PTSD can occur following exposure to a significant traumatic stressor that involves a threat to the physical integrity of oneself or others. Most cases of PTSD are seen in combat veterans and victims of sexual assault. Nearly 23% of female veterans reported being sexually assaulted while serving in the military. Onset of symptoms of PTSD typically occurs within 3 months of the exposure but can be delayed for months or even years. The classic symptoms of PTSD may include hyperarousal/hypervigilance, intrusive memories and re-experiencing (flashbacks), avoidance responses or withdrawal/distancing, trouble sleeping and/or concentrating, memory problems, relationship problems, aggression, self-destructive behavior (self-harm or substance abuse), and low self-worth and hopelessness. Emerging evidence also supports an association between PTSD and dementia in veterans.

Nurses need to be aware of what triggers a veteran's PTSD (Table 20.1). If they acknowledge having PTSD, inquire about triggers, symptoms, and how they manage their symptoms. Hospitalized trauma patients who are veterans may experience additional triggers, such as being in pain, intubated, restrained, or delirious. Engage with the trauma team to continue home medications or add as-needed agents to aid in symptom management (Table 20.2).

FAST FACTS

Pain, intubation, restraints, and/or delirium can trigger PTSD in the hospitalized veteran.

SUBSTANCE USE IN VETERANS

Veterans with PTSD commonly self-medicate to alleviate their symptoms, using alcohol, opioids, sedatives, marijuana, and other illicit substances. Thus, substance use disorder is common among veterans. Veterans should

TABLE 20.1

PTSD Stressors and Triggers

PTSD Stressors	PTSD Triggers
Physical: - Injury/blast wave/head injury - Noise - Toxic agents - Temperature - Sleep deprivation - Diet - Austere conditions - Infectious agents - Multiple immunizations **Psychological:** - Anticipation of combat - Combat trauma - Deprivation - Noncombat trauma - Separation from family/home **Psychosocial:** - Marital and/or parenting issues - Social functioning - Occupational/financial concerns - Risk of redeployment - Spiritual	- Lack or loss of power and/or control - Transitions and routine/schedule disruption - Feelings of rejection and vulnerability - Feeling threatened - Sensory overload - Sights, sounds, smells, physical surroundings, and situations (e.g., fireworks) - Emotional state of mind (e.g., terror, rage, grief, and adrenalin rush) - Exposure to traumatic events that include an element of victimization, racism, or catastrophic losses - Anniversary dates (i.e., holidays, time of the year that have meaning from time in war zone) - Media exposure to war zone–like events - Music that elicits feelings related to those experienced during wartime - Significant losses, such as death of a loved one, divorce, separation, financial or job losses, serious illnesses, loss of bodily functions or parts, or imminent death - Conflicts with authority figures including medical, governmental, religious, or supervisors

PTSD, posttraumatic stress disorder.
Source: Used with permission from Carpenter, Fast Facts for the Adult-Gerontology Acute Care Nurse Practitioner (AGACNP).

routinely be screened for substance use disorder and referred for treatment (see Chapter 21).

FAST FACTS

Almost 20% of service members reported binge drinking on a weekly basis. This figure was higher in veterans who were exposed to combat.

SUMMARY

In summary, trauma patients who are veterans of the armed forces have unique needs and may not have accessed treatment through the VHA system. Thus, the highest priority for nurses is to identify which patients are

TABLE 20.2

Interventions to treat PTSD

Outpatient	Inpatient
■ Cognitive therapy, cognitive behavioral therapy* ■ Exposure therapy* ■ Stress inoculation training* ■ Present-centered therapy ■ Interpersonal psychotherapy ■ Psychoeducation* ■ Narration (oral, written, and fictional)* ■ Eye movement desensitization and reprocessing ■ Complementary and alternative modalities (meditation, acupuncture, reiki, and yoga) ■ Pet/dog therapy ■ Benzodiazepines are contraindicated	■ Restart PTSD home medications as soon as possible ■ Coordinate care with PCP's office ■ Recommended treatment options for PTSD: sertraline and paroxetine (FDA approved); fluoxetine and venlafaxine also recommended but off-label ■ Prazosin (Minipress) for treatment of nightmares ■ Avoid benzodiazepines, divalproex, tiagabine, guanfacine, risperidone, and D-cycloserine ■ Benzodiazepines are strongly discouraged unless they cannot be avoided due to severe hypoxic respiratory failure or alcohol withdrawal ■ Consider dexmedetomidine (Precedex) for sedation needs ■ Consider psychiatry consultation

FDA, Food and Drug Administration; PCP, primary care provider; PTSD, posttraumatic stress disorder.

*A-level recommendation.

Source: Used and modified with permission from Carpenter, Fast Facts for AGACNP.

veterans and discuss their specific service-related healthcare needs. Nurses should customize their care in the context of these needs.

REVIEW QUESTIONS

1. The first question a nurse should ask a patient about military service is:
   a. Were you wounded, injured, or hospitalized?
   b. Were you assigned to a hostile or combative area?
   c. Have you or has someone close to you ever served in the military?
   d. Did you experience enemy fire, see combat, or witness casualties?
2. Which medication should be avoided in veterans?
   a. Paroxetine (Paxil)
   b. Sertraline (Zoloft)
   c. Lorazepam (Ativan)
   d. Dexmedetomidine (Precedex)

References

Juergens, J. (2021, March 24, 2021). *Veterans and addiction*. Addictions Center. https://www.addictioncenter.com/addiction/veterans/

Platoni, K. (n.d.). *Warning signs, triggers, and coping strategies for Iraqi war veterans: Patriot outreach*. https://patriotoutreach.org/warning-signs.html#1

Ritchie, K., Cramm, H., Aiken, A., Donnelly, C., & Goldie, K. (2019). Posttraumatic stress disorder and dementia in veterans: A scoping literature review. *International Journal of Mental Health Nursing, 28*(5), 1020–1034.

The Management of Posttraumatic Stress Disorder Work Group. (2017). *VA/DOD clinical practice guideline for the management of posttraumatic stress disorder and acute stress disorder.* https://www.healthquality.va.gov/guidelines/MH/ptsd/VADoDPTSDCPGFinal012418.pdf

U. S. Department of Veterans Affairs. (2018, June 1). *Gulf war veterans' medically unexplained illnesses.* http://www.publichealth.va.gov/exposures/gulfwar/medically-unexplained-illness.asp

U. S. Department of Veterans Affairs. (2019, October 18). *PTSD: National center for PTSD.* http://www.ptsd.va.gov/professional/index.asp

Substance Use and Toxicology
Dawn Carpenter

Substance use in the trauma population creates unique and challenging situations for nurses to recognize and manage. Trauma patients commonly have alcohol or other substances in their system at the time of injury that may have contributed to their injuries. They can experience alcohol withdrawal symptoms and delirium tremens, which may complicate and prolong the hospital course. They may also be using various illicit substances, especially fentanyl and heroin, which cause the patient to develop tolerance, making adequate pain control challenging.

In this chapter, you will learn:
1. To recognize alcohol intoxication.
2. Terminology associated with opioid use.
3. To contrast toxidromes.
4. To identify antidotes for a variety of toxins/drugs.

INTRODUCTION

Trauma patients typically have severe acute pain associated with their injuries. Treatment of acute pain from injuries commonly includes use of opioids, which can be the nidus for developing opioid dependence and subsequently lead to misuse or abuse. Trauma patients also can experience intentional or unintentional toxic ingestions or overdoses. Additionally, many trauma patients require general anesthesia and/or conscious sedation, which may precipitate oversedation. Thus, the astute trauma nurse must be able to promptly recognize intoxications, toxidromes, and oversedation and be able to rescue the patient with the proper antidote.

ALCOHOL USE

Alcohol use is a common factor triggering patients to be traumatically injured. Alcohol use can lead to a vicious circle of trauma and alcohol abuse.

History of traumatic experiences and previous traumatic injuries, especially those resulting in chronic pain or posttraumatic stress disorder, can lead to an alcohol use disorder (AUD). The increased alcohol use then can precipitate additional traumatic injuries.

Signs of clinical intoxication include rambling, incoherence, slurred speech, incoordination, staggering or unsteady gait, and nystagmus. Behavior may be overly friendly, annoying, rude, offensive, aggressive, or even violent. Critical signs of intoxication requiring medical interventions include stupor, loss of consciousness, vomiting, bradypnea, bradycardia, and seizures.

All trauma patients should be screened for alcohol use (see the "Screening, Brief Intervention and Referral to Treatment" [SBIRT] section). A serum blood alcohol level is drawn for medical purposes. These differ from legal blood alcohol levels, but the medical alcohol levels can be subpoenaed for use in court. Medical blood alcohol levels are considered protected health information and, as such, should not be shared with family if the patient is older than 18 years. Do not share with police or legal representatives, because sharing this information may constitute a Health Insurance Portability and Accountability Act violation.

Screening for AUD is standard of care for trauma patients. AUD is a medical condition categorized as an inability to control or stop alcohol use despite adverse health, occupational, or social consequences. Patients with AUD are at risk for alcohol withdrawal, delirium tremens, seizures, and death if not promptly treated. Alcohol withdrawal symptoms include anxiety, headaches, nausea, vomiting, dry heaves, tremors, diaphoresis, agitation, visual disturbances, tactile disturbances, auditory disturbances, seizures, and delirium. The Clinical Institute Withdrawal Assessment—Alcohol Scale Revised tool should be used. Prophylactic administration of benzodiazepines, phenobarbital, or chlordiazepoxide (Librium) can reduce alcohol withdrawal symptoms. Refer to institutional policy and order sets for alcohol withdrawal prevention and treatment. Seizures require a rapid response team activation, treatment with benzodiazepines, and transfer to the ICU.

Trauma patients who have AUD are commonly malnourished and have electrolyte disturbances. Supplemental thiamine, folate, multivitamins, and magnesium may be prescribed. The enteral route is preferred if the gastrointestinal tract is intact and functional; alternatively, these supplements can be given intravenously. Malnourished patients are at risk for refeeding syndrome when adequate oral nutrition or tube feedings are initiated. Trauma patients have higher caloric needs for wound healing and should have a clinical nutritionist consulted. Signs of refeeding syndrome include electrolyte abnormalities such as hypophosphatemia, hypokalemia, and hypomagnesemia. Aggressive replacement of electrolytes, especially phosphorus, is a high priority to avoid respiratory insufficiency.

FAST FACTS

Trauma patients who have AUD or chronic illicit drug use are commonly malnourished. They are at risk for refeeding syndrome. The hallmark sign of refeeding syndrome is hypophosphatemia with hypokalemia and hypomagnesemia.

OPIOID USE DISORDERS

Traumatically injured patients will have acute pain. Differentiating between acute pain, chronic pain, and drug-seeking behaviors may be challenging. Nurses must recognize that patients may have a tolerance to opioids or an opioid use disorder (OUD), and thus require higher doses of opioids to achieve adequate pain control. The trauma team must treat the patient's acute pain in addition to the chronic pain medications that the patient may be taking. Collaboration among the trauma team, nursing, pharmacy, acute pain team, or anesthesiologist will yield best results.

The opioid epidemic has heightened awareness and broadened insights into acute and chronic pain management and the consequences of opioid misuse. Trauma nurses should use current terminology to recognize, treat, and document patients' pain conditions and conditions associated with opioid use.

- **"Opiates" versus "opioids":** Although similar; they are different:
    - **Opiates:** Are natural opioids, such as morphine and heroin.
    - **Opioids:** Include natural, semisynthetic, and synthetic opioids, such as fentanyl and oxycodone.
- **Tolerance:** Repeated drug use reduces the response to the drug.
- **Physical dependence:** The body's adaptation to a drug that when stopped, produces withdrawal symptoms.
- **Drug misuse:** Using prescription drugs in a manner other than as directed. Misuse includes taking greater amounts, more frequently, for longer periods than prescribed, or taking someone else's prescription.
- **Opioid use disorder:** A pattern of opioid use that significantly impairs the patient's ability to function in society. Diagnosis includes specific criteria including, but not limited to:
    - Inability to cut down or control use.
    - Use resulting in social problems and/or failure to satisfy work, school, or home obligations.

Patients may experience withdrawal from opioids while hospitalized. Clinical signs of opioid withdrawal include tachycardia, diaphoresis, restlessness, tremors, dilated pupils, bone or joint aches, rhinorrhea, nausea, vomiting, diarrhea, yawning, anxiety, irritability, or "goose bumps." Use of the Clinical Opiate Withdrawal Scale is recommended. Prevention and treatment of opioid withdrawal require use of opioids. Consult with the acute pain management team to achieve adequate analgesia and prevention or treatment of acute opioid withdrawal. If oversedation occurs, administration of naloxone (Narcan) to patients with chronic OUD may cause immediate withdrawal symptoms.

SCREENING, BRIEF INTERVENTION, AND REFERRAL TO TREATMENT

Every encounter with a trauma patient is an opportunity to affect their life. All trauma patients should be screened for drug and alcohol use on admission. These substances may be the reason or contributing factor for why the patient was injured. The use of the SBIRT approach is standard of care for all patients who have positive alcohol or drug screens. The three SBIRT components are discussed below.

Alcohol Screening

All trauma patients should be screened to identify unhealthy use of drugs and alcohol. Several screening tools are available for use. These may be integrated into the nursing admission questionnaire.

The Binge question is simple and consists of one question. Ask men, "Have you consumed five or more drinks on a single occasion?" Or for women, "Have you consumed four or more drinks on a single occasion?" A positive answer implies the patient may have a problem. The cut, annoyed, guilty, and eye-opener (CAGE) questionnaire is a four-question tool useful in identifying alcohol misuse with a simple yes/no format. The four questions are:

- Have you felt the need to **Cut** down on your drinking?
- Do you feel **Annoyed** by people complaining about your drinking?
- Do you ever feel **Guilty** about your drinking?
- Do you ever drink an **Eye-opener** in the morning to relieve the shakes?

Patient responses on the CAGE are scored 0 for no or 1 for yes. A higher score indicates an alcohol use problem. A total score of 2 or greater is considered clinically significant and should be referred to treatment. The trauma nurse should consult social work and discuss with the trauma providers who can implement Clinical Institute Withdrawal Assessment monitoring.

Although the CAGE is quick and easy to recall, the Alcohol Use Disorder Identification Test—Consumption screening tool can obtain more information and patient history than CAGE. Patients who screen positive are at high risk for acute consequences, such as trauma and/or illness. Risky drinking is considered:

- For healthy men up to age 65: More than four drinks/day AND more than 14 drinks/week.
- For all healthy women and men over 65: More than three drinks/day AND 7 drinks/week.

In the United States, one "standard" drink (or one alcoholic drink equivalent) contains roughly 14 g of pure alcohol, which is found in:
- 5 ounces of regular beer, which is usually about 5% alcohol.
- 5 ounces of wine, which is typically about 12% alcohol.
- 1.5 ounces of distilled spirits, which is about 40% alcohol.

Drug Screening

All trauma patients should also be screened for illicit drug use. The single-item drug screen can assess drug use. The single-item drug screen question is:
- How many times in the past year have you used an illegal drug or used a prescription medication for nonmedical purposes?

Greater than 1 is positive for both men and women. If positive, the patient requires further assessment by the team.

FAST FACTS

All trauma patients, regardless of age, race, gender, or socioeconomic status, should be screened to identify unhealthy use of alcohol and drugs.

Brief Intervention

For trauma patients with a positive screen, a brief intervention should be completed by providers or social work to provide feedback about the patient's unhealthy substance use. The brief intervention is a short conversation to increase awareness of their risks associated with drug or alcohol use. This is a collaborative conversation to assess the patient's motivation to reduce or stop alcohol and/or other drug use, to reduce the risk for additional traumatic injuries to themselves or others.

Referral to Treatment

Patients who are interested in decreasing or stopping use should be referred to substance use treatment. This referral increases access to addiction assessment and treatment by specialists. Consult social work or addiction medicine services to begin this process. Discharge options include:
- Acute inpatient treatment services if medical intervention is needed to manage withdrawal symptoms.
- Clinical stabilization services for those who have already been detoxified or do not require medical supervision.
- Local outpatient treatment.
- Always provide contact numbers to Alcoholics Anonymous and Narcotics Anonymous for peer support and Al-Anon for family members. www.samhsa.gov/find-help/national-helpline.
- The Substance Abuse and Mental Health Services Administration (SAMHSA) has tools available for local resources:

- SAMHSA's National Helpline, 1-800-662-HELP (4357) (also known as the Treatment Referral Routing Service), or TTY: 1-800-487-4889, is a confidential, free, 24-hours-a-day, 365-days-a-year information service, in English and Spanish, for individuals and family members facing mental and/or substance use disorders. This service provides referrals to local treatment facilities, support groups, and community-based organizations.
- Also visit the online treatment locator or send your zip code via text message to 435748 (HELP4U) to find help near you. Read more about the HELP4U text messaging service.

Inpatient treatment can be started and may include use of methadone to treat acute pain, or buprenorphine. Patients on these agents should be continued on them throughout the hospital stay. Providers or nurses should call the provider of the methadone directly to confirm the dosage. Suboxone should be avoided as it has naloxone combined with buprenorphine and will decrease the effectiveness of opioids that the trauma patient needs to control their pain.

Toxidromes

Trauma patients may have ingested other substances, either intentionally or unintentionally, including prescription medications. The trauma nurse must be astute in assessing for and differentiating between distinct patterns of symptoms. A toxidrome is a cluster of signs and symptoms that are classically associated with exposure to substances or a category of substances (Table 21.1).

Opioids and Sedatives

Trauma patients may develop oversedation or iatrogenic oversedation as they may have received narcotics for pain control, benzodiazepine for alcohol withdrawal, muscle relaxants, and other agents, all of which can cause respiratory depression. Many trauma patients require conscious sedation or general anesthetics for surgical procedures, increasing their risk for oversedation, especially in the older adult population. Furthermore, trauma patients may take their own prescription medications or illicit drugs in addition to what is prescribed while in the hospital. They may even crush, snort, or inject these agents into their IV, central line, or peripherally inserted central catheter line. Thus, trauma nurses need to closely monitor for oversedation and be ready to reverse these agents. Nurses need to ensure patient rooms are stocked with an Ambu bag and know how to provide ventilatory support for the patient. Patients may require noninvasive ventilation or intubation with mechanical ventilation.

FAST FACTS

Trauma nurses must be able to rescue hospitalized patients who develop respiratory depression from opioids and benzodiazepines. The reversal agent for opioids is naltrexone (Narcan), and the reversal agent for benzodiazepines is flumazenil (Romazicon).

TABLE 21.1 Clinical Presentations of Toxidromes, With Example Agents

Toxidrome	Vital Signs	Mental Status	Eye Exam	Additional Findings	Examples of Agents
Opioid	Hypothermia, bradycardia, hypotension, bradypnea	CNS depression, coma	Miosis+	Hyporeflexia, pulmonary edema	Opioids (morphine, oxycodone, hydrocodone, hydromorphone, fentanyl, codeine, methadone, and heroin)
Sedative/hypnotic	Hypothermia, bradycardia, hypotension, and bradypnea	CNS depression, confusion, and coma	Miosis+	Hyporeflexia	Alcohol, benzodiazepines, barbiturates, nonbenzodiazepine, GABA agonists, and chloral hydrate
Anticholinergic	Hyperthermia, tachycardia, hypertension, and tachypnea	Hypervigilance, agitation (mad as a hatter), and hallucinations	Mydriasis++ (blind as a bat)	Dry, flushed skin (dry as a bone, red as a beet), urinary retention	Scopolamine, atropine, antihistamines, TCAs, antispasmodics, jimson weed, and psychedelic mushrooms
Cholinergic	Bradycardia, tachycardia, and hypertension	Confusion, coma	Miosis+	SLUDGE	Organophosphates, carbamate pesticides, cholinesterase inhibitors, nerve agents, and physostigmine
Sympathomimetic	Hyperthermia, tachycardia, and tachypnea	Agitation, hyperalertness, and paranoia	Mydriasis++	Diaphoresis, tremors, hyperreflexia, and seizures	Cocaine, amphetamines, pseudoephedrine, phenylephrine, and ephedrine
Serotonergic	Hyperthermia, tachycardia, hypertension, and tachypnea	Confusion, agitation, and coma	Mydriasis++, ocular clonus	Tremor, myoclonus, diaphoresis, hyperreflexia, trismus, rigidity, and muscular hypertonicity	MAOIs, SSRIs, buspirone, tramadol, and dextromethorphan

(continued)

TABLE 21.1 (continued)
Clinical Presentations of Toxidromes, With Example Agents

Toxidrome	Vital Signs	Mental Status	Eye Exam	Additional Findings	Examples of Agents
Neuroleptic malignant syndrome	Hyperthermia, tachycardia, hypertension, tachypnea, and arrhythmias	Agitation, delirium	Oculogyric crisis (rare)	Trismus, dystonia, ataxia, parkinsonism, and neuroleptic malignant syndrome	Haloperidol, olanzapine, quetiapine, chlorpromazine, promethazine, prochlorperazine, fluphenazine, and perphenazine

CNS, central nervous system; GABA, gamma aminobutyric acid; MAOI, monoamine oxidase inhibitor; SLUDGE, salivation, lacrimation, urination, diaphoresis/diarrhea, gastrointestinal upset, and emesis; SSRI, selective serotonin reuptake inhibitor; TCAs, tricyclic antidepressants.

†Miosis: Constricted pupils; ††Mydriasis: Dilated pupils.

Source: Used with permission from Carpenter, Fast Facts for the Adult-Gerontology Acute Care Nurse Practitioners (AGACNP).

Toxins and Antidotes

Nurses may care for trauma patients who have purposely taken excess prescribed medications as a suicide attempt. Not all overdoses are admitted to the trauma service; however, it is not uncommon for patients to attempt suicide with several methods simultaneously, such as taking medications and driving into a tree or jumping off a building. Alternatively, an older adult may become delirious from an infection and unintentionally take excess medications, resulting in a fall with traumatic injuries. Thus, the trauma nurse must be prepared for such events and be familiar with the reversal agents and dosing to rescue the patient from untoward effects, including organ failure and possible death. Table 21.2 lists several common medications and their antidotes.

TABLE 21.2

Specific Drugs and Antidotes

Drug/Agent	Antidote
Acetaminophen	N-acetylcysteine
Anticholinergics	Physostigmine
Benzodiazepine	Flumazenil
Beta-blockers	Glucagon
Calcium channel blockers	10% Calcium chloride Dextrose and insulin
Cholinergic	Atropine Pralidoxime
Coumadin	Phytonadione Fresh frozen plasma PCC
Cyanide	Hydroxocobalamin* Sodium nitrite Sodium thiosulfate
Digoxin	Digibind
Ethylene glycol, methanol	Fomepizole
Heparin	Protamine sulfate
Insulin	Glucose
Iron	Deferoxamine
Isoniazid, hydrazine	Pyridoxine
Lead	Dimercapol CaNa2 EDTA

(continued)

TABLE 21.2 (continued)
Specific Drugs and Antidotes

Drug/Agent	Antidote
Methemoglobinemia	Methylene blue 1%
Methotrexate	Folinic acid (leucovorin)
Neuroleptics	Bromocriptine Dantrolene
Opioids	Naloxone
Organophosphates	Atropine Pralidoxine (2-PAM)
Sulfonylureas	Octreotide
TCAs	Sodium bicarbonate
Valproic acid	L-carnitine

CaNa₂ EDTA, edetate calcium disodium; PCC, prothrombin complex concentrate; TCAs, tricyclic antidepressants; 2-PAM, 2-pyridine aldoxime methyl chloride.

*Preferred.

SUMMARY

In summary, trauma nurses will encounter patients with substance use disorders on a regular basis. Ingestions, whether accidental or intentional, are common. Patients may also take their own medications in addition to those administered in the hospital and may receive anesthetics, sedatives, and other narcotics while hospitalized. Therefore, the trauma nurse must recognize signs of oversedation and know what medications to administer to reverse narcotics and benzodiazepines. The trauma nurse is an essential member of the healthcare team and, as such, engages resources and team members as needed to care for the patient.

REVIEW QUESTIONS

1. An older adult patient who fell and fractured their hip is now just back from having surgical repair. In the postanesthesia care unit, the patient received a total of 10 mg of morphine and 5 mg of oxycodone for 10/10 pain. The patient arrived at their room and is somnolent and has pinpoint pupils. Their heart rate is 60 beats per minute, respirations are 8 per minute, blood pressure is 100/60 mmHg, and oxygen saturation is 88% on 2 L of oxygen by nasal cannula. The nurse anticipates treatment with:
   a. Atropine
   b. Naloxone (Narcan)
   c. N-acetylcysteine (NAC)
   d. Flumazenil (Romazicon)

2. A patient received lorazepam (Ativan) to treat alcohol withdrawal and became somnolent. Heart rate is 60 beats per minute, respirations are 8 per minute, blood pressure is 100/60 mmHg, and oxygen saturation is 88% on 2 L of oxygen by nasal cannula. The nurse anticipates treatment with:
   a. Atropine
   b. Naloxone (Narcan)
   c. N-acetylcysteine (NAC)
   d. Flumazenil (Romazicon)
3. A patient presents after being stabbed in the chest. They are agitated, restless, and fidgeting. Heart rate is 120 beats per minute, respirations are 26 per minute, blood pressure is 180/100 mmHg, and oxygen saturation is 98% on room air. Extended focused assessment with sonography for trauma is negative. Blood alcohol level is .18. The laceration was sutured closed. The most likely cause of the patient's symptoms is:
   a. Cocaine intoxication
   b. Hemorrhagic shock
   c. Tension pneumothorax
   d. Alcohol withdrawal

References

Hargraves, D., White, C., Frederick, R., Cinibulk, M., Peters, M., Young, A., & Elder, N. (2017). Implementing SBIRT (screening, brief intervention and referral to treatment) in primary care: Lessons learned from a multi-practice evaluation portfolio. *Public Health Reviews*, *38*(1), 1–11.

Kuo, K. (n.d.). *Toxic ingestions.* http://www.learnpicu.com/toxidromes

Murray, E., Walthall, L., & Wise, K. R. (2017). Drug overdose and withdrawal. In S. J. McKean, J. J. Ross, D. D. Dressler, & D. B. Scheurer (Eds.), *Principles and practice of hospital medicine* (2nd ed., pp. 2057–2069). McGraw Hill Education.

National Institute on Alcohol Abuse and Alcoholism. (n.d.). *Alcohol's effects on health: What is a standard drink?* NIAAA. https://www.niaaa.nih.gov/alcohols-effects-health/overview-alcohol-consumption/what-standard-drink#:~:text=In%20the%20United%20States%2C%20one,which%20is%20about%2040%25%20alcohol

Rasimas, J., & Sinclair, C. M. (2017). Assessment and management of toxidromes in the critical care unit. *Critical Care Clinics*, *33*(3), 521–541.

Saunders, J. B., Aasland, O. G., Babor, T. F., De La Fuente, J. R., & Grant, M. (1993). Development of the alcohol use disorders identification test (AUDIT): WHO collaborative project on early detection of persons with harmful alcohol consumption-II. *Addiction*, *88*(6), 791–804.

Skinner, H. A. (1982). The drug abuse screening test. *Addictive Behaviors*, *7*(4), 363–371.

Smith, P. C., Schmidt, S. M., Allensworth-Davies, D., & Saitz, R. (2009). Primary care validation of a single-question alcohol screening test. *Journal of General Internal Medicine*, *24*(7), 783–788.

Sullivan, J. T., Sykora, K., Schneiderman, J., Naranjo, C. A., & Sellers, E. M. (1989). Assessment of alcohol withdrawal: The revised clinical institute withdrawal assessment for alcohol scale (CIWA-Ar). *British Journal of Addiction*, *84*(11), 1353–1357.

Vitesnikova, J., Dinh, M., Leonard, E., Boufous, S., & Conigrave, K. (2014). Use of AUDIT-C as a tool to identify hazardous alcohol consumption in admitted trauma patients. *Injury, 45*(9), 1440–1444.

Wesson, D. R., & Ling, W. (2003). The clinical opiate withdrawal scale (COWS). *Journal of Psychoactive Drugs, 35*(2), 253–259.

Disaster Readiness and Response
Alexander Menard

Disasters are unique situations that often occur with little or no notice. The World Health Organization defines the term disaster as a sudden phenomenon of sufficient magnitude to overwhelm the resources of a hospital, region, or location, requiring external support. Trauma care is distinctly different when responding to a disaster. Care shifts toward providing the greatest good for the greatest number of victims.

In this chapter, you will:
1. Discuss disasters and disaster management.
2. Compare internal and external disasters.
3. Define the four stages of disaster management.

INTRODUCTION

The incidence of declared disasters is increasing worldwide. Disasters are sudden incidents or events of sufficient magnitude to overwhelm the resources of a hospital, region, or location. Disasters can be broadly broken down into natural or man-made (Table 22.1).

Types of Disasters

Disasters are also delineated as either internal or external disasters. An internal disaster is an event that occurs within a hospital itself, such as an active shooter, power outage, or radiation exposure. External disasters occur outside the hospital and can range from motor vehicle and other transportation-elated events to natural disasters such as hurricanes, wildfires, and floods. Disasters are further categorized as acute or ongoing, with acute resulting in a rapid influx of patients arriving to the hospital in a relatively close timeframe to the event. Ongoing disasters are those in which there is a slower influx of patients to the hospital, but eventually, the influx overwhelms the available resources. An example of an acute disaster is that of a train crash, with many patients arriving to the hospital in a short amount of time for care, whereas an ongoing disaster example is that of a global pandemic, in which the hospital system gradually becomes overwhelmed with an increase in patient presentations.

TABLE 22.1

Disaster Examples

Disaster Type	Examples
Natural ■ Often associated with weather or geologic events	■ Earthquakes ■ Floods ■ Wildfires ■ Volcanic eruptions ■ Hurricanes ■ Epidemics or pandemics
Man-made ■ Often associated with criminal intent ■ May also be related to human-made large-scale events	■ Terrorism (weapons, explosives, and biologic/chemical agents) ■ Active shooter/mass shooting incident ■ Events related to transportation, storage, and use of hazardous materials* ■ Bridge collapse*

*Denotes potential man-made disasters that may not be due to criminal intent.

Nurses have a significant role in disasters as caretakers and rescuers, who can assist with triage, manage resources, and assist with communication and distribution of information. Nurses are key members of the healthcare workforce and can apply their skills and knowledge to disaster situations. Disaster management has four phases: preparedness, mitigation, response, and recovery.

FAST FACTS

Disasters are sudden incidents of sufficient magnitude to overwhelm available resources.

Disaster Mitigation

Disaster mitigation is the vulnerability assessment and activities that go into reducing the likelihood of disasters or the impact and severity that disasters can cause. Disaster mitigation informs how a healthcare facility can tailor its disaster preparedness plan. Ongoing threat assessments must be performed in collaboration with local, state, and federal political leaders and law enforcement agencies.

Disaster Preparedness

Disaster preparedness is a continuous cycle of anticipation of contingencies needed following a disaster, in turn, increasing a hospital's ability to respond during and after a disaster. Preparedness occurs at the national, state, and local levels. Hospital-based preparedness involves the determination of risks, ability to increase capacity in the event of a disaster, and identification of resources that can be leveraged based on the type of disaster (internal vs. external). The key to preparedness is the development of "all-hazards" plans. The all-hazards methodology focuses on developing one plan that can manage all disasters with specific pathways defined for specific types of disasters. Disaster preparedness includes staff education and disaster drills to improve proficiency.

Disaster Response

Disaster response occurs during an actual disaster, when efforts to prepare and train for a disaster are put into action. The coordination of the healthcare facility disaster response comes from the incident command system (ICS), a widely accepted format/structure. The ICS should be established and roles defined and assigned before a disaster (Figure 22.1). The ICS structure includes the following:

- An incident commander who sets objectives and priorities and is the overall leader during the disaster.
- An operations center that will direct resources (equipment, medical personnel, etc.).
- A planning core to collect/evaluate information and maintain resource status.
- A logistics core to support incident and responder needs.
- Administration staff to monitor costs, execute contracts, offer legal advice, and maintain records.

Triage

Triage is an important component of a disaster response and is different from triage of a trauma patient outside of disasters. The standard principle behind triage is to do the greatest good for the patient, compared with disaster triage, in which the goal is to do the greatest good for the greatest number of patients. Triaging patients is an aspect of a disaster response in which nurses can play a key role. There are two widely used triage methods: simple triage and rapid treatment (START) for adults (Figure 22.2) and JumpSTART, which is tailored for the pediatric population.

As part of the triaging process, determining whether hazardous materials or contaminants are present is important. In disasters in which hazardous materials are present, it is imperative to decontaminate the patient before they enter the care facility. If decontamination is not completed before patients enter the healthcare facility, there is the potential to contaminate the entire facility, rendering it an unsafe place to provide care and further reducing available resources.

FAST FACTS

Decontamination must be completed before patients enter the emergency department.

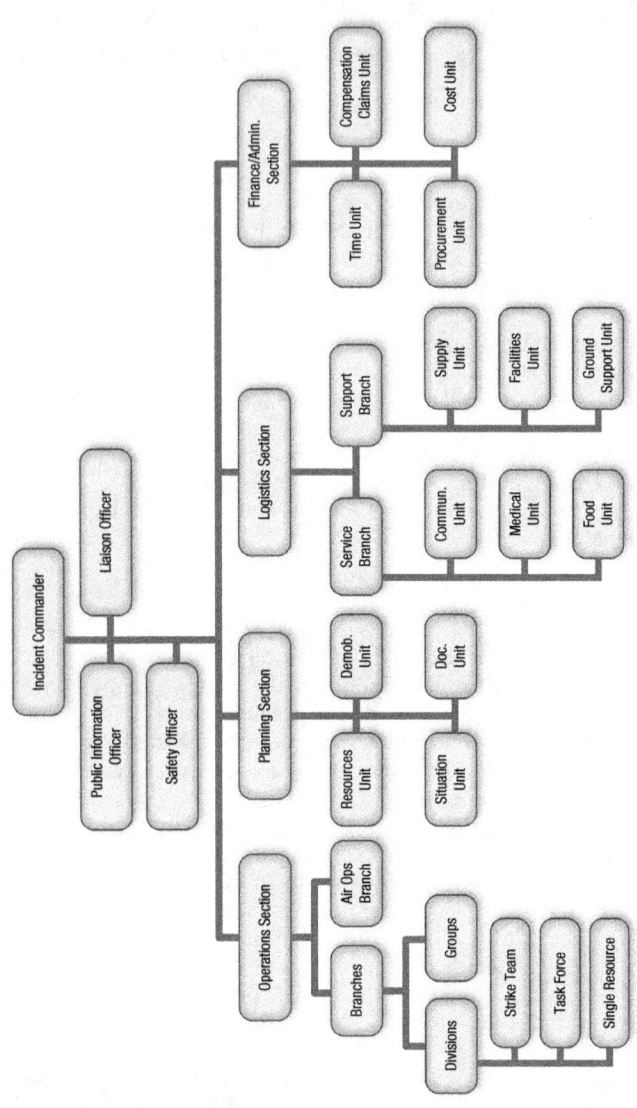

Figure 22.1 FEMA ICS-100 organizational chart.

Source: (IS-0100.c: An Introduction to the Incident Command System, ICS 100, 2018).

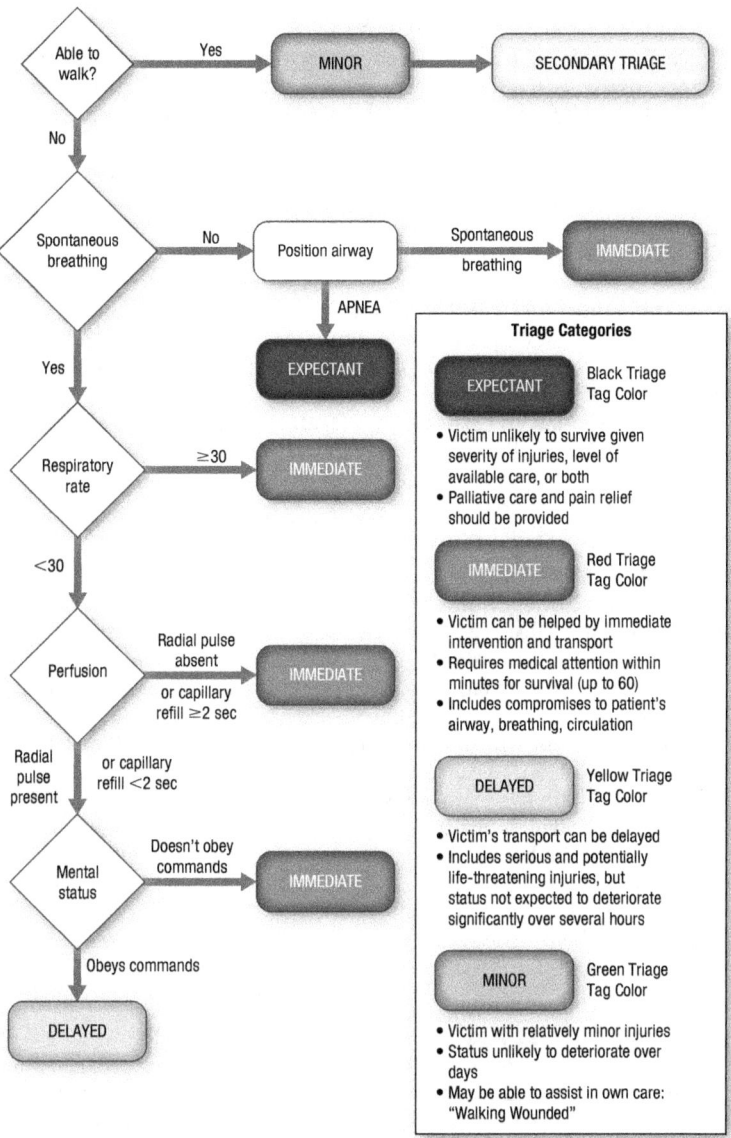

Figure 22.2 Start adult triage.

Source: https://chemm.hhs.gov/startadult.htm; Linking copyright statement from this website https://chemm.hhs.gov/about.htm#feedback.

Crisis Standard of Care

Crisis standard of care is defined as a substantial change from both usual healthcare operations and the level of care that is delivered, necessitated by a pervasive (e.g., pandemic influenza) or catastrophic (e.g., earthquake, hurricane) disaster. This change in the level of care delivery is justified by specific events and is officially declared by a state government. The formal declaration that crisis standards of care are in effect enables specific legal and regulatory powers with protections for healthcare providers to allocate limited medical resources and use alternative facility operations.

Once crisis standards of care have been enacted, rapid triaging protocols are implemented to evaluate and sort patients based on their clinical status and potential outcome. The START triage tool is widely used in the United States for mass casualty incidents. A common triage tool used in hospitalized patients is the sequential organ failure assessment score. Patients who score too high will not likely benefit from medical care, and those who score too low will likely survive without substantial care. There are several other triage tools and algorithms. These systems are designed based on criteria including vital signs, patients' chief problem/s, or the resources required to respond to patients' needs.

Ethical Issues in Disasters

Given the complexities of disasters, scarce medical resources are common, which can cause ethical issues for critically ill patients during a disaster. Clinicians' treatment standards may drastically change when crisis standard of care is implemented. Situations such as removing ventilator assistance from a patient or ceasing pediatric resuscitations in the field can cause ethical dilemmas and emotional distress for clinicians. Situations such as these have been known to cause a high rate of moral distress.

An interdisciplinary team consisting of a palliative care provider, a critical care provider, a surgeon, a nurse, a social worker, and an institutional leader can be helpful in determining if/when a patient is requiring too many resources. This team is also available to support the care team as well and has been shown to effectively decrease caregiver moral distress. If the patient is to be transitioned to palliative care, a social worker or mental health professional should be consulted to support team members.

Psychological First Aid

Psychological first aid is an evidence-informed modular approach to help children, adolescents, adults, relief workers, first responders, and families in the immediate aftermath of a disaster or terrorism. Psychological first aid is designed to reduce the initial distress caused by traumatic events and to foster long-term adaptive functioning and coping. The principles and techniques of psychological first aid meet basic standards; they are:

- Consistent with evidence-based research regarding risks and resilience following trauma.
- Applicable and practical in field settings.

- Appropriate for developmental levels across the life span.
- Culturally informed and delivered in a flexible manner.

Psychological first aid is delivered by mental health and other disaster response workers who provide early assistance to affected children, families, first responders, and adults as part of an organized disaster response effort. Providers may be present in a variety of response teams, including first responders, primary and emergency healthcare providers, school crisis response teams, faith-based organizations, community emergency response teams, medical reserve corps, and other disaster relief organizations. The goal of psychological first aid is to assist with current needs, decrease distress, and encourage adaptive functioning. Guidelines for delivering psychological first aid are as follows:

- First, observe the situation. Ask respectful questions to determine how you may help.
- Provide practical assistance; offer food, water, and blankets when appropriate.
- Initiate contact only after you have observed the situation and the person or family and have determined that contact is not likely to be intrusive or disruptive.
- Be prepared that survivors responses may include avoidance or over-contact.
- Speak in concrete terms; do not use acronyms or jargon.
- If survivors want to talk, be prepared to listen.
- Acknowledge the positive features of what the survivor has done to keep safe.
- Provide information that directly addresses the survivor's immediate needs.
- Provide information that is accurate and age appropriate.

Disaster Recovery

Each disaster can affect a community and its people in unique ways. The disaster recovery phase starts once it is determined that the situation is controlled. This is a time for leadership to direct efforts toward psychological first aid. A debriefing assesses the emotional and psychological impact the disaster has had on the staff and responders. This informs the decision to pivot resources to the support of these individuals.

Additionally, a timely debrief with leadership, staff, and responders needs to occur to understand best practices in the response and identify opportunities for improvement and notable actions from the response. The results of this debriefing should be documented and disseminated, and any action plan to address opportunities for improvement must be documented and instituted to prepare for future events.

SUMMARY

In summary, disaster preparedness requires communities to be in a constant state of readiness. This is done by ongoing assessment of risks and planning and training for a wide range of disasters based on an all-hazards approach. The goal of disaster management is to provide the greatest amount of good to the greatest number of patients. Trauma nurses are uniquely prepared to be part of disaster mitigation, preparedness, and response.

FAST FACTS

The goal of disaster care is to provide the greatest amount of good to the greatest number of patients.

REVIEW QUESTIONS

1. The goal of disaster care is to:
   a. Provide the greatest amount of good to the greatest number of people
   b. Reduce mortality and increase morbidity
   c. Distribute resources to everyone
   d. Increase disaster preparedness
2. The nurse is preparing to accept patients from a hazardous chemical plant explosion. What must occur before the patients enter the emergency department?
   a. Administration of pain medications
   b. Notification of family members
   c. Patient and responder decontamination
   d. Notification of authorities regarding a potential terrorist threat

References

American College of Surgeons: The Committee on Trauma. (2018). *ATLS: Advanced Trauma Life Support student course manual* (10th ed.). American College of Surgeons.

Bazyar, J., Farrokhi, M., & Khankeh, H. (2019). Triage systems in mass casualty incidents and disasters: A review study with a worldwide approach. *Open Access Macedonian Journal of Medical Sciences, 7*(3), 482–494. https://doi.org/10.3889/oamjms.2019.119

Brymer, M. J. A. (2006). *Psychological first aid: Field operations guide* (2nd ed.). NCTSN. https://www.nctsn.org/resources/psychological-first-aid-pfa-field-operations-guide-2nd-edition

Herstein, J. J., Schwedhelm, M. M., Vasa, A., Biddinger, P. D., & Hewlett, A. L. (2021, October 13). Emergency preparedness: What is the future? *Antimicrobial Stewardship & Healthcare Epidemiology, 1*(1), e29. https://doi.org/10.1017/ash.2021.190

Hougan, M., Nadig, L., Altevogt, B. M., & Stroud, C. (Eds.). (2010). *Crisis standards of care: Summary of a workshop series*. National Academies Press.

Klein, T. A., & Irizarry, L. (2022). *EMS disaster response*. StatPearls Publishing.

McQuillan, K. A., & Flynn-Makic, M. B. (2020). *Trauma nursing: From resuscitation through rehabilitation* (5th ed.). Elsevier.

Puryear, B., & Gnugnoli, D. M. (2023 January). *Emergency preparedness.* [Updated July 25, 2023]. StatPearls Publishing. https://www.ncbi.nlm.nih.gov/books/NBK537042/

Tussing, T. E., Chesnick, H., & Jackson, A. (2022, December). Disaster preparedness: Keeping nursing staff and students at the ready. *Nursing Clinics of North America, 57*(4), 599–611. https://doi.org/10.1016/j.cnur.2022.06.008

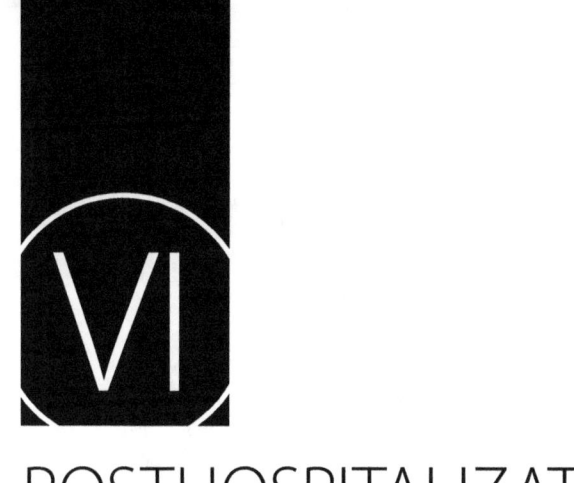

POSTHOSPITALIZATION

Discharge and Follow-Up
Dawn Carpenter

Discharge planning starts upon presentation. Nurses should consider discharge needs when the patient is still in the emergency department. Consider whether the patient can return home or whether the patient likely needs rehabilitation. Physical and occupational therapists play a key role in guiding recommendations for safe discharge and should be consulted early in the admission. Every patient who is discharged after experiencing traumatic injuries must leave the hospital with planned follow-up appointment(s) to reassess their injuries and assess for post-traumatic stress and post-ICU syndrome.

In this chapter, you will learn:
1. To differentiate between levels of postdischarge care options.
2. To differentiate between levels of the Rancho Los Amigos cognitive levels.
3. Discharge education for trauma patients.

INTRODUCTION

Discharge planning is an essential element for all trauma patients and families. Collaboration with the case manager is essential to ensure patients are discharged to the appropriate level of care. Nurses provide incredible care, information, and support to trauma patients and families during the time leading up to discharge. Nurses also need to have knowledge of the patient's needs and expectations in the postdischarge setting. Discharge options include discharge to home with self-care, home with outpatient services, and home with in-home care. If the patient is unable to safely go home, they may require inpatient rehabilitation, a long-term acute care hospital, subacute rehabilitation, or a long-term care nursing facility (Table 23.1).

Discharge to home with home health nurses and therapies requires the patient to be homebound, meaning they do not leave their home to go anywhere except for medical appointments. If patients are mobile and can leave the home, then they can travel to outpatient therapy.

TABLE 23.1

Post-Acute Care Discharge Options for Inpatient Rehabilitation

	Subacute Rehabilitation	Acute Rehabilitation	LTACH
Type of care provided	Daily skilled nursing or rehabilitation services for a short period in a facility after an inpatient stay of 3 or more days	Intensive rehabilitation therapy in an inpatient environment. Patient requires, and is expected to benefit from, 3 hours or more of therapy 5 days/week	Continued hospital level of care
Typical medical conditions	■ Heart failure ■ Hip and femur procedures ■ Joint replacement ■ Kidney and urinary tract infections ■ Infections	■ Brain injury ■ Lower extremity fracture ■ Major joint replacements ■ Neurologic disorders ■ Stroke	■ Complex medical conditions ■ Complex wound/burn management ■ Mechanical ventilation weaning
Daily therapy requirements	1 to 1.5 hours	>3 hours	NA
Average length of stay	27 days	13.1 days	26.6 days
Average cost for care per patient	$10,800	$17,100	$38,500

LTACH, long-term acute care hospital.

Discharge to home or inpatient hospice is also an option for medically complex and frail patients who happen to be near the end of life and become injured. Traumatic injuries may exacerbate medical conditions, causing acceleration of the dying process from their tenuous medical conditions rather than the traumatic injuries. Consultation with palliative care teams is valuable to assist with end-of-life conversations and family acceptance. Patients with uncontrolled symptoms may be discharged and readmitted to a general inpatient hospice service as an option. Alternatively, for patients whose symptoms are controlled, discharge home with family can be coordinated. Nurses need to educate families that home hospice care is similar to a home health nurse, where the nurse visits a few times per week. The hospice nurse does not provide 24-hour coverage. Patient care primarily depends on the family providing the hands-on care.

DISCHARGE OPTIONS

Most patients desire to be discharged to the comfort of their home. Many trauma patients need rehabilitation services. Physical therapy and occupational therapy aid the team in determining discharge recommendations. Rehabilitation services can be provided on an outpatient basis, where the patient lives at home and regularly travels to receive therapy services at an outpatient center. Alternatively, for patients who are homebound, meaning they cannot leave their home except for physician appointments, home therapies may be ordered by providers in addition to home health nursing evaluation.

Some trauma patients require inpatient rehabilitation services, especially those who are weak, medically frail, older, or have more than one extremity that has been injured. Trauma patients may be reluctant and even resistant to going to a rehabilitation facility. Thus, the trauma nurses play a key role in educating patients and families about the risks of going home before being physically ready and educating them on the benefits of rehabilitation. Nurses must also be able to articulate the differences among the various levels of care postdischarge.

LEVELS OF CARE POSTDISCHARGE

Nurses must be familiar with the various discharge options, which include long-term acute care hospitalization; acute rehabilitation; and subacute rehabilitation, also referred to as short-term rehabilitation (see Table 23.1). Nurses play a key role in explaining the differences to patients and their families.

Some patients require specialized services such as traumatic brain injury (TBI) or spinal cord injury rehabilitation. Admission to TBI rehabilitation is guided by a patient's cognitive functioning. Both speech and occupational therapists are educated to perform cognitive evaluations. Any patient who has had a loss of consciousness should have a formal cognitive evaluation. Most patients with concussions can, if required, receive outpatient cognitive therapy. Patients with severe TBIs are graded on the Rancho Los Amigos Scale (Table 23.2).

FOLLOW-UP CARE

Trauma patients should ideally have follow-up appointments established prior to discharge. All patients should have a follow-up appointment with their primary care provider within 1 to 2 weeks.

Trauma patients with multiple systems injured require follow-up appointments with the trauma providers. Isolated injuries may only require specialty follow-up at the interval per their recommendations, which can vary from 1 to 4 weeks. Specialty services may include orthopedics, neurosurgery, ear/nose/throat, plastic surgery, and so forth. Instructions for care

TABLE 23.2

Rancho Los Amigos Levels of Cognitive Functioning

Level	Response	Assistance Required
I	No response to pain, sound, touch, or sight	Total
II	Generalized response, reflex to pain	Total
III	Localized response, withdrawal or vocalization to painful stimuli, blinks to light, turns toward/away from sounds, and inconsistent response to commands	Total
IV	Agitated, alert, very active; may have aggressive or bizarre behaviors, performs motor activities but behavior is not purposeful, and very short attention span	Maximal
V	Confused, inappropriate, nonagitated, gross attention to environment, highly distractable and requires constant redirection, difficulty learning new tasks, agitated with too much stimulation, and may engage with social behaviors but has inappropriate verbalizations	Maximal
VI	Confused, appropriate, inconsistent orientation to time and place; retention and short-term memory is impaired, consistently follows simple directions, has goal-directed behavior with guidance	Moderate
VII	Automatic, robot-like, appropriate, performs ADLs in familiar environments, and skills noticeably deteriorated in unfamiliar environments	Minimal with ADLs
VIII	Purposeful, appropriate, consistently oriented to person, place, time; initiates and completes familiar household tasks and leisure activities and can modify the plan with assistance	Standby
IX	Purposeful, appropriate, able to think of consequences of decisions with assistance, and independent with personal and household tasks and leisure activities in a familiar environment and can perform same in unfamiliar environment with assistance	Standby on request
X	Purposeful, appropriate, able to perform daily routine but may require more time or adaptive strategies	Modified independent

ADLs, activities of daily living.
Source: Lin, K., & Wroten, M. (2023, January). *Ranchos Los Amigos*. [Updated August 22, 2022]. StatPearls Publishing. https://www.ncbi.nlm.nih.gov/books/NBK448151/#.

of all injuries should be in the discharge summary and discharge instructions. Nurses should review in detail the discharge instructions with both the patient and family. Written and verbal discharge instructions should include:

- No driving or operating motorized vehicles or equipment while on opioids or muscle relaxers.

- Opioids can cause dependence.
  - Do not allow other family members to take the patient's prescriptions.
  - Keep opioids locked up and educate on proper disposal of unconsumed pills.
  - Opioids can cause opioid-induced constipation. Patients should be advised to take a bowel regimen, such as senna, MiraLAX, fiber, and so forth.
- Provider or clinic phone number to call with questions.

Nursing and provider education should include anticipatory guidance that patients may experience signs and symptoms of posttraumatic stress disorder (PTSD) and post-ICU syndrome (PICS).

Signs of PTSD Include
- Difficulty recalling the event
- Reliving the experience, flashbacks, intrusive images or memories, and nightmares
- Overwhelming emotions with the flashbacks, images, memories, or nightmares
- Not feeling emotions or feeling "numb" worried, depressed, or guilty
- Insomnia
- Dissociation or feeling "out-of-body" experiences
- Avoidance behaviors, include staying away from specific places or items that remind the patient of the traumatic event
- Hypervigilance, such as being intensely startled by stimuli that resemble the trauma
- Angry outbursts

PTSD can occur immediately after the traumatic experience or may occur weeks, months, or up to years later. Depression, anxiety, and/or increased alcohol or other substance use or abuse often accompany symptoms of PTSD. Patients should be assessed for these symptoms at follow-up appointments.

Signs of Post-ICU Syndrome
Some trauma patients require prolonged time in the ICU to recover from life-threatening injuries. They are at risk for PICS, which includes an array of physical, cognitive, and functional changes and symptoms.

Physical Problems
- Decreased interest/pleasure in activities and/or hobbies, decreased appetite
- Difficulty falling or staying asleep or increased sleeping
- Feeling depressed, hopeless, anxious, nervous, tense, fearful, and panicky
- Resists help from others, agitated at those trying to help
- Impulsive behaviors without thought to consequences, wandering
- Believing others are planning to harm or steal from them

Cognitive Problems
- Difficulty with memory and/or thinking, that is, forgetting the correct month and/or year
- Difficulty remembering appointments
- Difficulty with judgment or decision-making
- Repeating things over (stories, questions)
- Inability to handle finances, such as balancing a checkbook, paying bills or taxes

Functional Problems
- Difficulty learning how to use a tool or appliance
- Difficulty planning, preparing, or serving meals
- Problems taking medications at the right time/dose
- Difficulty ambulating, falling, tripping, and difficulty bathing
- Unable to shop for personal items and/or groceries
- Problems with housework, chores
- Decreased quality of life
- Unable to be left alone, decreased safety

FAST FACTS

Families should be educated to monitor for signs and symptoms of PTSD and PICS.

Special Situations

Patients who attempted suicide should have already been seen by psychiatry during the inpatient admission and have an established follow-up plan for either inpatient or outpatient follow-up care in place prior to discharge. Patients who had alcohol or illicit substances in their system at the time of admission should have a screening and brief intervention performed by either social work or the providers and offered substance use rehabilitation (refer to Chapter 21). This could be in the form of written resources, referral to outpatient therapies, or even admission to an inpatient facility. Laws and regulations vary by state regarding involuntary commitment for both suicide attempts and substance use disorders.

SUMMARY

Knowledge of discharge requirements and facility capabilities can aid in efficient patient discharges to appropriate facilities. Be aware of your hospital's readmission rates and advocate mobilizing resources to safely discharge patients to the most appropriate levels of care.

REVIEW QUESTIONS

1. A patient with severe multisystem injuries who has spent the last 13 days in the ICU now has a trach and feeding tube and is being discharged to a long-term acute care hospital. Upon return to the follow-up appointment, the patient should be screened for:
   a. Alcohol use disorder
   b. Substance use disorder
   c. Post-ICU syndrome
   d. Post-admission syndrome
2. A patient is being discharged with a prescription for oxycodone. Nursing discharge instructions should include:
   a. Do not allow others to take the prescription.
   b. Properly dispose of unconsumed pills.
   c. Opioids can cause opioid-nduced constipation.
   d. All of the above.

References

Bisson, J. I., Cosgrove, S., Lewis, C., & Robert, N. P. (2015). Posttraumatic stress disorder. *British Medical Journal (Clinical Research Edition), 351*, h6161. https://doi.org/10.1136/bmj.h6161

Liang, S., Wang, X., Li, C., & Shao, L. (2023). Screening for postintensive care syndrome: Validation of the healthy aging brain care monitor self-report Chinese version. *Nursing in Critical Care*. https://doi.org/10.1111/nicc.12949

Lin, K., & Wroten, M. (2022). *Ranchos Los Amigos*. StatPearls Publishing.

Stefanacci, R. (2015). Admission criteria for facility-based postacute services. *Ann Long-Term Care Clinical Care Aging, 23*, 18–20.

Injury Prevention
Alexander Menard

Injury prevention is a priority. Injury prevention is the collaboration of all trauma team members with the community. The American College of Surgeons plays a critical role in the certification of trauma centers in the United States, outlining and providing resources for injury prevention. All level I trauma centers must have a dedicated injury prevention coordinator. At lower-level trauma centers, the injury prevention coordinator may be combined with the trauma program manager. Many injuries are predictable and thus preventable. This chapter discusses the basic tenets of injury prevention and describes how nurses play a critical role in injury prevention.

In this chapter, you will learn:
1. The history of injury prevention.
2. To define contributing factors of injury/trauma.
3. Nursing interventions to prevent injuries.

INTRODUCTION

The World Health Organization reports that both unintentional and violence-related injuries take the lives of 4.4 million people around the world yearly and are responsible for 8% of all deaths. In the United States, unintentional injuries are the leading cause of death in children, adolescents, and adults aged 45 years and younger. Motor vehicle crashes and falls account for most unintentional injuries, whereas physical assaults and gun violence account for many intentional injuries. Of note, drug overdoses are the leading cause of injury deaths in the United States.

Injury prevention focuses on the most common causes of injuries in local/regional communities, including the top three mechanisms of injury and interventions implemented based on this epidemiologic data. Principal concepts of an effective injury prevention program include:

- Focus on the community—identify the leading causes of injury and/or death.
- Work upstream—that is: determine the root cause and contributing factors.

- Choose preexisting proven programs.
- Partner with other organizations (law enforcement, schools, prehospital, etc.).
- Embrace the media—be a reliable source of prevention information.
- Become politically savvy—engage elected officials.
- Use data—develop surveillance and monitoring tools.

Injury prevention is divided into three main types of prevention: primary, secondary, and tertiary prevention (Table 24.1). Nurses can make an impact in their everyday work.

FAST FACTS

Injury prevention is focused on populations at risk and mitigating those risk factors.

The goal of injury prevention is to intervene early to prevent or reduce the impact of an injury. Four main concepts determine strategies for interventions: education, engineering, enforcement, and economic approaches, commonly referred to as the "four E's."

Education
Education is a major contributor to injury prevention. Informing an individual and the population can reduce injuries by teaching the risk factors and strategies to avoid injury. Providing knowledge to populations can also influence society as a whole, leading to changes in policy, laws, and social norms.

Engineering
Engineering plays a large role in reducing or preventing injuries. First, engineering can be implemented to stop an injury from occurring by removing

TABLE 24.1

Levels of Prevention

Level of Prevention	Description	Examples
Primary	Preventing injury before it occurs	Gun control laws
Secondary	Reduce impact of injury that has occurred by means of early detection	Use of seat belts
Tertiary	Limit the impact of injury after it has occurred	Emergency response systems (such as 911 system)

a causative or contributing factor to the injury. An example of this is removing hazardous building materials that are known to cause fires, or engineering to reduce or absorb energy that is transferred during an impact. Examples of this include engineering of helmets, restraint systems, or a roll cage on an off-roading vehicle.

Enforcement

Adhering to laws, policies, and regulations is required to meet the goals of injury prevention. Without enforcement of injury prevention, adherence is less likely to occur. Examples of this include:

- Laws that require motor vehicle occupants to wear a seat belt and receiving a ticket if not compliant.
- Regulations mandating motor vehicles have/meet certain safety standards, such as seat belts or lane departure technology.
- Policies that support school-aged children receiving fire safety training.

Economic Approaches

Economic approaches apply both incentives and disincentives to motivate adherence. Incentivizing injury prevention encourages an individual or population to benefit from reducing risk of injury. Examples include firearm buyback programs or lower insurance premiums for safe driving. Disincentives are designed to encourage individuals or groups to adopt safe practices. Examples include fines for traffic violations or for unsafe work environments.

The Nurse's Role

Nurses play a crucial role in injury prevention. Nurses' influences span from the bedside to the community and policy making and government settings. Nurses often spend the greatest amount of time with patients while they are hospitalized. This presents a unique opportunity for nurses to educate patients and families on methods of injury prevention (Table 24.2).

FAST FACTS

Nurses play a crucial role in injury prevention.

SUMMARY

In summary, the concept of injury prevention has evolved and will continue to evolve over time. New technology can improve injury prevention but can also create new contributing factors for injury. New initiatives for trauma/injury prevention must continue to evolve in efforts to reduce preventable trauma/injury. Nurses are uniquely positioned to provide guidance and education to patients to prevent injury.

TABLE 24.2

Injury Prevention Examples, With Nursing Interventions

Injury Prevention Topic	Nursing Interventions
Motor vehicle	Education and encouragement regarding protective equipment use: ■ Wearing seat belts ■ Refraining from impaired driving (alcohol and/or drug) ■ Refraining from distracted driving (cell phones)
Motorcycle	■ Helmet ■ Gloves ■ Full coverage leather riding clothes ■ Proper footwear
Bicycle	■ Wearing a helmet ■ Not applying stickers that prevent the helmet from skidding on the pavement ■ Proper operation (walking bike across traffic lanes)

Fire	■ Discuss fire prevention:
	   ■ No extension cords under rugs
	   ■ Safe candle use
	   ■ Gas stoves
	   ■ Fire and carbon monoxide detectors
	■ Need for a home evacuation plan and ongoing drills

Falls	■ Home assessments (particularly important for older adult patients) to reduce fall risk
Firearms	■ Safe storage, gun locks, storage of ammo and weapons separately, and so forth
Drowning	■ Water safety: "Feet first, first time" ■ Provide or take swimming lessons
Intimate partner violence	■ Signs of intimate partner violence ■ Reporting when mandated by state or local law ■ Referral to services as applicable

REVIEW QUESTION

1. Educating elementary students about the benefits of wearing a helmet when riding a bicycle is an example of what type of prevention?
   a. Primary
   b. Secondary
   c. Tertiary
   d. Quaternary

References

American College of Surgeons: The Committee on Trauma. (2018). *ATLS: Advanced Trauma Life Support student course manual* (10th ed.). American College of Surgeons.

Dukleska, K., Borrup, K., & Campbell, B. T. (2022, October). Childhood injury prevention: Where we've been and where we need to be. *Seminars in Pediatric Surgery*, *31*(5), 151220. https://doi.org/10.1016/j.sempedsurg.2022.151220

McQuillan, K. A., & Flynn Makic, M. B. (2020). *Trauma nursing from resuscitation through rehabilitation* (5th ed.). Elsevier.

Moore, K. (2016, September). Injury prevention and trauma mortality. *Journal of Emergency Nursing*, *42*(5), 457–458. https://doi.org/10.1016/j.jen.2016.06.015

Scholl, L., Seth, P., Kariisa, M., Wilson, N., & Baldwin, G. (2019). Drug and opioid-involved overdose deaths—United States, 2013–2017. *Morbidity and Mortality Weekly Report*, *67*(5152), 1419–1427. https://doi.org/10.15585/mmwr.mm675152e1

Sidwell, R., Matar, M. M., & Sakran, J. V. (2017, October). Trauma education and prevention. *Surgical Clinics of North America*, *97*(5), 1185–1197. https://doi.org/10.1016/j.suc.2017.06.010

World Health Organization. (2021). *Injuries and violence*, World Health Organization. www.who.int/news-room/fact-sheets/detail/injuries-and-violence.

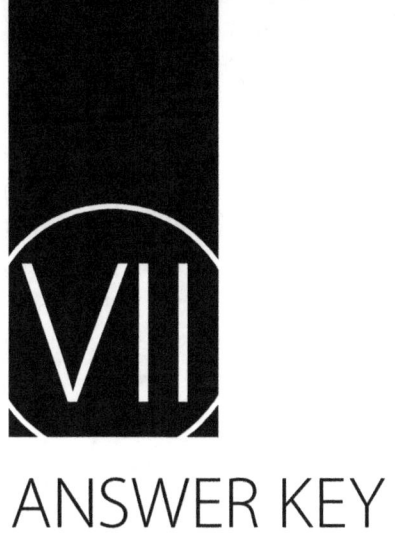

ANSWER KEY

Study Question Answers and Rationales

ANSWERS AND RATIONALES

Chapter 1
1. Answer: c. Reduce mortality rates
   Rationale: National certification ensures compliance with evidence-based practice.
2. Answer: c. Mechanism of injury
   Rationale: D-MIST = Demographics, Mechanism of Injury, Inspection/injury/illness, Signs and Symptoms, Treatment.
3. Answer: b. Be quiet
   Rationale: A quiet room allows for the team leader and documenter to hear the closed-loop communication.

Chapter 2
1. Answer: b. Polyvictimization
   Rationale: Trauma and violence are socially contagious, linking multiple trauma and violence exposure to trauma, more commonly reported by the term *polyvictimization*. A mass casualty event occurs when victims presenting to the hospital exceed current resources. *Multisystem trauma patient* refers to the multiple physiologic systems that may be injured.
2. Answer: c. Preventable
   Rationale: Much evidence exists regarding trauma and trauma prevention. The common statement is that "If something is predictable, then it is preventable." Although caring for critically injured trauma patients can be exhilarating for staff, knowing they've made an impact on the outcomes, it is not exciting for the patient or family.
3. Answer: b. Growing up in an urban area in a single-parent home
   Rationale: Risk factors for trauma include social factors such as the composition of the family and location where people live, with noted increase in trauma risk for living in an urban area and living in a single-parent home.

Chapter 3

1. Answer: True
   Rationale: Trauma can have multiple types of injuries depending on the mechanism of injury.
2. Answer: d. Four
   Rationale: There are four impacts: The vehicle impacts another object. The occupant (driver or passenger) collides with the interior of the vehicle or other object. Internal tissues collide with ridged structures within the body. Secondary impacts (passengers within a car collide with each other or other objects).
3. Answer: b. Radiation
   Rationale: A burn due to prolonged exposure to ultraviolet rays of the sun or to other sources of radiation results in a radiation burn.
4. Answer: a. Mechanism of injury
   Rationale: Mechanism of injury is a key component for first responders and the trauma care team to decide the level of care (facility capabilities) and diagnostic workup and interventions that are warranted. Patient and family preferences are important, but meeting the immediate life-threatening needs of the patient and matching with facilities that are capable of managing these injuries is a higher priority to improve mortality. Alcohol level is not a factor in deciding where to transport a patient.

Chapter 4

1. Answer: b. Perform a rapid assessment of the patient's vital functions
   Rationale: The focus of the primary survey is identification of life-threatening injuries, intervening on those injuries deemed critical, and prioritizing the plan of care for the patient.
2. Answer: a. Hemorrhagic shock
   Rationale: Hemorrhagic shock is the leading type of shock affecting trauma patients. The source of shock in a trauma patient is always "bleeding until proven otherwise."
3. Answer: a. Acidosis, hypothermia, and coagulopathy
   Rationale: The tenets of the "lethal triad" include acidosis, hypothermia, and coagulopathy. Patients who are acidotic, hypothermic, and coagulopathic are at a much greater risk of coagulopathy from alteration in the clotting cascade and death.

Chapter 5

1. Answer: c. Palpate the chest wall for tenderness
   Rationale: The other options are part of the primary survey.
2. Answer: b. Allergies
   Rationale: Allergies are the first part of the mnemonic for AMPLE history. Airway is part of the primary survey. Atrial fibrillation is an important medical history that belongs to P for past medical history. Adjunctive testing is done during the secondary survey.

3. Answer: d. A CT scan of the brain
   Rationale: CT is needed to assess for traumatic brain injury. Patients may be combative due to head injury, drug, or alcohol ingestion. Obtaining a CT scan to diagnose a brain injury is the highest priority in absence of a brain injury sedation may be indicated. Sedation and analgesics may mask a traumatic brain injury. Urine drug screen is needed but is not the highest priority.

Chapter 6
1. Answer: c. Identify occult injuries
   Rationale: Both answers A and B are completed in the primary survey, and answer D is not part of the tertiary survey. The tertiary survey is used to detect any injuries that may not have been initially detected.
2. Answer: a. Reevaluation of the patient and all testing
   Rationale: The tertiary survey is used to detect any injuries that may not have been initially detected or reported on patient testing. The other options are all part of the primary survey.

Chapter 7
1. Answer: d. Ensure the HOB is >30 degrees
   Rationale: Ensuring the HOB is elevated will optimize passive venous drainage in an attempt to reduce ICP. The other options are for medications and would require a medication order from a provider. Interventions should be completed in a stepwise fashion from least invasive (elevation of HOB) to more invasive (giving intravenous medications).
2. Answer: b. Suggest they place a subclavian line
   Rationale: In the setting of traumatic brain injury, it is important to not impede venous drainage. The risk for DVT formation increases with a jugular central venous catheter. A subclavian central venous catheter reduces that risk.
3. Answer: b. Notify the provider
   Rationale: The patient has sustained ICP elevation despite optimal medical management. The provider must be made aware that current interventions are not adequate to control the ICP elevation.
4. Answer: a. Tell the neurosurgeon
   Rationale: If a nurse observes violation of a sterile field during a sterile procedure, it is that nurse's responsibility to notify the proceduralist. Filling out an incident form, reporting to the charge nurse, and changing the cables will not prevent an infection.
5. Answer: c. Epidural hematoma
   Rationale: The classic presentation of a patient with an epidural hematoma includes a head strike with loss of consciousness, a "lucid period," and then rapid neurologic deterioration. A concussion and subdural and subarachnoid hemorrhages do not typically present with unequal pupils.

Chapter 8

1. Answer: b. HOB elevation and direct pressure
   Rationale: The nurse's role in managing epistaxis includes elevation of the head of bed and applying direct pressure. The other interventions all require provider-level interventions or orders.
2. Answer: a. Ocular pain, b. Sudden loss of sight, and d. Sudden sectorial vision changes
   Rationale: Blurred vision that does not clear with blinking is a red flag.
3. Answer: a. Upper airway narrowing
   Rationale: Stridor is caused by narrowing of the upper airway, indicating impending airway emergency. An increased oxygen requirement indicates a problem in the lower airways and lungs due to impaired gas exchange. A cuff leak indicates insufficient air in the endotracheal tube or that the tube has slid out of the airway. A temporal bone fracture will not cause stridor.

Chapter 9

1. Answer: b. Cardiac tamponade
   Rationale: These are the classic signs of cardiac tamponade: muffled heart sounds, JVD, and hypotension. These three symptoms are commonly referred to as the Beck triad.
2. Answer: b. Tricuspid
   Rationale: The tricuspid area is at the left sternal border, fourth intercostal space. The aortic area would be at the right sternal border, second intercostal space. The mitral area is at the fifth left intercostal space, midclavicular line. The pulmonic area is at the left sternal border, second intercostal space.
3. Answer: a. Ventricular fibrillation cardiac arrest
   Rationale: Commotio cordis occurs as a result of significant direct impact to the anterior chest wall, which can precipitate ventricular fibrillation cardiac arrest.

Chapter 10

1. Answer: b. Tension pneumothorax
   Rationale: Signs of tension pneumothorax include tracheal deviation and distended neck veins.
2. Answer: d. Respiratory acidosis
   Rationale: Low pH in the setting of increased CO2 and normal bicarb indicates respiratory acidosis.
3. Answer: b. Narrowed airway
   Rationale: Narrowing of the upper airway can cause increased air speed through the passage, resulting in an abnormal sound: stridor.

Chapter 11

1. Answer: c. Passing flatus
   Rationale: Passing flatus and stool is a sign that the bowel function has returned following trauma or surgery. The presence of bowel sounds does not always indicate the bowel is fully functioning. Hyperactive

bowel sounds can be present with a bowel obstruction. Patients do not always have nausea, and it is not a reliable sign of bowel function.
2. Answer: d. Overwhelming postsplenectomy infection
Rationale: Patients who have had a splenectomy are at risk for overwhelming postsplenectomy infection (OPSI). Although they may develop renal failure due to hypovolemia and contrast use during CT scans, renal failure is not due to the splenectomy. Patients with spleen injuries may develop left upper quadrant pain that can radiate to the left shoulder (Kehr sign); STEMI is less likely to be the cause. Patients who have a splenectomy may develop bowel obstruction from adhesions, the greatest risk being from OPSI, and require vaccinations to prevent these infections.
3. Answer: b. Challenge the order
Rationale: The nurse should challenge the order because the patient may have a urethral injury that can be made worse with catheter insertion. The trauma team or urologist should insert the Foley catheter. The trauma team should call the urology team once diagnostic testing is complete to discuss the injuries. A coude catheter may be needed but is not the best course of action by the nurse.
4. Answer: a. Bowel injury
Rationale: Patients involved in head-on collisions may develop bowel injuries from the abdomen impacting the steering wheel. Bowel injuries are difficult to detect on initial CT scan unless there is bleeding in the area. Thus, bowel ischemia or perforation causing peritonitis may take hours to a day to present. Liver and spleen injuries are readily apparent on CT scan. Delayed rupture is possible but does not present with peritonitis. Pancreatic injuries typically present with epigastric rather than RLQ pain.
5. Answer: d. Abdominal compartment syndrome
Rationale: Abdominal compartment syndrome (ACS) may occur as a result of increased pressure in the abdomen from the presence of blood from hemorrhage. Pancreatic injuries can result in pancreatitis and inflammation, requiring IVF from third-spacing of fluids, thus increasing intra-abdominal pressures. A bowel injury is possible, but the scenario does not indicate the patient developed peritonitis. An acute kidney injury may be present from hypotension, contrast, or ACS, but the symptoms presented are consistent with ACS.

Chapter 12

1. Answer: b. Refer to social work
Rationale: Social work can offer support to the patient and ensure a safe discharge plan, which may require other family support or discharge to a shelter. The patient must agree to call the police, unless the patient is a minor or an elder. In that situation, the provider would call psychiatry if the patient has conditions that would warrant psychiatry's expertise.

2. Answer: d. Notify the trauma team leader
   Rationale: The nurse should notify the team leader of the finding because it may represent a urethral injury and require specialized diagnostic testing. The team leader would decide if urology consultation were required and would place that order and contact the on-call provider. The nurse should not place a Foley or three-way Foley, because it could cause further injury.
3. Answer: c. Assess the urine output for color, quantity, and presence of clots
   Rationale: The nurse is responsible for assessing and monitoring the urine output for quantity, color, and presence of clots. Although continuous bladder irrigation may be required to keep it free from clots, a specific order is required. In this instance, catheter removal should be performed at the direction of the providers, typically urology, and not via a nurse-driven protocol. Although traction may be required, the urologist would have likely applied the traction at the time of surgery.

Chapter 13
1. Answer: b. Acute compartment syndrome
   Rationale: The patient presents with a crush injury and three of the six P's suggestive of acute compartment syndrome. A spinal cord injury and nerve root injury may present with paresthesia and paralysis but would not present with the pallor or taught leg. A DVT would not cause pallor or paresthesia.
2. Answer: c. Creatine phosphokinase
   Rationale: A CPK level five times that of normal is diagnostic for rhabdomyolysis and is effective in evaluating whether the treatment for rhabdomyolysis is working. Sodium levels can indicate dehydration. Hemoglobin levels can indicate anemia or dehydration. ALT monitors for ischemic or toxic injuries to the liver.
3. Answer: d. Erythema, edema, and pain
   Rationale: Although all of these may represent potential for DVT, the most reported symptom combination is redness, swelling, and pain. Ecchymosis, pulselessness, paresthesias, and muscle spasms are not signs of DVT.
4. Answer: b. Pelvic binder
   Rationale: A pelvic binder can be placed around the greater trochanter to stabilize the pelvic ring and help control/tamponade internal bleeding. A tourniquet and pressure bandages are applied to extremities not the pelvis. A knee immobilizer is not effective for pelvis fractures.

Chapter 14
1. Answer: b. Parkland formula
   Rationale: The Parkland formula is used to calculate the total amount of fluid resuscitation needed in the first 24 hours following a burn. Wells criteria are a risk stratification score and clinical decision tool to estimate the probability that a patient has an acute pulmonary embolism.

The Harris-Benedict equation is a calorie formula using the variables of height, weight, age, and gender to calculate basal metabolic rate. The heat equation calculates how heat diffuses through a given region.

2. Answer: a. Respiratory compromise
   Rationale: Stridor is a sign of respiratory compromise. With a known inhalation injury, stridor is very concerning for ongoing tissue swelling and airway narrowing. Signs and symptoms of carbon monoxide poisoning include malaise, shortness of breath, headache, nausea, chest pain, irritability, ataxia, altered mental status, and loss of consciousness, up to and including coma. Clinical signs include tachypnea, tachycardia, and hypotension. Signs of cyanide poisoning include confusion, headache, nausea/vomiting, dyspnea, tachypnea, tachycardia, and hypotension. Signs of inadequate resuscitation include tachycardia, hypotension, and oliguria.

3. Answer: d. Avulsion
   Rationale: A degloving injury is when a piece of skin and the layer of soft tissue below are partially or completely separated from the body. This is a type of avulsion injury. Puncture wounds result from a sharp or pointed object that pierces the skin and penetrates beyond deeper layers. Laceration results in a linear separation of skin, or blunt impact results in a more jagged-appearing wound and wound edges. Abrasion results from friction and varies in depth (superficial, partial-thickness, or full-thickness abrasion).

4. Answer: c. 1.5 to 2 g of protein per kilogram of body weight
   Rationale: Burn injuries can induce a hypermetabolic state that is proportional to the extent of the burn. This state can persist for months after the injury. The goal for daily protein intake is 1.5 to 2 g of protein per kilogram of body weight.

Chapter 15

1. Answer: c. Assess, resuscitate, and stabilize the trauma patient
   Rationale: In the instance when a trauma patient is brought to a facility that does not provide a high enough level of care, the initial hospital is required to assess, resuscitate, and stabilize the patient.

Chapter 16

1. Answer: d. Have the patient perform incentive spirometry
   Rationale: Incentive spirometry can help resolve atelectasis, which occurs from inadequate pain relief. Applying oxygen will make the atelectasis worse. Ordering a chest x-ray is out of the nurse's scope of practice. Call the provider if the hypoxia doesn't resolve after performing incentive spirometry.

2. Answer: b. Dilaudid .5 mg IV
   Rationale: The patient is in severe pain and is imminently going to the operating room. Dilaudid has a short onset, whereas both Tylenol and oxycodone are oral and thus have an onset of 30 minutes. The fentanyl patch onset is hours.

3. Answer: c. Pepcid for SUP
   Rationale: The patient is at risk for Curling ulcer and likely will be intubated for over 48 hours. Lovenox should be started 24 hours after a stable head CT, not on admission, until cerebral bleeding has stabilized. In head injuries, heavy sedation should be avoided to obtain neurologic exams. Other agents can treat ICPs. Family is encouraged at the bedside, but in the setting of uncontrolled ICPs, the nurse should maintain a low-stimulation environment.

Chapter 17

1. Answer: b. Institute a sleep protocol
   Rationale: Ativan is a benzodiazepine, which can worsen delirium. Delirium can prolong the hospital stay and increase mortality. Treating with an analgesic is not appropriate because it can also worsen delirium. Turning on the lights can also impede sleep, which can worsen delirium.
2. Answer: d. All of the above
   Rationale: This patient may be experiencing elder mistreatment. Either the patient is being injured or, if the patient is falling frequently, they may be being neglected and need additional care and supervision. Social work can discuss with family the amount of support available at home and caregiver stress. The providers can investigate for other healed fractures or old fractures that did not receive treatment and can help discern between abuse and neglect. Elder services should be engaged to perform an investigation.

Chapter 18

1. Answer: a. Place on left side
   Rationale: The inferior vena cava (IVC) runs parallel to the spine on the right side. Thus, lifting the right side of the backboard or placing the patient in the left lateral recumbent position will shift the fetus off the IVC and augment venous return to the heart. Fluid and blood may be indicated, but the first step is to optimize the current status by shifting the fetus.
2. Answer: d. Rh immunoglobulin
   Rationale: All pregnant Rh-negative trauma patients should receive Rh immunoglobulin within 72 hours of injury, unless the injuries are minor and far from the fetus.

Chapter 19

1. Answer: b. Report the suspected maltreatment to the appropriate authorities
   Rationale: Nurses are mandated reporters, and thus when child maltreatment is suspected it must be reported. It is not the nurse's job to make a formal determination of child maltreatment, rather to report the suspicion.

2. Answer: c. Weight
   Rationale: Patient weight is a key data point when resuscitating a pediatric trauma patient. Initial fluid management requires 20 mL/kg.

Chapter 20

1. Answer: c. Have you or has someone close to you ever served in the military?
   Rationale: This is an initial open-ended question to elicit their service. Do not presume someone has served based on tattoos. Building trust among veterans is an important tenant of trauma-informed care. Immediately asking about injuries or combat or experiences does not allow for the nurse to build trust.
2. Answer: c. Lorazepam (Ativan)
   Rationale: Avoid benzodiazepines in the veteran population, because they are at an increased risk for adverse effects, including death from drug overdose. Paroxetine and sertraline are recommended treatment for PTSD. Dexmedetomidine is a strong recommendation for sedation for veterans with PTSD.

Chapter 21

1. Answer: b. Naloxone (Narcan)
   Rationale: The patient is experiencing opioid overdose/oversedation. The reversal agent of opioids is Narcan. Flumazenil is the reversal agent for benzodiazepines. N-acetylcysteine is the reversal agent for acetaminophen (Tylenol). Atropine is not warranted because the heart rate is 60 beats per minute and is not unstable.
2. Answer: d. Flumazenil (Romazicon)
   Rationale: The treatment for benzodiazepine overdose is flumazenil (Romazicon). Naloxone reverses opioids. N-acetylcysteine is the reversal agent for acetaminophen (Tylenol). Atropine is not warranted because the heart rate is 60 beats per minute and is not unstable.
3. Answer: a. Cocaine intoxication
   Rationale: This patient has signs and symptoms consistent with cocaine intoxication. Hemorrhagic shock and tension pneumothorax have been ruled out. Alcohol withdrawal would not occur this early in their stay, with a positive alcohol level on admission.

Chapter 22

1. Answer: a. Provide the greatest amount of good to the greatest number of people
   Rationale: Disaster care has unique characteristics. When an influx of patients can overwhelm the health care system, resource utilization shifts to providing the greatest good for the greatest number of people.
2. Answer: c. Patient and responder decontamination
   Rationale: Decontamination from hazardous material must occur prior to patients or responders entering the emergency department. Failure to

decontaminate can force the healthcare facility to close or be unable to take patients because of internal contamination and the risk to current and future patients.

Chapter 23
1. Answer: c. Post-ICU syndrome
   Rationale: The patient should have been screened for alcohol and substance use on admission. The patient should be screened for PICS.
2. Answer: d. All of the above
   Rationale: These are all instructions that should be given to the patient to avoid opioid tolerance, misuse, and abuse.

Chapter 24
1. Answer: a. Primary
   Rationale: Educating about the benefits of wearing a helmet while riding a bicycle is aimed at preventing injury before it occurs.

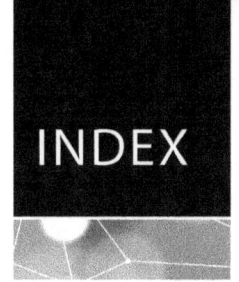

INDEX

abdominal assessment
  auscultation, 150
  inspection, 150
  palpation, 150
  percussion, 150
abdominal compartment syndrome (ACS). *See* intra-abdominal hypertension (IAH)
ACEs. *See* adverse childhood experiences
acidosis, 38
acute respiratory distress syndrome (ARDS), 144
AD. *See* autonomic dysreflexia
admission and transfer criteria, triage
  institutional resource limitations, 212
  prioritizing ICU patients, 213, 214
  therapeutic capabilities, 212
  tips for, 214–215
  transfer out of ICU, 215
  types of inpatients, level of care, 213
advanced trauma life support (ATLS), 11, 137
adverse childhood experiences (ACEs), 18–19
airway, breathing, circulation, disability, and exposure (ABCDEs), 11, 33–38
airway (A) evaluation
  jaw-thrust maneuver, 35
  nasal trumpet, 35
  primary survey of, 33, 34
  restriction of cervical spine motion, 35
airway management
  airway obstruction, 137
  extubation criteria, 142–144
  intubation, 137–138
  ventilator management, 139–141
airway obstruction, 137
alcohol use disorder (AUD), 266
AMPLE history, 47–48
analgesia
  multimodal pain regimen strategies, 219–221
  post-intensive care syndrome, 221
  sedation, 221
  types of pain, 217–219
anaphylactic shock, 108
anisocoria, 86
ARDS. *See* acute respiratory distress syndrome
arterial blood gas interpretation
  noninvasive positive pressure ventilation, 135–137
  oxygen delivery options, 135, 136
  values and normal ranges, 134
  ventilation assessment, 134–135
aspiration, 145
atelectasis, 79
ATLS. *See* advanced trauma life support
autonomic dysreflexia (AD), 80

BCI. *See* blunt cardiac injury
BCVI. *See* blunt cerebral vascular injuries
Beers criteria, 238–239

INDEX

best practices
  A to J bundle elements, 217–230
  study question answers and rationales, 311–312
blunt cardiac injury (BCI), 114–115
blunt cerebral vascular injuries (BCVI), 81
blunt trauma
  falls, 24, 26
  motor vehicle crashes, 24, 25
bowel injuries, 155
brain death
  definition, 74
  nursing care, 75
  organ procurement organization (OPO), 74
brachial plexus, 188–189
breathing and ventilation (B) evaluation, 36
brown bag approach, 230
burn injuries, 28, 29
  burn wound care, 200
  classification of, 198, 199
  methods to estimate TBSA in adults, 198
  Parkland formula and example, 198, 200
  skin grafting, 201

cardiac contusions, 115
cardiac rupture, 115
cardiac tamponade, 116–117
cardiogenic shock, 108–109
cardiovascular assessment
  arterial injuries—Great Vessels, 118–119
  auscultate heart sounds, 98
  blunt cardiac injury (BCI), 114–115
  chest palpation, 97–98
  end points of resuscitation, 112, 114
  hemodynamic monitoring, 98–103
  penetrating cardiac injury, 115–117
  shock, 103–112
  study question answers and rationales, 308
  unequal blood pressures (BPs), 98
CEN. *See* certified emergency nurse
certified emergency nurse (CEN), 10

chest tubes
  air leak identification, 129
  dry suction chest tube system, 127, 128
  patient position, 129
  pigtail catheters, 128–129
  preferred medication, 129
child maltreatment, 230, 256–257
circulation-bleeding, monitoring, deep vein thrombosis prophylaxis, and anticoagulation
  for atrial fibrillation, 224
  deep vein thrombosis prophylaxis, 224
  initial resuscitation, 223
  postresuscitation, 223–224
circulation with hemorrhage control (C)
  early and continued resuscitation, 37–38
  hemorrhage, 37
  shock types, 36, 37
clavicle fracture, 180
coagulopathy, 38
commotio cordis, 114–115
compartment syndrome, 188–189, 205–206
constipation, 80
contractures, 205

deep vein thrombosis (DVT), 79–80, 183
delirium prevention, 224–225
diagnostic peritoneal lavage (DPL), 151
diagnostic testing
  decision to transfer, 52
  initial laboratory testing, 48–51
  radiologic studies, 51
disability (D), 38–39
disaster management
  crisis standard of care, 282
  ethical issues, 282
  mitigation, 278
  natural or man-made, 276, 277
  preparedness, 278–279
  psychological first aid, 282–283
  recovery, 283
  response, 279–281
  study question answers and rationales, 313–314
  types of disasters, 277–278

discharge planning
  follow-up appointments, 291–294
  levels of care postdischarge, 291, 292
  palliative care team consultation, 290
  post-acute care discharge options, inpatient rehabilitation, 289, 290
  rehabilitation services, 291
  study question answers and rationales, 314
disfigurement, 205
distributive shock, 108
D-MIST approach, 12
DPL. *See* diagnostic peritoneal lavage
DVT. *See* deep vein thrombosis

early mobility, 225
elder mistreatment, 230, 240
emergency medical services (EMS)
  hospital preparation, 7
  mnemonic for, 12
  prearrival huddle, 8
  prehospital, 7
  trauma bay, 7
EMS. *See* emergency medical services
esophageal perforation, 133–134
EVD. *See* external ventricular drains
exposure/environmental control (E), 39–40
external ventricular drains (EVD), 70

falls
  injury patterns with, 24, 26
  risk factors for, 24, 26
  versus syncope, 239–240
fatal traumatic injuries, 16
fat embolism, 187
femur fracture, 183
fevers, 100
flail segment, 131, 132
flight-or-fight response, 19
fluids, foley, and family, 225–226
focused assessment with sonography for trauma (FAST), 37
follow-up care
  post-ICU syndrome, signs of, 293–294
  PTSD, signs of, 293

  special situations, 294
  written and verbal discharge instructions, 292–293
foot and ankle fractures, 183–184

gastric/stress ulcer prophylaxis, 226–227
gastrointestinal assessment
  abdominal, 149–150
  adrenal injuries, 156
  diagnostic testing, 151
  diaphragm injuries, 156
  hollow organ injuries, 154–155
  nasogastric tube assessment, 150–151
  pancreatic injuries, 156
  rectum, 150
  serial abdominal exams, 151
  solid organ injuries, 152–154
  study question answers and rationales, 308–309
  surgical intervention, 156–158
  trauma complications, 158–161
genitourinary assessment
  adjuncts to assessment, 166
  diagnostic testing, 166
  extraperitoneal injuries, 168
  inspection, 165–166
  intraperitoneal injuries, 168
  palpation, 166
  penile injury, 169–170
  renal trauma, 167–168
  scrotal injury, 170
  study question answers and rationales, 309–310
  testicular injury, 170
  ureteral injuries, 168
  urethral injuries, 168–169
Glasgow Coma Scale (GCS), 38, 39
golden hour, after injury, 16
gynecologic assessment
  inspection, 166–167
  vaginal and vulvar injuries, 171

head, eyes, ears, nose, and throat (HEENT) assessment
  anisocoria, 86
  auscultation of neck, 87
  hemotympanum, 85

head, eyes, ears, nose, and throat (HEENT) assessment (*cont.*)
  maxillofacial fractures, 88–89
  nasal fracture patterns, 91–93
  nasal speculum exams, 87
  ocular injury classification, 89–90
  otorrhea, 85
  rhinorrhea, 86
  scalp lacerations, 88
  strangulation injuries, 93–94
  study question answers and rationales, 308
  sudden hearing loss, 91
  Weber test, 87
head-to-toe examination
  assessment by system, 43–46
health disparities, 18
hematuria, 169
hemodynamic monitoring
  blood pressure, 101
  continuous pulse oximetry, 102–103
  patient's temperature, 99–100
  permissive hypotension, 101–102
  respiratory rate, 100–101
  telemetry, 99
  vital signs interpretation, 99
hemorrhagic shock, 36
hemotympanum, 85
high-velocity penetrating trauma, 26–27
hip fracture, 181–183
hospital stay, 228
humerus fracture, 80, 178
hypothermia, 38
hypovolemic shock, 107

ICP. *See* intracranial pressure
infections, 229
injury prevention
  economic approaches, 299
  education, 298
  enforcement, 299
  engineering, 298–299
  levels of prevention, 298
  principal concepts of, 297–298
  role of nurse, 299, 300
  study question answers and rationales, 314

integumentary assessment
  burn injuries, 197–201
  cold injuries, 202–203
  complications related, 203–207
  hypothermia, 201–202
  inhalation injury, 201
  inspection, 193–194
  layers of skin, 195
  palpation, 194–195
  study question answers and rationales, 310–311
  traumatic wounds and soft tissue injuries, 195–197
  wound healing, 203
intimate partner violence (IPV), 18, 229–230, 249
intra-abdominal hypertension (IAH)
  clinical signs of, 159, 160
  measurement of pressure, 159–160
  risk factors for, 158, 159
  treatment of, 161
intracranial pressure (ICP)
  analgesics, 72
  carbon dioxide, 73
  cerebral perfusion pressures (CPP) monitoring, 69–70
  cerebral spinal fluid drainage, 73
  clinical signs of, 69
  complications, 74
  Cushing's triad, 70
  monitor types, 70
  nursing care of, 70–71
  osmolar therapy, 73
  positioning, 72
  refractory elevated, 73
  seizure prophylaxis, 73
  sodium management, 73
  tiered management strategies, 71–72
  venous access, 73
intubation, 137–138
IPV. *See* intimate partner violence

jaw-thrust maneuver, 35

knee injury, 183

lower extremity injury
  femur fracture, 183
  foot and ankle fractures, 183–184
  hip fracture, 181–183
  knee injury, 183
  pelvic fracture, 180–181
  tibia/fibula, 183
low-velocity penetrating trauma, 27, 28

maxillofacial fractures, 88–89
mechanical ventilation, 144–145
mechanism of injury
  blunt trauma, 24–26
  burn injuries, 28, 29
  study question answers and rationales, 306
  penetrating trauma, 25–28
mediastinitis, 145
medication reconciliation, 230, 238
MODS. *See* multiple organ dysfunction syndrome
motor testing, 63
motor vehicle crashes (MVCs), 24, 25
multiple organ dysfunction syndrome (MODS), 16
musculoskeletal (MSK) assessment
  circulation, sensation, and movement assessment, 176–178
  complications of, 184, 186–189
  fractures, 178, 179
  inspection, 176
  lower extremity injury, 180–184
  palpation, 176, 177
  spinal fractures, 184–186
  study question answers and rationales, 310
  upper extremity injury, 178, 180
muzzle blast, 27
MVCs. *See* motor vehicle crashes

nasal trumpet, 35
nasogastric tube (NGT) assessment, 150–151
National Institutes of Health Stroke Scale (NIHSS), 65
nerve injury, 188, 205

neurogenic shock, 108
  nursing care, 77–79
  vasopressor options for, 77, 78
neurological assessment
  blunt cerebral vascular injuries (BCVI), 81
  brain death, 74–75
  cranial nerve function and testing, 63–65
  dermatome levels, 63, 66
  increased intracranial pressure, 69–74
  motor testing, 63
  National Institutes of Health Stroke Scale, 65
  sensation testing, 65
  spinal cord injuries (SCI), 75–80
  study question answers and rationales, 307
  traumatic brain injuries (TBI), 65–69
NIHSS. *See* National Institutes of Health Stroke Scale
NIPPV. *See* noninvasive positive pressure ventilation
nonhemorrhagic hypovolemic shock, 107–108
noninvasive positive pressure ventilation (NIPPV), 135–137
nutrition, 226–227

obstructive shock, 109
occupational therapy, 228
older adult trauma patients
  Beers criteria, 238–239
  elder mistreatment, 240
  falls *versus* syncope, 239–240
  medication reconciliation, 238
  physiologic changes with aging, 235–238
  study question answers and rationales, 312
opioid use disorder (OUD), 269
OPO. *See* organ procurement organization
organ procurement organization (OPO), 74
otorrhea, 85

pediatric patient assessment
  anatomic and physiologic, 253–255
  assessment, 255–256
  child maltreatment, 256–257
  interpreting behavior, 256
  resuscitation, 256
  study question answers and
      rationales, 312–313
  vital signs by age/weight, 255–256
pelvic fracture, 180–181
penetrating trauma
  definition, 25
  high-velocity, 26–27
  low-velocity, 27, 28
permissive hypotension, 38
physical therapy (PT), 228
pneumonia, 79, 145
positive end-expiratory pressure
      (PEEP), 222
post-ICU syndrome (PICS), 293
post–intensive care syndrome (PICS),
      221
posttraumatic stress disorder (PTSD),
      261, 293
pregnant trauma patients
  analgesics and sedatives, 249
  anatomic changes, 244
  intimate partner violence, 249
  monitoring, 248–249
  obstetric urgencies and emergencies,
      249–250
  physiologic and anatomic changes,
      243–248
  study question answers and
      rationales, 312
  supine position, 243–244
  traumatic injuries, 248
pressure injuries, 80
problems and associated medications,
      230
primary survey
  airway, breathing, circulation,
      disability, and exposure
      (ABCDEs), 11, 33–38
  study question answers and
      rationale, 306

pulmonary assessment
  breath sounds types, 124, 125
  chest tubes injuries, 127–130
  hemothorax, 127
  inspect, 124
  open pneumothorax, 127
  palpation, 124
  percussion sounds, 125, 126
  pneumothorax, 126–127
  pulmonary contusion, 130
  pulmonary laceration, 130
  study question answers and
      rationales, 308
  tension pneumothorax, 127
  thoracic cage, 131–146
pulmonary hygiene, 222–223
pulmonary sequelae, 145–146

radius and ulnar fractures, 180
Rancho Los Amigos levels of cognitive
      functioning, 291, 292
rectal injuries, 155
restriction of cervical spine motion, 35
resuscitation, 37–38
rhabdomyolysis, 189, 206–207
rhinorrhea, 86
rib fractures, 131
Richmond Agitation Sedation Scale,
      221
Riker Sedation-Agitation Scale goal,
      221

scalp lacerations, 88
scapula fracture, 132–133, 180
SCI. *See* spinal cord injuries
screening, brief intervention and
      referral to treatment (SBIRT),
      266
  alcohol screening, 268–269
  discharge options, 269–270
  drug screening, 269
  feedback, 269
  opioids and sedatives, 270
  specific drugs and antidotes, 273–274
  toxidromes, clinical presentation of,
      270–272

secondary survey
  AMPLE history, 47–48
  decision to admit, 54
  diagnostic testing, 48–52
  head-to-toe examination, 43–47
  reassessment and monitoring, 52–53
  specialty consultation, 53–54
  study question answers and rationales, 306–307
sedation awakening trial (SAT), 221
sensation testing, 65
septic shock, 108
shock
  compensatory mechanisms, 103–104
  definition, 103
  hemodynamic monitoring devices and methods, 110
  laboratory findings, 110–112
  physical assessment, 105
  physical examination, 109
  treatment of, 112–114
  types of, 105–109
  vital signs, 109–110
speech therapy, 228
spinal cord injuries (SCI)
  complications, 79–80
  key terminology for, 75, 76
  neurogenic shock, 75–79
  postoperative care, 79
  spinal cord syndromes, 75–77
spinal fractures, 184
spontaneous breathing trials (SBTs), 222
stab wounds, 27, 28
sternal fracture, 131–132
strangulation injuries, 93–94
stress ulcers, 205
Substance Abuse and Mental Health Services Administration (SAMHSA), 269
substance use and toxicology
  alcohol use, 265–267
  opioid use disorders, 267–268
  screening, brief intervention, and referral to treatment, 268–270
  study question answers and rationales, 313

TBI. *See* traumatic brain injuries
tetanus, 187, 204–205
tertiary survey
  documentation and communication, 58
  missed or occult injuries identification, 58
  patient reassessment, 58
  study question answers and rationales, 307
thoracic cage
  airway management, 137–144
  esophageal perforation, 133–134
  fractures, 131–133
  mechanical ventilation, 144–145
  oxygenation and ventilation, 134–137
  pulmonary sequelae, 145–146
  traumatic diaphragmatic injury, 133
tibia/fibula fractures, 183
toxidromes, 270–272
tracheostomy, 144
trauma
  adverse childhood experiences, 18–19
  age spectrum, 17
  fatalities, 16
  intimate partner violence (IPV), 18
  pattern of injury, 17
  risk-taking behaviors, 17
  social determinants of, 18
  study question answers and rationales, 305
  trauma centers preparedness (*See* trauma centers preparedness)
trauma bay
  airway equipment availability, 7
  member roles and responsibilities in, 8–10
  patient arrival, 12–13
  vital equipment for, 7
trauma centers preparedness
  advanced trauma life support, 11
  emergency medical services (EMS), 5, 7–10
  key team members, 5
  level of, 4

trauma centers preparedness (*cont.*)
  study question answers and rationales, 305
  triage criteria, activation by injury and patient status, 5, 6
trauma certified registered nurse (TCRN), 10
traumatic brain injuries (TBI)
  dark quiet environment, 69
  definition, 65
  elevate head of bed, 67
  hypnotic fluids avoidance, 68
  management of, 67
  severity of, 66, 68
  types of, 66, 67
traumatic diaphragmatic injury, 133
traumatic toxic stressors (TTS), 19
triage
  admission and transfer criteria
    institutional resource limitations, 212
    prioritizing ICU patients, 213, 214
    therapeutic capabilities, 212
    tips for, 214–215
    transfer out of ICU, 215
    types of inpatients, level of care, 213
  mode of transport, 212
  study question answers and rationales, 311

upper extremity injury
  clavicle fracture, 180
  humerus fracture, 178–180
  radius and ulnar fractures, 180
  scapula fracture, 180
urine retention, 80

venous thromboembolism (VTE), 186–187, 204
Veterans Health Administration (VHA), 259
veterans health and trauma
  assessment, 260
  illness syndromes by war, 260–261
  posttraumatic stress disorder, 261–263
  study question answers and rationales, 313
  substance use, 261–262
VTE. *See* venous thromboembolism

Weber test, 87
WOCN. *See* wound ostomy continence nurse
wound ostomy continence nurse (WOCN), 228–229

young male syndrome, 17

FAST FACTS FOR EMERGENCY NURSING

Choose from 50+ Titles!

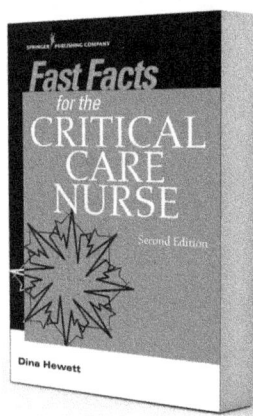
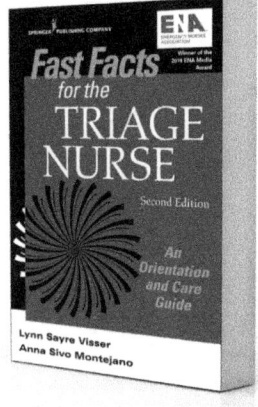
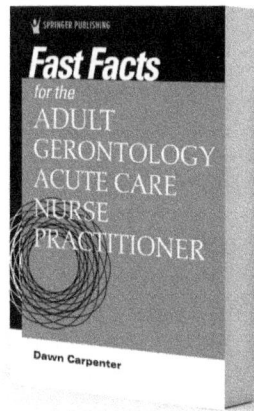
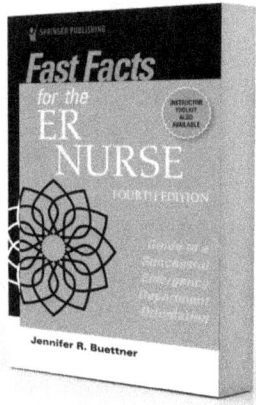

Pocket-sized and affordable, this series of must-have reference books provide quick access to information you need to know and use daily in a clear, precise format.

springerpub.com/FastFacts

www.ingramcontent.com/pod-product-compliance
Lightning Source LLC
LaVergne TN
LVHW010253260326
834688LV00044B/1265